The Clinical Approach to the Patient

WILLIAM L. MORGAN, Jr., M.D.
Professor of Medicine
The University of Rochester
School of Medicine and Dentistry

GEORGE L. ENGEL, M.D.
Professor of Psychiatry and Professor of Medicine
The University of Rochester
School of Medicine and Dentistry

ILLUSTRATED BY EVELYN LIPMAN ENGEL

W. B. SAUNDERS COMPANY
Philadelphia · London · Toronto

W. B. Saunders Company: West Washington Square
                          Philadelphia, PA 19105

                          1 St. Anne's Road
                          Eastbourne, East Sussex BN21 3UN, England

                          1 Goldthorne Avenue
                          Toronto, Ontario M8Z 5T9, Canada

Listed here is the latest translated edition of this book together with the language of the translation and the publisher.

Spanish — NEISA — 1st ed.
Il Pensiero Scientifico — Rome, Italy — 1st ed.

The Clinical Approach to the Patient   ISBN 0-7216-6550-0

Print No.:   15   14   13   12   11

*Dedicated to
Our Students*

Contents

Introduction

This is not a textbook of physical diagnosis in the traditional sense. It is a book designed to guide the beginning student in the steps used to acquire, analyze, and report clinical data derived from the patient. These successive steps are organized into seven chapters:

1. The setting and circumstances in which the student meets his first patients.

2. A consideration of the diagnostic process.

3. The methods involved in establishing a relationship with the patient and eliciting the history of his illness.

4. The sequence and flow of the physical examination.

5. The proper recording of the clinical information and its diagnostic evaluation.

6. The principles of medical order writing.

7. The requirements for effective presentation of the patient on teaching rounds.

Appendices include (A), a verbatim interview with running commentary to illustrate how the interview proceeds, how interview data are organized into the written history, and how such information is evaluated diagnostically; and (B), an example of a complete case write-up. In brief, this text deals with the unique and distinctive techniques common to all clinicians, regardless of their specialty. The procedures described are the basic clinical skills the medical student is called upon to use daily in the course of his work with patients. Facility, efficiency, and sensitivity in the execution of these procedures are the hallmark of an effective clinician, a goal to which every student should aspire.

This book is also concerned with issues traditionally considered as belonging to "the art of medicine." The student in transition from the role of a biological scientist to that of a clinician must recognize that the development of clinical competence is not dependent exclusively upon his knowledge of the biological principles underlying disease. He must also have insight into the human experience of being a patient and an understanding of the psychological factors determining how the patient and physician relate to each other. It is such knowledge which enables the clinician to create the optimal conditions for the study and care of his patient. This book also points out how the behavior and personal approach of the student may enhance the patient's motivation to cooperate, whether it be in giving a history, undergoing a physical examination, or submitting to disagreeable diagnostic or therapeutic procedures. Above all, the text emphasizes respect for the individuality of each patient and for the uniqueness of his experience with illness.

The need for this book arose during a revision of the clinical curriculum at the University of Rochester. For some years, a number of the faculty had been increasingly concerned at the casualness, if not the neglect, with which students were being instructed in the basic clinical skills.[1] In one study of the clinical teaching carried out at a number of first-rank schools, it was found that the students rarely were called upon to demonstrate how they elicited the historical or physical data which they reported on rounds. Indeed, in one fourth of such exercises the patient was not even seen by the instructor.[2] It is well known that the instruction of the physical examination is often relegated to junior staff members who are the least experienced teachers. In many, if not most schools, there is no systematic instruction in interviewing. Among our own students ready to graduate, not to mention interns coming from other schools, we have encountered many individuals who were seriously deficient in their ability to elicit a history or to perform a physical examination. Actually many students are completing their undergraduate medical education at present without ever having these techniques directly supervised by a senior clinician.

On the strength of such observations, the University of Rochester revised its clinical curriculum to place greater emphasis on the teaching of the basic clinical skills. After five years of experience with different methods of instruction, a 3-month General Clerkship at the beginning of the third year was inaugurated in the fall of 1966. This program is run by an interdepartmental committee of which both authors are members and one (W.L.M.) is the chairman. Teaching guides in the

[1]Engel, G. L.: Clinical Observation. The Neglected Basic Method of Medicine. J.A.M.A., *192*:849, 1965.
[2]Reichsman, F., Browning, F. E., and Hinshaw, J. R.: Observations of Undergraduate Clinical Teaching in Action. J. Med. Ed., *39*:147, 1964.

form of mimeographed material had been developed by the authors over the course of years, culminating in 1966 in a manual, "Examination of Patients," specifically designed for the use of students in the General Clerkship. The present text is a revision and elaboration of that manual, based on the experience of the third year students during 1966 and 1967.

Inherent in the philosophy of the General Clerkship is the fact that the transition from preclinical to clinical work involves for the student both the development of clinical skills and the achievement of the role of a physician. This takes time. In order to facilitate the transition, several important principles have been followed in the design of the General Clerkship:

1. Students are assigned in small groups to a given ward and to given instructors. Thus, from the outset the students are placed in the environment of the ward and begin to learn the role of the physician by precept and example. There is also no competing course work.

2. The teachers are drawn from all clinical services and are selected on the basis of their interest and enthusiasm in transmitting basic clinical methods, regardless of their clinical discipline. In this way, the student comes to appreciate which clinical skills are common to every physician and under what circumstances the experienced physician asks a specialist to elaborate or check his observations.

3. Student responsibility progresses in the course, beginning with partial interview experience and regional physical examination, advancing to complete work-ups and the presentation of the patient on rounds. There is adequate time and repeated opportunities for students to practice their techniques of interviewing and physical diagnosis under direct observation of instructors. This makes it possible for the student to develop reasonable technical facility without being overwhelmed by details.

4. Teaching is organized around the patient, with whom a relationship can be initiated and developed. The approach and method of examination is emphasized, rather than the demonstration of abnormalities of disease.

5. The procedures of data gathering, analysis, and reporting are taught in the sequence in which the physician usually approaches a clinical problem.

By the completion of the General Clerkship, students are able to carry out with reasonable competence all the procedures recorded in this text. As we observe our students move into their departmental clerkships, what is most notable is their poise and self-confidence. They are sufficiently comfortable in their new but still emerging roles as physicians and technically proficient enough so that they can collect data and make observations without being excessively preoccupied with their own techniques. With such a foundation, not only is the student in a position to improve his basic clinical skills, but also, in the course of time, he is able to develop the refinements and techniques of the specialist. Obviously, the methods and organization of instruction for the beginning clinical student vary greatly from one medical school to another. Although this book was designed to meet the needs of one curriculum, it should be of value to all students. Physicians will find it useful as well. However, as with the learning of any skill, there is no substitute for precept and practice. A book can serve only as a guide.

Recognition is owed to members of the Medical-Psychiatric Liaison Group at the University of Rochester, especially to Dr. William A. Greene, Dr. Franz Reichsman, Dr. Arthur H. Schmale, Jr., and Dr. Sanford Meyerowitz, who not only contributed to the material on the techniques of interview in the former manuals and ultimately to the conceptions enunciated in this book, but also were among the first to introduce into the clinical curriculum a systematic approach to interview instruction.[3] We are indebted to Dr. Daniel O. Levinson for his help and advice, especially with respect to the chapter on the diagnostic process. Appreciation is also gratefully acknowledged to those who contributed to or reviewed parts of the text: Dr. Edward C. Atwater, Dr. John C. Donovan, Dr. Paul F. Griner, Dr. Robert J. Joynt, Dr. Milton N. Luria, Dr. Harry C. Miller, Dr. John H. Morton, Dr. William A. Peck, Dr. Bernard F. Schreiner, Jr., Dr. Albert C. Snell, Jr., Dr. James S. Williams, and Dr. Lawrence E. Young. Shirley Kinsella, R. N., Dr. Stanley L. Minken, Dr. Michael B. Mock, Dr. Dennis S. O'Leary, and Patricia M. Pye, R. N., gave helpful advice on the writing of medical orders. Students George T. Conklin, III, Dominic M. Erba, and Paul J. Mayer served as subjects in the preparation of the illustrations. A special debt of gratitude is owed to Mrs. Nina B. Crosier for her typing of the former manual, and to both Mrs. Crosier and Miss Angela Filippi for the burdensome task of typing and retyping the present manuscript. Miss Ann Hamilton also helped considerably with the final typing. Grateful appreciation is owed to Mrs. William L. Morgan, Jr., for her dedicated help with editing.

The illustrations were prepared by a gifted artist, Evelyn Lipman Engel, whom one of the authors met when he was a medical student and she was learning medical illustrating under the guidance of the late Max Brodel in the Department of Art as Applied to Medicine at the Johns Hopkins University School of Medicine.

The Commonwealth Fund has provided support for the General Clerkship. One of the authors (G.L.E.) is a Research Career Awardee of the National Institute of Mental Health (MH 14151).

---

[3]Engel, G. L.: Medical Education and the Psychosomatic Approach. A Report on the Rochester Experience, 1946-1966. J. Psychosom. Res., *11*:77, 1967.

REFERENCES

Engel, G. L.: Clinical Observation. The Neglected Basic Method of Medicine. J.A.M.A., *192*:849, 1965.
Engel, G. L.: Medical Education and the Psychosomatic Approach. A Report on the Rochester Experience, 1946-1966. J. Psychosom. Res., *11*:77, 1967.
Reichsman, F., Browning, F. E., and Hinshaw, J. R.: Observations of Undergraduate Clinical Teaching in Action. J. Med. Ed., *39*:147, 1964.

Chapter 1
INTRODUCTION TO THE PATIENT

BEGINNING CLINICAL WORK

The education of the clinical student is conducted in a setting entirely different from the preclinical years. For the first time other human beings are the direct objects of study, and his work with them includes responsibility for their well-being. No longer can the student determine the conditions under which his material will be studied, as was the case in the physiology laboratory or the autopsy room. Clinical education is founded upon a unique human bond, the physician-patient relationship, without which the patient is unable or unwilling to share the information necessary for the student to understand and learn about disease.

The purpose of this book is to help the student undertake clinical responsibilities and assume the role of the physician. It explains how the doctor-patient relationship is established and outlines how the interview and the physical examination are performed. The method of organizing clinical data in the medical record is described. Finally, the book discusses how this information is analyzed in terms of the differential diagnosis of disease, the evaluation of the patient, and the planning of future studies and management.

THE ROLE OF THE PHYSICIAN

Role refers to the rights and obligations regulating the relationship between two people. The prescribed role of the physician entitles him to make personal inquiries of the patient, to examine his body, and to carry out treatment; but at the same time, the physician is obliged to be medically competent and to provide help and comfort. Correspondingly, a person in the role of patient is entitled to ask for a physician's help, to submit to examination without fear of exploitation, and to share in confidence his personal feelings and thoughts. Such a role confers upon him the obligation to cooperate with the physician and to accept the restrictions required for adequate study and treatment.

1

The codification of these roles provides the basis for the ethical and moral standards of medical practice. So basic are the principles regulating the relationship between physician and patient that many of the rules set forth in the Hippocratic Oath, though formulated almost 2500 years ago (460 B.C.), still have relevance for the physician today:

> I swear by Apollo Physician, by Asclepius, by Health, by Panacea and by all the gods and goddesses, making them my witnesses, that I will carry out, according to my ability and judgment, this oath and this indenture. To hold my teacher in this art equal to my own parents; to make him partner in my livelihood; when he is in need of money to share mine with him; to consider his family as my own brothers, and to teach them this art, if they want to learn it, without fee or indenture; to impart precept, oral instruction, and all other instruction to my own sons, the sons of my teacher, and to indentured pupils who have taken the physician's oath, but to nobody else. I will use treatment to help the sick according to my ability and judgment, but never with a view to injury and wrong-doing. Neither will I administer a poison to anybody when asked to do so, nor will I suggest such a course. Similarly I will not give to a woman a pessary to cause abortion. But I will keep pure and holy both my life and my art. I will not use the knife, not even, verily, on sufferers from stone, but I will give place to such as are craftsmen therein. Into whatsoever houses I enter, I will enter to help the sick, and I will abstain from all intentional wrong-doing and harm, especially from abusing the bodies of man or woman, bond or free. And whatsoever I shall see or hear in the course of my profession, as well as outside my profession in my intercourse with men, if it be what should not be published abroad, I will never divulge, holding such things to be holy secrets. Now if I carry out this oath, and break it not, may I gain for ever reputation among all men for my life and for my art; but if I transgress it and forswear myself, may the opposite befall me.[1]

Clearly, the oath recognizes the power of the physician inherent in the doctor-patient relationship and serves as a warning to him against its abuse. Fundamental to this relationship is the need of the patient to be able to place himself under the care of the physician with complete trust and confidence. Indeed, so potent is this need that patients commonly ascribe qualities and capabilities to their physicians which they do not, in fact, possess. Experience shows that the physician who is primarily motivated by concern for the welfare of his patient is not only less likely to abuse this trust, but he is also more likely to provide conditions conducive to an effective relationship. Francis Peabody aptly summarized this essential quality of a physician in his classical article, by saying, "the secret of the care of the patient is in caring for the patient."[2]

The desire to help others and to alleviate suffering which underlies the career choice of most medical students also helps them to assume the role of a physician as they begin their clinical work. When a student feels concern for the patient, he is already beginning to act like a physician. This is true even at a time when he has few skills and even less knowledge. It is common for patients to ascribe the role of a physician to the

---

[1]Jones, W. H. S.: Hippocrates. William Heinemann, London; G. P. Putnam's Sons, New York, 1923, Vol. 1, pp. 298-301. (In Greek with English translation.)

[2]Peabody, F. W.: The Care of the Patient. J.A.M.A., *88*:877, 1927.

student, simply because he wears the familiar white coat, carries a stethoscope, and is seen in the company of physicians. *However, most important of all is the student's expression of genuine, sustained interest in the problems and well-being of the patient.* This is what provides a realistic basis for the patient's feeling of confidence and his consequent willingness to cooperate. It is mainly through such interactions that the rights and obligations of the physician and patient are defined for the student.

THE DOCTOR-PATIENT RELATIONSHIP

The general consideration of the roles of the physician and patient does not define the nature of the relationship between any one physician and patient. This is determined more by the circumstances of the illness, the personal characteristics of the physician and of the patient, and the previous experiences of each. By no means are all of these determinants either conscious or rational on the part of either. The attitude of each toward the other may be based as much on personality characteristics, prejudices, or unconscious mental attitudes as upon the reality of the situation. Hence, consideration must be given to some of the factors that affect the first meeting of the student and patient and that influence the subsequent relationship.

Factors Influencing the Patient's Behavior

HIS NEED FOR HELP

When a person admits to himself that he is sick, he is conceding that he is no longer as self-sufficient as before. It is this acknowledged need for help which places him in the role of a patient and provides the opportunity to establish a doctor-patient relationship. People differ in their ability and willingness to accept the patient role. Some can accept dependency with ease and readily initiate a relationship with the student. But, if the dependent needs of such a person are abnormally great, he may also have unreal expectations of the student-physician, and may become anxious, angry, or depressed when such expectations are not fulfilled. Other people find the passive, dependent role threatening. For them it is very difficult to be a patient and to place themselves in the hands of a physician. They are prone to minimize or deny symptoms, to refuse to accept the usual hospital regulations, and may even display hostile behavior when the physician attempts to interview and examine them. Familiarity with the varieties of personality structure is of considerable aid in understanding how different patients relate to a physician.

HIS PAST EXPERIENCES IN THE PATIENT ROLE

Previous experiences with physicians, good and bad, will obviously influence how the patient relates to a new doctor. Yet, even when the patient's reactions are based primarily on the incompetent or tactless behavior of a former physician, it is notable how readily he will respond to the more adequate behavior of a new physician.

HIS PAST EXPERIENCES IN RELATING TO OTHER PERSONS

Very basic attitudes about accepting a physician's help originate from the patient's experiences with important persons in his childhood. The patient who as a child had confidence in his parent's capacity to provide help usually can place himself in the physician's hands with trust and confidence. On the other hand, a childhood experience with unreliable, rejecting, or neglectful parents may seriously interfere with the patient's capacity to have confidence in even the most dedicated physician. Such a patient may remain aloof, suspicious, and be only indifferently cooperative. Patients with an unfulfilled need for parental approval may try to gain the physician's acceptance, even by omitting or distorting facts.

It is, therefore, important for the physician to inquire about the patient's early and current relationships. By understanding how he interacts with others, the physician can anticipate the form that the patient's relationship will take, and he can modify his own behavior accordingly.

HIS FEARS CONCERNING THE ILLNESS

Some patients have major fears about the nature of the illness or of hospital procedures. Whether such concerns are realistic or not, the physician must recognize their existence and encourage the patient to speak of them. This often serves to overcome what might have been a serious barrier to communication. For instance, the patient who is afraid that his symptoms of cough and expectoration mean cancer will more readily talk if the physician discreetly inquires about his fears.

SOCIAL, CULTURAL, EDUCATIONAL, AND ECONOMIC DETERMINANTS

These factors may all significantly influence the patient's expectations of the physician. Especially when the student-physician's background differs from that of his patient, it behooves him to learn about the patient's upbringing and current life situation. The most immediate and practical means of so doing is through proper attention to the patient's personal and social history. (See Chapters 3 and 5.) Students who have had experience with people of backgrounds different from their own are at a decided advantage in this regard.

Factors Influencing the Student-Physician's Behavior

HIS INSECURITY IN THE NEW ROLE

A serious obstacle to the student's initial efforts to relate to his patient is his feeling of insecurity because of inexperience. Commonly, this leads to inappropriate diffidence on his part. The beginning student need not behave as if it is an imposition to inquire into the patient's illness or to perform a physical examination. He need not approach the patient apologetically to ask permission to carry out necessary tasks or to thank the patient for cooperating. *The student should appreciate that his personal educational goals and the patient's need for help are complementary, not antagonistic!* In fact, the opportunity for the patient to tell his story, to share his concerns, and to be examined by an understanding clinical student often is of therapeutic value to the patient. The student should also recognize that his ready access to other members of the clinical staff is an important means of communication for the patient. Further, the student is likely to spend more time with his patient and to know more about him than do many members of the staff. Blumgart illustrates the high degree of confidence a patient may develop in a student with the story of a patient who refused to consider surgery for severe gastric hemorrhage despite the advice of the Chief of Medicine and other specialists.[3] Only when the patient had a chance to talk it over with the fourth year clerk, did he consent to surgery! *The obvious lesson is that most patients regard the student as an important source of help. When the student acts accordingly, he will be more successful in establishing the type of relationship that will further his own learning and will provide the patient with the best type of care.*

HIS YOUTH AND INEXPERIENCE

This is not as much of a barrier in establishing a relationship as many students might think. There are some patients who, because they fear authority, may confide even more readily in a student than in an

---

[3]Blumgart, H. L.: Caring for the Patient. New Eng. J. Med., *270*:449, 1964.

older physician. A subtle factor that sometimes influences the patient's response to the youth of the student may be his relationship with his own children. For example, an occasional older patient may treat the student as a son whom he helps by providing the history and cooperating in the examination. A patient may even take pleasure in his young doctor's performance. An adolescent patient may perceive the student as an older sibling to whom he more readily can relate than to the older physician. On the other hand, it must also be appreciated that irrational attitudes on the part of a patient may derive from conflicts with his own children or with younger siblings, a fact which may become evident from how the patient speaks of his own children.

HIS PERSONAL ATTITUDES AND PSYCHOLOGICAL PROBLEMS

Each student will quickly discover that there are certain categories of patients with whom he readily gets along, and therefore likes, and others with whom he has difficulties, and dislikes. These attitudes involve such varied aspects of the patient as his age, sex, educational background, physical attractiveness, racial origin, and behavior. Predisposition to such biases on the part of the student is embedded in his own background and involves his personality, his unresolved psychological conflicts, and his prejudices. Such characteristics can be diminished through understanding and self-discipline, but usually can not be totally eliminated. When a student becomes aware of difficulty with a particular type of patient, it is well for him to try to understand what it is about the patient that disturbs him, so that he can attempt to modify his own reaction. For example, the student may find himself becoming irritated with a patient whose slowness and inattention hinder his obtaining a good history. Appreciation that such "stupidity" or "resistance" on the patient's part may actually reflect depression or organic brain disease, and is really not directed toward him as an individual, enables the student to overcome his feeling of irritation and to modify appropriately his approach to the patient.

While positive feelings toward a patient generally facilitate the establishment of a relationship, they should be questioned if they are exceptionally intense or if they are repetitively aroused by a certain type of patient. Under these circumstances, there is a risk of inappropriate involvement with the patient. Generally, such intense involvements have as their source some unresolved problem in the student. One is well advised to remember that no human being is free of the capability of behaving irrationally. Hence, when he finds himself intensely involved with a patient or when an instructor calls his attention to the inappropriateness of his reaction, the student should give some thought to what might be responsible and, if necessary, seek advice. Many times the problem is alleviated by discussing the situation with a more experienced physician.

THE CLINICAL SETTING

The student's first experience in the study and care of patients generally takes place on a hospital ward. Later he has opportunities to see patients in other settings, such as the out-patient department, the emergency ward, the community clinic, and even in the patient's home or the physician's office. The ward has many advantages for the introduction to clinical work. Patients are readily available, they are usually hospitalized long enough for unhurried study, and there is an ever-present professional staff for guidance and instruction. William Osler, the master clinician, may be credited with bringing the student from the lecture room to the patient's bedside in the teaching of clinical medicine.[4]

The Ward as a Clinical Laboratory

The student on the ward learns through actual experience and practice the role and functions of a physician as well as the nature, manifestations, and treatment of disease. He learns something of how illness and hospitalization affect patients and their families. He sees how doctors, nurses, nursing assistants, physical therapists, occupational therapists, social workers, technicians, and clergymen work with each other and with the patient toward the common goals of diagnosis and treatment. The student learns how to fit into this complex social structure. Above all, he learns how the physician makes observations and how he collects, records, and analyzes the information obtained from the patient, the family, and the laboratory. He also learns how such data are used to gain an understanding of the patient and his illness, which provides the basis for a plan of treatment.

The student discovers quickly enough that patients admitted to a hospital are likely to have serious or complicated illnesses. Even though he is a beginner, he no longer has the advantage of starting with the elementary and progressing to the complex. His first patients may be as difficult and as obscure as any he will encounter in the future, taxing the ingenuity and knowledge of his most experienced teachers. Often the

---

[4]Osler, W.: Aequanimitas with Other Addresses. The Blakiston Co., Philadelphia, 1952.

student will find serious disagreement among the staff as to the findings, their interpretation, and the management of the case. The thoughtful student appreciates the educational value of such disagreements. He attempts to learn the reasons for the conflicting opinions by inquiring of the staff and by studying the hospital record. He follows closely the subsequent course of events, attempting to form his own judgments. He observes his patients daily; he takes note of new findings; he follows his patient to the operating room or to the autopsy table; and when the occasion permits, he inquires about his patient's condition after discharge.

At the same time, the student will discover that often the hospital ward is a difficult place in which to work. There may be inadequate space around the bed. There may be poor lighting, interruptions by ward personnel, and noise from neighboring patients or low-flying airplanes. The patient may be away from the ward for tests. A student must learn to be flexible and adjust to such variable and frustrating conditions.

The Ward as a Social Structure

For both the patient and the student, introduction to a hospital ward requires adjustment to the rules, customs, and organization of an unfamiliar social structure. The new student adapts more quickly to the hospital setting if he is assigned to a specific area for a number of weeks. It is helpful for him to be conducted about the ward by a member of the staff and to be introduced to the personnel. He should also inform himself concerning the regulations and ward staffing routines, such as meal times, nursing shifts, and visiting hours. Some of this information may be posted on bulletin boards. Beyond that, the observant student, by tactfully observing the conduct of the various professional staff, quickly becomes familiar with the organization and his place in it. As this is accomplished, he finds himself in a position to observe what being in a hospital means to the patient.

Hospitalization is by no means a uniform experience for all patients. Some see it as a haven to which they come for help and the relief of symptoms; others see it as a strange and frightening place where they may be hurt or even die. But for all patients, admission to the hospital, especially for the first time, requires a major adjustment. They are separated from home and family; for some this may be distressing; for others, a relief. Patients are deprived of certain personal liberties and freedom of action, yet are relieved of many responsibilities. They are often confined to bed, and clothing and personal possessions are taken away. The schedule of meals and sleep is altered; there is a limited choice of diet. Unpleasant or painful procedures are anticipated, and distressing sights and sounds may be witnessed. At the same time, patients are provided with care and service; and are supported by the hope that their distress will be relieved and their problems solved.

In addition, patients find they must relate to a bewildering number of people. Even the active, well person in everyday life is not ordinarily called upon to meet, recognize, and relate to so many others and in such rapid succession. The nursing staff shifts three times a day; the house staff, medical students, and nursing students are rotated away from the ward; and consultants, dietitians, and technicians come and go. Anxiety, depression, irritability, anger, or other psychological disturbances may at times reflect the patient's inability to identify who is responsible for his care. It is in this area that the student may be particularly helpful. Because of the time he spends with the patient, often he is the most consistent person to whom the patient can relate.

The nurses, doctors, and students all share a responsibility for helping the patient adjust to the ward routine. *The basic principle involved is to reduce uncertainty as much as possible for the patient.* By being thoroughly familiar with the organization of the ward and knowing the names of the head nurse, the house staff, and the attending staff, the student can assist appreciably in orienting the patient to his new environment. *The student should also be sure to clearly identify himself and explain his own role in the future study and care of the patient.* As best he can, the student learns in advance what procedures, examinations, or consultations are planned, since, on occasion, he must inform the patient and explain the studies to him. Such preparation spares the patient the distress of the unexpected and often enables his questions to be answered or his fears to be resolved. The student also has the responsibility to inform his patient when he is to be presented on teaching rounds, to explain to him what is involved, and to answer any questions he may raise.

A subtle and often overlooked influence in a hospital ward is the effect patients may have on each other. Particularly in multibed units, the newly arrived patient may be indoctrinated by his roommates, not always appropriately. Patients come to know one another and often are distressed when their fellow patient gets sicker, is discharged, or dies. A patient's loneliness may be increased when his roommates have attentive visitors; or he may become upset when the others behave inappropriately. *The student must be attentive to the impact that other patients and their visitors have on his patient.* He should know the medical condition of others in the room, should observe how the patients interact, and pay attention to what each says about the other.

THE RESPONSIBILITIES AND OBLIGATIONS OF THE CLINICAL STUDENT

The primary objectives of the medical student are to learn the substance and methods of medicine and to achieve the professional role of the physician. These are best accomplished through graduated and carefully supervised engagement in the care of the sick, an activity which imposes additional responsibilities and obligations on the beginning student.

Obligations to the Patient

Under all circumstances, the well-being and comfort of the patient take precedence. He must be treated with respect and consideration in a professional, not in a diffident or apologetic manner. This means that the student has the right to interview, to examine patients, and to carry out certain procedures; and he should proceed to do so without apology. He must be aware that observations he makes do have relevance to the care of the sick, and that the great majority of patients expect him to carry out his duties in a business-like fashion. Most patients appreciate that the young doctor has to learn and are tolerant of the student's slowness or awkwardness. For the student, the factors which facilitate his work with the patient are sensitivity and concern for the patient's well-being. This, coupled with a professional attitude, does much to help the patient accept necessary but disagreeable procedures.

The professional attitude literally means that the student behave in a manner which patients expect of a physician. This includes attention to such matters as personal dress, grooming, cleanliness, language, and decorum, the standards for which are well established in the minds of patients. It means that gum chewing, smoking, horseplay, laughing, joking, sitting on the patient's bed, and other behavior quite permissible in other settings is unacceptable and, indeed, may seriously interfere with the patient's ability to establish a relationship and cooperate in the examination. The professional attitude calls for dignity, seriousness, conscientiousness, and the exhibition of a genuine intellectual effort to understand the patient's problems. It requires that personal interests and feelings not be permitted to interfere with the immediate task at hand, the relief of the suffering of another human being.

At all times, the student must be aware that the sick person is preoccupied with himself and may subjectively interpret or misinterpret whatever the student may say or do. The student must be thoughtful in his choice of language when speaking with the patient and must be alert to what the patient may overhear, whether at the bedside or in a totally unrelated corridor conversation. Confiding to the patient one's own personal problems or concerns is inappropriate.

Strict observance of the patient's right to privacy and confidentiality requires that information be shared only with other professionally qualified persons. At times, the patient needs to be reassured that his statements will be kept in confidence. Demonstration of sexual interest or expression of personal disapproval have no place in the behavior of the student-physician. *Basic to professional conduct is respect for the patient, regardless of how deviant his behavior may appear to be.* Such an attitude on the part of the physician is not only in the highest ethical tradition of medicine, but it is also essential if he is to effectively carry out his functions. One must be reminded that in times past, victims of epilepsy, venereal disease, and mental illness were regarded as objects of moral opprobrium and beyond the province of the physician. Even now, the role of the physician in the care of patients with such problems as alcoholism, drug addiction, and sexual deviancy is only beginning to be clarified.

Obligations to the Patient's Family and Visitors

Consideration for the family and friends of the patient is also important. They are often anxious in the hospital setting and may have made the visit at considerable personal inconvenience. Their presence can do much to help the patient adjust to the hospital as well as maintain a link with the outside world. When the student finds a visitor at the bedside, he should introduce himself, establish the identity of the visitor, and learn how long he has been with the patient. If it is only a short time and the student's business is not urgent, he should arrange with the patient and visitor to return later at a specific time. On his return, the student informs the visitor of the approximate duration of the examination, asks him to wait in the visitor's lounge, and notifies him when he has finished seeing the patient.

The student may also be asked questions by visitors. When these involve issues about the patient's illness they should, in general, be referred to the physician primarily responsible for the patient's care, either the house officer or the personal physician. It is his responsibility to keep the family informed concerning the patient's condition. Should an unforeseen complication arise, the physician-in-charge immediately notifies the family. On the other hand, it is quite appropriate for the student to respond to inquiries that do not directly concern the patient's condition, such as information about hospital routine.

Because visitors may be disturbing as well as helpful to his patient, the student should make a point to learn who visits and who does not. The effect of family and friends on the patient's feelings is noted. *The student should also make it a practice to interview important family members, not only for additional information concerning the patient, but also because it often is helpful for the relative to be able to speak of his concerns about the patient.* Further details on the technique of interviewing relatives are covered in Chapter 3.

Obligations to Ward Personnel

Others on the ward play a vital role in patient care. Consideration for them and their responsibilities is of utmost importance. For example, to delay a patient's dinner in order to finish a lengthy examination disrupts the work of the Dietary Department and results in the patient's receiving a cold meal. Interruption of the nurses' chart rounds or of drug administration at the bedside are only justified in urgent situations. When planning an interview or a physical examination, the student should check with the head nurse or the ward secretary to learn when the patient will be unavailable because of diagnostic or therapeutic procedures. Nonetheless, interruptions by nurses to administer medications, by technicians to perform tests, or by house staff to carry out procedures are unavoidable.

The student should understand that the information he obtains from his observation of the patient or family may be of great importance. If he has any reason to suspect that he has discovered something not known to the staff, it is his responsibility to bring it to the attention of the house officer or nurse-in-charge. A new symptom or sign, the inadequate functioning of drainage or intravenous tubing, an urgent question or complaint by the patient, all should be reported promptly. By serving as a channel of communication between the patient and other personnel, the student performs a service for the patient and enhances his relationship.

THE RIGHTS AND PRIVILEGES OF THE CLINICAL STUDENT

Along with responsibilities and obligations go rights and privileges. The student's role in patient care is well recognized. The legal responsibility for his supervision is assumed by the educational institution in the form of his preceptors, who are licensed physicians. The following are some of the rights and privileges of the clinical student:

1. *To interview.* This includes access to personal, family, and social data that are not ordinarily proper subjects of inquiry in a nonprofessional setting.

2. *To perform a physical examination.* The student has the right to perform a complete physical examination, including the rectal and pelvic examination.

3. *To carry out minor procedures.* When a student has attained competence through supervision, he may perform such procedures as venipunctures, throat cultures, or the passage of nasogastric tubes.

4. *To ask for help.* It is essential for the patient's well-being and the student's education that he feel free to seek help from interns, residents, nurses, and attending physicians.

5. *To examine his patient's charts and records.* These include records from other hospitals, for which authorization from a responsible faculty member is usually required.

6. *To speak with other personnel responsible for the care of the patient.* Should the student need additional information, he should speak with such staff as the house officer, the consultant, the social worker, the physiotherapist, the occupational therapist, or the dietitian. The patient's private physician is an important source of information, with whom the student should not hesitate to communicate in person or by a phone call.

7. *To observe special procedures or examinations.* When others carry out procedures on an assigned patient, including surgery, the student may be in attendance. Courtesy, however, requires that permission be obtained from the physician carrying out the procedure.

8. *To request access to laboratory material for personal examination.* This includes the privilege of examining such material as x-ray films, electrocardiograms, electroencephalograms, and pathological specimens. With this privilege goes the right to ask for assistance in interpretation. On the other hand, it is not the student's prerogative to *order* such procedures.

THE QUALITIES OF THE IDEAL PHYSICIAN

There is no agreement as to the qualities of the ideal physician or how such qualities are to be developed. Medicine is a broad and varied field. There is a place in it for persons of many different persuasions. Undergraduate medical education should produce an undifferentiated physician; that is, one who has grasped what is basic and essential to all medicine, yet who has had the opportunity to apply such principles in a variety of more specialized areas. Such a physician can then develop in whatever direction his personal inclination and talents indicate. Regardless of the ultimate career choice, the following are offered as the qualities that best exemplify the characteristics of the ideal physician:

He is first and foremost humane. The ideal clinician deals not simply with the abstraction, disease, but with a fellow being in distress. He relates to his patient with empathy, which implies the ability to understand and appreciate how the patient feels without being distressed himself. The physician appreciates that all that bears on his patient's life, comfort, and happiness is properly a subject for scientific inquiry and observation. To deal with the disease alone and forget the patient is to fail as an able physician.

He is constantly observant. From the time the doctor first meets the patient, or walks into the room, he is studying him and his surroundings to learn clues to his disease, his personality, and the sources of his distress.

He uses a systematic approach. He trains himself in the interview and physical examination, as well as in his thinking, to follow an orderly sequence and not to omit important findings. Yet, he is not inflexible; he is prepared to meet the new or unexpected and to adapt his approach.

He knows and understands basic principles. He has learned that comprehension of the basic reasoning behind medical concepts and techniques greatly enhances his capacity to apply knowledge and to devise approaches to new and unfamiliar situations.

He uses reason in all his actions. Each step in diagnosis and management is thoughtfully considered. He knows that the physician who approaches a problem automatically, or routinely, may fail to help the individual patient.

He is aware of the limitations of his own knowledge and of knowledge in general. He constantly strives to extend his knowledge and to learn for himself the boundaries of generally established knowledge. He is at all times ready to seek the counsel and help of the more experienced and is not afraid to say "I don't know." He learns to think logically and to commit himself to a diagnosis. However, he appreciates that any commitment he makes to diagnosis or treatment is subject to revision on the basis of new information, and he does not hesitate to change his views under such circumstances. The welfare of his patient takes precedence over his personal pride.

He respects the information that comes from the patient. While appreciating variation in patient reliability, he recognizes that the patient is likely to be the best source of information concerning his own condition, with close family members or friends as important supplementary sources. He knows that data derived from the interview and the physical examination provide the basis upon which further laboratory and other diagnostic procedures are selected, and that ordinarily such procedures are used to *confirm, not make,* diagnoses. He has learned that the indiscriminate use of laboratory procedures is not only uneconomical, but also may be misleading.

He is a perpetual student. He has developed the sequence of *see-think-read*, then think and see again. He interviews and examines a patient, then reads about the issues bearing on his observations. He returns to the patient to extend and clarify his findings which he uses to plan further diagnostic and therapeutic procedures. He never underestimates his own ability to make a new and original observation.

References

Blumgart, H. L.: Caring for the Patient. New Eng. J. Med., *270*:449, 1964.
Jones, W. H. S.: Hippocrates. William Heinemann, London; G. P. Putnam's Sons, New York, 1923, Vol. 1, pp. 298-301. (In Greek with English translation.)
Osler, W.: Aequanimitas with Other Addresses. The Blakiston Co., Philadelphia, 1952.
Peabody, F. W.: The Care of the Patient. J.A.M.A., *88*:877, 1927.

Chapter 2

THE DIAGNOSTIC PROCESS

Diagnosis has two major objectives. One is to characterize the nature of the pathologic processes in scientific, impersonal terms. The other is to evaluate the consequence of these processes in the individual patient. Feinstein has proposed that the first be referred to as the disease and the second as the illness.[1] The diagnostic process ultimately leads to the classification of disease and the evaluation of a patient's illness, both of which provide a rational basis for estimating his prognosis and planning for his care. For example, the term "diabetes mellitus" refers to the *disease* present in all patients so diagnosed. But the term gives relatively little information concerning an individual's experience with diabetes. In order to understand an individual's *illness*, one must learn about the severity, duration, stage, and course of diabetes in that patient; the influence of his particular biological or psychosocial disposition on the diabetes; and the impact of the disease on his way of life.

The diagnostic process is the mental operation through which the disease is identified and the illness evaluated. The procedures utilized by the physician are the interview, the physical examination, and various technical diagnostic procedures. The interview, whether directed to the patient or to an informed observer, yields information, such as the patient's subjective sensations (e.g., pain, nausea, or shortness of breath), his feelings (e.g., apprehension, despair, or irritability), changes in appearance (e.g., swellings, pallor, or skin lesions), and alterations in function (e.g., constipation, paralysis, or inability to work). The interview also provides information concerning the past health of the patient and his family, his development and relationships, and the setting in which the illness arose. In the physical examination, the physician evaluates the condition of the patient's body and his behavior. Diagnostic studies, such as blood and urine tests, endoscopy, electrocardiography, or roentgenography, are used to extend the range of the physician's observations.

The clinical manifestations of illness are classified as symptoms and signs. *Symptoms* are the subjective sensations and changes in body or mental function which the patient or the inquiring physician regards

---

[1]Feinstein, A. R.: Clinical Judgment, Williams and Wilkins Co., Baltimore, 1967, pp. 24-25.

as abnormal. Such information is obtained through the interview. *Signs* are the abnormal findings that are detected by the physician in the physical examination.

The diagnostic process involves a systematic analysis of symptoms, signs, and related clinical data. The physician must decide first which findings are abnormal by comparing them to accepted standards and to the individual's previous status. He then attempts to interpret the symptoms and signs in terms of underlying morphologic, biochemical, physiologic, microbiologic, or psychosocial factors to make the diagnosis of the disease. Finally, he evaluates the personal experience of the patient in relationship to the disease to gain an understanding of his illness.

The diagnostic process involves six separate but interrelated considerations:

1. The identification of the abnormal findings.
2. The localization of the abnormal findings in anatomic terms.
3. The interpretation of the abnormal findings in structural and functional terms.
4. The consideration of etiology.
5. The classification of the disease.
6. The evaluation of the patient's illness.

THE IDENTIFICATION OF THE ABNORMAL FINDINGS

The physician's first task is to identify which symptoms and signs are abnormal for the patient under study. From the patient's perspective, a symptom always signifies an abnormal state. In some instances, his interpretation is obviously correct, as when the complaint is shortness of breath, nausea, bloody diarrhea, or memory loss. In other instances, the symptoms are based on misinterpretation of physiologic variants, as when a patient anxiously expresses concern about a minor skin blemish. Persistence of such concern, in spite of reassurance, constitutes a symptom in its own right usually indicative of a psychologic disturbance. But not all patients report even obvious changes. For psychological reasons some minimize or even deny symptoms which are alarming to other patients. Such symptoms must be elicited by the physician. For example, a patient may deny that he is short of breath, but upon questioning may reluctantly acknowledge that he no longer takes his customary walks because he does not enjoy them. Further inquiry may reveal that it is because he gets "a little winded." Here, the doctor's experience enables him to identify a subjective abnormality not acknowledged by the patient, which must then be evaluated by objective examination. Some abnormalities are not experienced by patients as unpleasant or as a source of concern. An obese person, for instance, who has wished to slim down, may not report a loss of weight caused by developing diabetes; or the progressive symptoms of a cough due to bronchogenic carcinoma may be dismissed as a cigarette cough.

Changes in the patient's way of life may also reflect an abnormality. A patient may alter his pattern of eating because it makes him feel better; for example, he may find that frequent meals alleviate his hunger pangs, not recognizing these as ulcer symptoms. A patient may change his job because the work imposes too great a physical or psychological demand; or he may marry or separate in an effort to resolve a personal conflict. Thus, different life patterns may not only reflect a patient's response to some underlying physical or psychological disturbance, they may also constitute an attempt to alleviate or resolve the difficulty. The knowledge and the experience of the physician enable him to recognize when such changes in behavior are manifestations of disease.

Abnormal signs are observed by the physician during his examination. If obvious, the patient may also be aware of an abnormality that is asymptomatic, such as the growth of a mole or the swelling of his ankles. In general, the patient's symptoms alert the physician to look for abnormal signs. Once a physical finding is discovered, the physician must decide whether it is a physiologic variant or the product of disease; and whether it is related to the patient's present problem. For example, the enlarged thyroid of a patient raised in the iodine deficient goiter belt is of far less significance than an enlarged gland in a patient with symptoms of thyrotoxicosis; or the elevation of blood pressure on an initial physical examination has less meaning compared to the finding of sustained hypertension on repeated examinations.

Finally, other abnormalities are neither reported by the patient (symptoms) nor become apparent to the physician on observation (signs) but are discovered by means of laboratory tests or special diagnostic procedures. For example, red blood cells may be seen in the urine on microscopic study, a polyp in the sigmoid colon upon sigmoidoscopy, or an unsuspected lung lesion found in a roentgen film of the chest.

THE LOCALIZATION OF THE ABNORMAL FINDINGS IN ANATOMIC TERMS

Here the physician considers whether the abnormal symptoms and signs can be localized in terms of anatomic subdivisions of the body. It is convenient to think in terms of several different levels of organization:

1. A region of the body (e.g., the abdominal cavity or thorax).

2. An organ system (e.g., the gastrointestinal tract or a subdivision, as the terminal ileum).

3. An organ (e.g., the liver or heart).

4. Multiple systems (e.g., cellular structure or a tissue component, as the red blood cell, blood vessels, or connective tissue).

In general, one can readily assign symptoms and signs to the larger anatomic categories; namely, a region of the body, an organ system, or a specific organ. Symptoms or signs deriving from cellular or tissue abnormalities involving several organs or systems may be more difficult to recognize from the interview and physical examination alone. Special laboratory procedures may be required in such diseases as polyarteritis nodosa, hemolytic anemia, or multiple myeloma.

Once the physician decides on the gross anatomic location responsible for signs or symptoms, he progressively explores the finer morphologic divisions. For example, the patient may complain of chest pain. By appropriate questioning, the physician will attempt to localize the pain to a given organ or organ system. Does chest pain originate in the chest wall (related to body movement), the esophagus (aggravated by swallowing), or the heart (brought on by exertion)? If he determines that the pain is pleuritic by demonstrating its relationship to breathing, the physician will then try to determine the exact location by physical examination. For example, he will look for a pleural friction rub and underlying pulmonary findings. A chest film may help to pinpoint the diagnosis.

It must be appreciated that psychologic symptoms may also be expressed in bodily terms. The physician may suspect that the chest pain is psychologic in origin, such as a conversion symptom. He will then attempt to demonstrate that the pain does not fit any anatomic pattern and will investigate what psychologic factors are responsible for the choice of the chest as the location of the pain in that particular individual.[2] Whether the underlying basis is physical or psychologic, the location of a symptom or a sign does not necessarily correspond to its source of origin. Paralysis of an arm may not be a result of injury to the arm itself, but may be due to conversion or brain injury; vomiting may be caused by an emotional disturbance or by digitalis intoxication with no organic gastrointestinal basis.

Finally, it must be appreciated that some clinical manifestations, such as fever, generalized weakness, and weight loss, have no localizing significance. Such symptoms in themselves are of little help in making a specific diagnosis, but they do serve to indicate generalized or systemic involvement and may be a measure of the severity of the illness.

---

[2]Engel, G. L.: Conversion symptoms. In MacBryde, C. M.: Signs and Symptoms. Applied Pathologic Physiology and Clinical Interpretation. 5th Ed., J. B. Lippincott Co., Philadelphia, 1969, Chap. 26.

THE INTERPRETATION OF THE ABNORMAL FINDINGS IN STRUCTURAL AND FUNCTIONAL TERMS

The symptoms experienced by the patient and the signs observed by the physician derive ultimately from alterations in structure and function. Accordingly, the physician must analyze the relationships between signs and symptoms and interpret them in terms of underlying pathologic anatomy (e.g., inflammation, neoplasia, degeneration); pathophysiology (e.g., left ventricular failure, renal insufficiency, hepatic failure); or psychopathology (e.g., conversion, delirium, psychosis). This step in the diagnostic process carries the thinking of the physician from the primary clinical data to an explanatory level. The clinician must infer from symptoms and signs the abnormalities in function and structure. For example, from the findings of dyspnea, orthopnea, and rales at the lung bases he infers pulmonary edema.

Necessary for such diagnostic thinking is a thorough grasp of the preclinical disciplines and continued familiarity with advances in clinical science. It is most important to appreciate that the patient's account of his illness represents an attempt to put into words his awareness of changes in his body, in his mind, or in the external environment. As the physician listens to the patient's story, he attempts to visualize what is going on in terms of his own scientific knowledge. For example, a sudden pain increasing within 15 or 20 seconds to a peak intensity that is maintained for a minute or two, that then subsides, only to recur again in another minute, should evoke in the listener's mind the image of a peristaltic contraction meeting resistance. The ability to visualize mentally this physiologic process is dependent on the physician's knowledge of the innervation and motor behavior of smooth muscle in the walls of hollow viscera. From the location and radiation of the pain, he is also able to infer which hollow organ is the most likely site of the obstruction. Knowledge of the natural history of pathologic processes is then brought to bear on the clinical data in order to reach a conclusion concerning the underlying abnormality — whether, for instance, the obstruction is more likely due to a stone, a neoplasm, or a fibrous band.

Not only must the patient's symptoms be understood in structural and functional terms, but so must the abnormal physical findings. For example, the signs of neck vein distention, rales, and ankle edema, together with the symptoms of dyspnea and orthopnea, are interpreted to mean abnormal cardiac function or congestive heart failure. Physical examination can also pinpoint a structural abnormality, such as a heart murmur, that may not be known to the patient, and hence, not mentioned in his story. Finally, laboratory studies are introduced to confirm and quantitate abnormalities in functional and structural terms. Cardiac catheterization, for instance, will measure the degree of restriction of cardiac output, and angiocardiography will visualize valve thickening and immobility.

THE CONSIDERATION OF ETIOLOGY

In the final analysis, disease may be conceptualized as a failure of the organism to cope with forces originating within itself or its environment which disrupt its dynamic steady state.[3] The abnormal signs, symptoms, and laboratory findings may reflect damage as well as attempts to prevent or repair damage. The combination of forces which are ultimately responsible for such reactions of the organism may be considered to be the causes or the etiology of disease.

In considering the problem of causes, the distinction between the disease and the illness assumes particular importance. With respect to the abstraction, disease, it is often possible to make definitive statements about etiology. Indeed, the names of certain diseases are based on specific etiologic factors. For example, the disease, tuberculosis, is named after the tubercle bacillus, and the diagnosis is based on the isolation of the organism or the demonstration of the characteristic pathological changes. One is justified in saying that the cause of the disease, tuberculosis, is the tubercle bacillus. But such a statement would be inadequate in defining the etiology of the illness, tuberculosis, which is the experience of an individual infected with tubercle bacilli. The analysis of causes, therefore, must include not only the identification of specific pathogenic agents, but also an evaluation of the factors responsible for the patient's exposure and vulnerability to such agents. The latter may range from genetic or constitutional factors to social conditions. With respect to the causes of illness, medical knowledge is still very limited. It is easier, for example, to identify the tuberculosis organism and diagnose the disease, than to answer why the organism is localized to a given area of the body, such as the lungs, kidneys, or meninges, or to explain why the patient developed the disease at a specific time in his life. But it must also be appreciated that medicine not only is imperfect in its knowledge of factors accounting for the patient's illness, but that it also lacks knowledge to explain the specific etiology of many diseases as well, such as diabetes mellitus, hypertension, or peptic ulcer.

Since the physician deals with an individual patient, he must attempt to

---

[3]Engel, G. L.: Psychological Development in Health and Disease. W. B. Saunders Co., Philadelphia, 1962, Chap. 23 to 25.

elucidate the causes of the illness, not simply of the disease. In practical terms, this means that he evaluates all possible factors which might play a role in the illness. He inquires into genetic predispositions; early injury or developmental failures; exposure to microorganisms, toxic materials, or physical agents; and any underlying factors that may alter resistance, such as age, nutrition, alcoholism, or other disease processes. He learns of the condition of the patient's life and evaluates it for possible psychological stresses that may ensue from real or threatened losses, conflicts, or personal frustrations.[4] In a case of pulmonary tuberculosis, for example, a full statement of the causative factors might include a strong family history of tuberculosis with frequent exposure in childhood; and a current setting of depression, alcoholism, and malnutrition, precipitated by the patient's reaction to the death of his wife.

THE CLASSIFICATION OF THE DISEASE

Once consideration has been given to etiology, the physician attempts to classify the disease process. Because of imperfect knowledge, the nomenclature and taxonomy of diseases are quite arbitrary. The lack of knowledge is admitted in the names of some diseases, such as essential hyperlipemia or idiopathic thrombocytopenic purpura. Vague terminology may derive from historical tradition. Raynaud's disease, Hodgkin's disease, or Parkinson's disease are named after the men who first described the condition. On the other hand, Christmas disease (Factor IX deficiency) is named after the first patient in whom the disease was recognized. Initial colorful descriptive nomenclature has been retained in other diseases: lupus erythematosis (the condition of the red wolf), named after the reddish facial skin lesions; pernicious anemia (deadly anemia), because of the former uniformly fatal course; or gout (drop), because it was once believed that a noxious agent dripped into the joint to cause the disease.

In the past, characteristic symptoms and signs of diverse etiology were grouped together as clinical syndromes. With more precise diagnosis, the number of syndromes have declined. A few are still popular, such as Horner's syndrome, the nephrotic syndrome, or the chronic brain syndrome. Even the major divisions of systems of classification are heterogeneous and imprecise. Some diseases are listed according to the organ system (diseases of the cardiovascular system, liver, or kidneys); others are classified in functional terms (metabolic diseases, nutritional diseases, or demyelinating diseases); and still others according to eti-

---

[4]Engel, G. L.: Psychological Development in Health and Disease. W. B. Saunders Co., Philadelphia, 1962, Chap. 26 and 27.

ology (infectious diseases, diseases due to chemical agents, or hereditary disorders).

Obviously, such terminology is highly confusing. The student is best guided in the classification of disease by his textbook reading or special publications.[5] When making a diagnosis, he should try to be as precise and specific as possible. Syndromes or functional abnormalities, such as congestive heart failure, uremia, or anemia, must be defined further as to cause. When descriptive terms are used, they should be clear and complete; and if alternative nomenclature is available, the use of historical names should be avoided. Known specific etiologic agents are also included. For example, instead of saying Addison's disease, it is better to state "chronic adrenal insufficiency due to adrenal tuberculosis"; or "acute pneumococcal pneumonia of the right lower lobe" is more specific and preferable to "pneumonia."

THE EVALUATION OF THE PATIENT'S ILLNESS

The final step in the diagnostic process is to understand the effect of the disease on the individual patient. The severity of an illness makes it unique for that individual. In order to estimate severity, the abnormal findings are evaluated in quantitative terms and are compared to those of a person in a normal state of health. Symptoms, such as pain, dyspnea, or anxiety, are estimated with regard to intensity, rate of development, and duration. Physical findings are measured against accepted standards (e.g., the size of a mass is expressed in centimeters; or cyanosis is described as mild, moderate, or severe). The degree of structural or functional impairment is estimated in absolute terms (e.g., the range of motion at an arthritic joint), or in relation to the patient's previous capabilities (e.g., the amount of activity possible without fatigue or dyspnea). For certain diseases, standards have been established by committees of experts. For example, cardiac function ranges from Class I, with no symptoms, to Class IV, with symptoms at rest.[6] Important, too, are the character and magnitude of the etiologic factors (e.g., the virulence of the organism or the amount of radiation) and the condition of the patient at the time the disease develops (e.g., the degree of malnutrition or the presence of depression). One must not only evaluate findings in

---

[5]Thompson, E. T., and Hayden, A. C., Eds.: Standard Nomenclature of Diseases and Operations. Published for the American Medical Association by the Blakiston Division of the McGraw-Hill Book Co., New York, 1961.

[6]Criteria Committee of the New York Heart Association, Inc.: Nomenclature and Criteria for Diagnosis of Diseases of the Heart and Blood Vessels. P. F. Mallon, Inc., New York, 1955.

quantitative terms, but must also be aware of any discrepancies in the severity of symptoms and signs. For example, is the dyspnea out of proportion to the demonstrated findings in the cardiac and respiratory systems? Is the patient's professed inability to carry on his job as a carpenter in keeping with the demonstrated degree of anemia? Attention to such discrepancies is important, for it encourages the physician to consider alternative explanations.

Especially important, and often disregarded, are psychological and social factors. Knowledge of them is essential for a full understanding of an illness in order to insure proper management. Included are the patient's feelings about being ill, about being hospitalized, and about his physician; his concerns about finances, his family, or job; and the availability of family or friends for emotional support. Knowledge of the patient's personality structure is also important in order to determine what program of care will best meet his needs. For example, a diabetic whose life has been marked by planning, orderliness, and attention to detail can be expected to follow a rigid schedule of treatment by himself; he may be contrasted to the basically dependent, overdemanding, and helpless diabetic who will need continuing guidance and supervision from his physician. Or a cardiac patient, whose life pattern has been characterized by independent activity, may respond to an overly strict regimen of bed rest with so much restlessness and anxiety that he defeats this plan of care.

Information bearing on psychosocial factors is derived from the doctor's direct observations of the patient as well as from the reports of the patient and others that describe his manner of dealing with comparable circumstances in the past. For example, a patient's relationship to his physician may be predicted from knowing how he relates with others when he is in a dependent role. The patient who has had unrealistic expectations of his parents, his wife, or his boss is likely to expect magic from his physician; the patient who generally has been suspicious and lacking in trust in all of his relationships may be expected to display a similar attitude toward his physician.

*****

The diagnostic process is one of the greatest challenges in medicine. It tests the physician's power of logic and reasoning, and should be as scientific as isolating an enzyme in the laboratory. With the advance in medical knowledge and a better understanding of the etiologic factors in a patient's illness, the steps in the diagnostic process will become more explicit. Regardless of the future developments in medicine and therapeutics, the management of the patient extends far beyond the inoculation, the administration of a drug, or the transplantation of an organ. Essential to the patient's proper care is an understanding of the personal and environmental factors in his illness, which will always be a major responsibility of the physician.

References

Criteria Committee of the New York Heart Association, Inc.: Nomenclature and Criteria for Diagnosis of the Heart and Blood Vessels. P. F. Mallon, Inc., New York, 1955.

Engel, G. L.: Conversion Symptoms. *In* MacBryde, C. M.: Signs and Symptoms. Applied Pathologic Physiology and Clinical Interpretation. 5th Ed., J. B. Lippincott Co., Philadelphia, 1969, Chap. 26.

Engel, G. L.: Psychological Development in Health and Disease. W. B. Saunders Co., Philadelphia, 1962, Chap. 23 to 27.

Feinstein, A. R.: Clinical Judgment. Williams and Wilkins Co., Baltimore, 1967, pp. 24-25.

Thompson, E. T., and Hayden, A. C., Eds.: Standard Nomenclature of Diseases and Operations. Published for the American Medical Association by the Blakiston Division of the McGraw-Hill Book Co., New York, 1961.

Chapter 3

THE APPROACH TO THE MEDICAL INTERVIEW

The purpose of the medical interview is to obtain the historical information which the physician needs to make a diagnosis of disease and to understand the patient's illness.[1] Equally important, the interview serves to establish a relationship between the physician and patient. The information obtained by the interview is ultimately organized into the following five major categories:

1. *Present Illness* refers to the recent changes in health that led the patient to seek medical attention.

2. *Past Health* constitutes an overall appraisal of the patient's general health prior to the Present Illness. It includes descriptions of all illnesses and diagnosed diseases in the past.

3. *Family Health* covers the health of the entire family, living and dead, with particular attention to possible genetic and environmental determinants of disease.

4. *Personal and Social History* includes information on the development, life experiences, and personal relationships of the patient.

5. *The Systems Review* summarizes, in terms of body systems, miscellaneous symptoms that are not included in the Present Illness or Past Health.

The full content of these divisions and how they are derived from the interview data are discussed in Chapter 5. The physician uses the order of the written history only as a rough guide in conducting his interview. He keeps in mind the necessity to obtain information relevant to each of the five major categories but follows the patient's associations in the interview, exploring each manifestation as it is introduced, regardless of which category it will ultimately be assigned to in the write-up. Only after all the information has been obtained is it organized in the format of the medical record.

This chapter outlines the order in which an interview usually develops and describes the procedures to be followed to yield the most

---

[1]See Chapter 2 for the distinction between disease and illness.

complete information from the patient and other informants. The chapter also considers commonly encountered technical difficulties and how the interview need be modified according to the patient's illness.

The principles of interviewing are illustrated in Appendix A, including a verbatim transcribed interview and a running commentary on procedure.

THE CONDUCT OF THE INTERVIEW

No two interviews follow precisely the same course. Nevertheless, there is a common basic pattern, as follows:

Step 1: The physician greets the patient, introduces himself, and defines his professional role.

Step 2: He explores how the patient is feeling at that moment and takes any appropriate measures to make him as comfortable as possible before proceeding further.

Step 3: He invites the patient to mention all symptoms and complaints leading to the hospitalization (Present Illness).[2]

Step 4: He examines in detail the manifestations of the current illness, including the sequence of development of each of the symptoms, their characteristics, and their interrelationships (Present Illness). At the same time he listens for and follows-up the patient's spontaneous references to concurrent life circumstances, illnesses in the past, and issues of family health and relationships (Past Health, Family Health, Personal and Social History).

Step 5: He inquires in detail into the patient's past health, beginning with items already mentioned (Past Health).

Step 6: He inquires in detail about the family members, beginning with those already mentioned, and explores their health as well as their past and current relationships with the patient (Family Health, Personal and Social History).

Step 7: He explores the patient's current life situation and past development, beginning with items the patient has already mentioned (Personal and Social History).

Step 8: He systematically surveys symptoms on a regional basis (Systems Review).

Step 9: He inquires whether the patient has anything to add or questions to ask, checks the accuracy of certain important details, and informs the patient of the next step in the work-up.

The logic of this sequence derives from the psychology of the sick person who seeks medical assistance. (See Chapter 1.) For the patient,

---

[2]The term in parenthesis indicates the category in the written history under which information in this phase of the interview will be organized.

the goal is the alleviation of distress and the restoration of health. To accomplish this, he must first establish a relationship with the person who is to care for him. He must satisfy himself that this person is not only professionally competent, but is also interested in him as an individual. For the physician, the primary objective is to secure the information needed to understand the illness and to institute appropriate treatment. To achieve this, he too must initiate a relationship and gain the confidence of the patient. This he does by actively demonstrating his professional concern for the patient and by willingly listening to the patient's personal and medical problems. Until the patient feels sure of the physician, he may withhold or even distort important information lest it jeopardize the physician's opinion of him. For this reason, giving the patient the opportunity to express himself freely at the beginning of the interview assures fuller and more accurate information. These principles are evident in the sequence of the interview:

Steps 1 and *2* are designed to clarify the professional role of the physician and to communicate from the outset a genuine concern for the comfort and well-being of the patient.

The relatively unstructured inquiry of *Step 3* permits the patient to express himself in his own words, which gives the physician an opportunity to learn something of the patient's personality, as well as to hear what is of most concern to him. It also provides a general overview of the scope and variety of the patient's problems.

In *Step 4* the physician begins to make explicit the kinds of information he wishes, while still remaining responsive to the spontaneous associations of the patient. It is during this phase of the interview that both parties usually achieve an understanding of what each seeks from the other, and the detailed sequential history of the current illness is obtained.

The fuller exploration of Past Health, Family Health, and Personal and Social History *(Steps 5, 6,* and *7)* is pursued as the patient's confidence in the physician becomes established. The physician initiates his inquiry about more personal matters by referring to the patient's earlier spontaneous associations. In this way he respects the patient's right to speak of such issues in his own way and at his own time. The physician thereby avoids being intrusive yet demonstrates his interest in whatever the patient has volunteered about his personal or family life.

Finally, *Steps 8* and *9* bring the interview to a close and cover items which may have been either overlooked or misunderstood by the patient or physician.

Before discussing the actual procedure involved in each of these steps, a few words about note taking and tape recording are indicated. Each person will develop his own technique of note taking. As long as the patient feels he has the student's complete attention, taking notes does not interfere with the interview. It should be done as unobtrusively as possible. On occasion, it is helpful to explain to the patient why notes are being taken and to ask his permission.

Beginning students will find note taking an invaluable aid. By jotting down the salient points, the student will find it easier to keep the material straight in his mind. Especially when the history is complex, note taking makes it easier to listen to the patient's account without feeling overwhelmed, since the student can always quickly refer to his notes to remind himself of the material that has been covered. Notes need only be fragmentary, just enough to refresh one's memory when writing the history. Only occasionally are specific quotations called for. The seven dimensions provide the most practical guide for note taking (see p. 35). One records symptoms and events with the corresponding dates and times. Chronology is the most practical framework around which to organize notes. It enables the interviewer to see at a glance which periods of time have been covered and which remain to be explored. Key words or phrases may be used to designate the other dimensions. The names of important people and places are jotted down, along with ages or associated symptoms and events. If a sensitive area is being discussed, it is wise to discontinue note taking temporarily. A few minutes later, when the patient is on more neutral ground, notes can be made about the earlier material. Once a relationship with the patient has been established, the student should not hesitate to stop and scan his notes; this is less disturbing to the patient than to repeat questions already answered or to refer to inaccurate information. By and large, patients respect this as an effort to be complete and accurate.

In some of the teaching sessions, use may be made of the tape recorder. *The patient's consent must always be obtained before the interview begins.* He should be informed that the interview is to be tape recorded to make it possible to review the interview in detail later, perhaps with a senior doctor. He should also be assured of confidentiality. Only very exceptionally do patients object. Questions usually are concerned with who will have access to the tape. The microphone should be placed as close to the patient as possible, while the recorder itself is located so that the patient is not distracted by the moving reels. Should the student sense that the tape recording is interfering with the interview, its use should be discontinued and the patient so informed.

Step 1: Introducing One's Self to the Patient

Before meeting his patient the student first learns his name and proper title, whether Mr., Dr., Mrs. or Miss. He then introduces himself by name and explains that he is a student doctor helping the staff care for patients on the ward. He informs the patient that he is one of the group responsible for his care and wishes to speak with him about his illness. The beginning clinical student often finds it awkward to assume such a professional role. However, he can be assured that most patients readily accept him as a member of the professional staff and are more than willing to cooperate. Indeed, it is through this repeated experience of being accepted as a physician that the student's professional identity begins to evolve. It is neither necessary nor appropriate for a student to ask the patient's permission to be interviewed or examined.

After having introduced himself, the student should inquire whether it is a convenient time for the patient to be seen. It may be necessary to postpone the interview briefly if the patient has just been examined by the intern, is about to eat or go to the bathroom, or if he is awaiting medication for a distressing symptom. Aside from being common courtesy, such an inquiry is evidence of the student's concern for the patient's comfort and facilitates his acceptance of the student as a professionally responsible person. The introduction may be accompanied by a handshake. If the patient is too ill, the student may place his hand on the patient's arm or hand, which will initiate a physical contact and indicate personal concern. The patient's response to the introduction and to the handshake often imparts important clinical information as well (e.g., the cold, moist hand of the anxious person, the feeble grasp of the seriously ill person, the hearty handshake of the person who is denying illness, or the bewildered expression of the demented person).

Step 2: Putting the Patient at Ease

The first consideration is to be sure that both the patient and the interviewer are as comfortable as possible. The student assists the patient to get settled and then locates himself so that the patient can easily see and talk with him. Lights and window shades are adjusted so as not to shine in the patient's or student's eyes. In a multibed unit the curtains are drawn around the bed to give more privacy. It should be recognized that even with the curtains drawn, other patients in the room may be listening and the patient's confidences may be jeopardized. Therefore, when personal information is being discussed, it may be necessary to take him to another room or to postpone this part of the interview. If necessary, other patients in the unit are asked to turn down their radios or to speak more softly. Throughout the interview the student watches for the development of patient fatigue or other discomfort in order to intervene appropriately.

The patient is often preoccupied with his own immediate distress and will be gratified to know that the interviewer also shares this concern. Hence, the student's first questions should determine how the patient is feeling at that time: "How are you feeling?" or "How are you?" The inquiry is not intended to be a social amenity, and the patient is encouraged to respond accurately. He may answer by saying "Fine" or "Pretty good," which is rather inappropriate for someone who is sick. The interviewer's echoing, mildly disbelieving question "Fine?" or "Pretty good?" or "How do you mean that?" generally will lead to further elaboration by the patient. Whatever the patient's response, he should be encouraged to go into more detail. He may mention a symptom of his illness or may report that he has some unrelated discomfort, such as pain from an intravenous needle, or that he is cold, thirsty, or needs to void. He may refer to some aspect of being a patient, perhaps voicing concern about his family or his fear of the hospitalization. The student demonstrates his concern and interest by paying serious attention to what the patient reports. Whenever possible, he should make the patient more comfortable, perhaps by adjusting the intravenous tubing, by providing a blanket, or by offering the patient a glass of water.

The patient's response to the initial inquiry may indicate the degree of his physical discomfort and often tells something about his personality. His response is a guide to the further conduct of the interview. If he is in distress, he should be advised to keep the interviewer informed how he is feeling as the interview proceeds, so that it may be interrupted, shortened, or even postponed. When in doubt about the advisability of proceeding with a patient who is very uncomfortable, the inexperienced student should consult a house officer. An occasional patient, when asked how he is feeling, will generate a barrage of complaints about the hospitalization or express concern about his family or his job, which he had to leave without adequate planning. The patient should be given the opportunity to voice his concerns. Not only does this indicate the student's interest in the patient's problems, but also what is said is likely to include important information about the patient's personality and life situation. Failure to take the time to listen may be interpreted by the patient as a lack of interest on the part of the interviewer, and the result may be a perfunctory and uninformative interview. The student should also be alert to any discrepancy between the patient's answer and his appearance. Such discrepancies must be taken into account in evaluating the accuracy of the patient's story. For example, an obviously ill patient with a need to deny weakness or disability may answer "I'm fine." In his further reporting of the history, he may omit or distort symptoms and mislead the interviewer. Or, another patient may be smiling as he states he is suffering excruciating pain. This may be the response of an hysterical patient or of a patient who is exaggerating the pain to impress the doctor with his courage.

Step 3: Establishing the Major Areas of Complaint

This is a gross screening process which is best initiated by a general question, as "Will you tell me what led you to come to the hospital?" or "What has been the problem that brought you here?" The initial response to this type of question varies widely. It may be a defensive "What would you like to know, doctor?" "My doctor sent me" or "I don't know." It may be a single word or phrase, as, "pneumonia," "pain," "shortness of breath," or "nervousness." It may be a detailed account of an illness or simply a repetition of what the referring physician told him.

Whatever the response, the primary objective is to get the patient to indicate his immediate problem in broad outline. No attempt is made at this juncture to elicit the details. These will be fully investigated later. The student's first questions are designed to encourage the patient to speak freely. Whenever the patient hesitates or stops, he is invited to continue by echoing his last word or phrase in a questioning tone, e.g., "You felt nauseated? Uh-huh" or by saying "Yes?" or "And then?" or "Anything else?" The student is particularly attentive to the patient's report of symptoms and indicates his interest by a nod or by repeating the patient's phrase, as "Pain in your leg, yes. . ." When the patient finally appears to have completed his preliminary account, he is asked "Are there any other problems?" or "Do you have any other symptoms (or troubles)?" Such questions are repeated until the patient has nothing further to add. At some point early in the inquiry the patient's age should also be determined.

Obtaining this initial information may be compared to locating the major landmarks on a map or blocking out the rough outlines of a painting, the finer details of which are filled in later. Ordinarily this phase of the interview occupies 5 to 10 minutes and yields the following:

1. A list of all the symptoms and complaints which the patient considers to be important. Occasionally an articulate and well-organized patient will give an accurate and virtually complete account of his illness.

2. A demonstration of the patient's capability to express himself when given relatively little guidance by the interviewer. For example, he may be lucid, garrulous, inarticulate, or disorganized.

3. An indication of the patient's personality and how he relates to the interviewer. For example, he may be self-assured, independent, helpless, aggressive, shy, or evasive.

The initial list of symptoms and the patient's manner of reporting indicate to the student how he should proceed with the interview. At the same time, this nondirective approach assures the patient that he is free to discuss his problems. *To begin questioning about details before this phase of the interview has been completed may seriously interfere with the further conduct of the interview.* Until the student has an overall view of the patient's problems, he has little basis on which to judge how symptoms are related or which are the most important. This is particularly true when symptoms are due to more than one disease. For example, a patient may have two kinds of abdominal pain, one due to an active peptic ulcer and the other to liver congestion secondary to heart failure. The unwary student, inquiring prematurely about the details of the "pain," may not realize that the patient is confusing two types of pain. When later he discovers this, he has to go back and repeat the questioning in order to resolve the confusion.

An even more serious consequence of premature questioning is that the patient may be so distracted by the questioning that he forgets to report certain symptoms or assumes the student is not interested. For example, a patient coming for surgical repair of a hernia may have planned to say that he is also having a recurrence of peptic ulcer symptoms. If the student immediately focuses on the hernia problem, the patient may forget to describe his ulcer symptoms and go to the operating room with this fact unknown to the staff.

The manner with which the student approaches the interview will determine the way the patient responds. If the interviewer begins with numerous, detailed questions, patients may respond by waiting silently for the next question and provide little spontaneous elaboration of their own. This places the entire burden on the student who struggles to think what next to ask the patient. Such interviews commonly degenerate into unproductive question-and-answer sessions. Students who make this error sometimes describe these patients as being uncooperative or uninformative, when in fact it is the student's technique that has inhibited the patient's spontaneity. It is far more efficient to encourage the patient to speak freely at the very beginning of the interview, using the material he mentions as the basis for further questioning. In practice, it is easier to guide a talkative patient into productive channels than one who is reticent. The entire course of the interview may be determined by how successful the student is in encouraging a free flow of information in these first few minutes. At the same time, it is important to recognize that the very talkative patient who wanders, or who provides excessive and minute detail, will need to be guided back to the pertinent issues. Also, other patients with a poverty of associations will need considerable encouragement to elaborate upon their problems. Some overly talkative or silent patients may be psychotic or suffering from organic brain disease.

Step 4: Delineating the Present Illness

The opening phase of the interview will have established the basis for communication between physician and patient and will have indicated the general areas for diagnostic consideration. Complaints such as shortness of breath, vomiting of blood, fever, anxiety, or headache, bring to mind possibilities as to where the underlying abnormalities may be located; what the disturbances in function or structure may be; and even what some of the etiologic factors may be. The interviewer will note that the reported symptoms tend to group together, constituting episodes of illness. He now has the task of characterizing each of these episodes and analyzing the relationship of one to another. He first tries to identify which episode is responsible for the patient's current clinical problem (Present Illness). This calls for a detailed and *sequential* reconstruction of the patient's most recent symptoms with careful attention to their development and characteristics. In the course of pursuing the interview, it will ultimately become clear which episodes properly belong in the Present Illness, and which represent past illnesses. When dealing with a well-circumscribed disease in a previously healthy individual, this presents no problem. However, a great variety of clinical situations may be encountered which are more complex, making it difficult to define the Present Illness. For example, the presenting symptoms may reflect: (1) more than one disease, such as pneumonia in a diabetic or acute appendicitis in a patient with cancer; (2) an exacerbation of a recurring disease, such as a flare-up of rheumatoid arthritis or of peptic ulcer; (3) a complication in a pre-existing disease, such as the occurrence of a pathological fracture and spinal cord compression in multiple myeloma or an intestinal obstruction in chronic regional enteritis; (4) a complication of treatment, for example, Cushing's syndrome in a patient being treated with corticosteroids or a hypersensitivity reaction to penicillin; or (5) a psychological reaction, such as depression or conversion in a patient being treated for some organic disease.

Because of this complexity of illness, the exploration of the presenting symptoms will commonly extend into the patient's current life circumstances, his past health, and the health of important family members. Thus, although the main objective is to elucidate the Present Illness, this part of the interview may contribute importantly to many other aspects of the medical history. Indeed, the subsequent investigation of the Family Health and the Personal and Social History is facilitated when the interviewer is able to refer to items the patient has already mentioned. Also, the patient's spontaneous association of his symptoms to life events may contribute to a better understanding of the present illness. For example, a patient's reference to his father's recent heart attack, while describing his own shortness of breath, may alert the listener to the possibility of a psychic origin of the symptom, namely conversion; or a patient with fever and abdominal pain, who comments that he has recently been in Mexico, raises the possibility of an amebic liver abscess.

Before discussing in more detail the interview techniques that are useful in delineating the present illness, it is necessary to describe how symptoms are characterized for diagnostic purposes and how the physician directs the interview yet simultaneously follows the patient's associations.

THE CHARACTERIZATION OF SYMPTOMS FOR DIAGNOSTIC PURPOSES

Symptoms, as elicited by the interviewer, are the patient's verbal expression of perceived changes in his body or mind. The physician's task is to reconstruct from the patient's words the bodily or mental processes underlying the symptom. To accomplish this, symptoms are considered in seven dimensions, as follows:

1. *Bodily location.* Where is the symptom located?
2. *Quality.* What is it like?
3. *Quantity.* How intense is it?
4. *Chronology.* When did the symptom begin and what course has it followed?
5. *Setting.* Under what circumstances does it take place?
6. *Aggravating and alleviating factors.* What makes it worse or better?
7. *Associated manifestations.* What other symptoms or phenomena are associated with it?

These seven dimensions are central to the diagnostic process. They provide the information which enables the physician to decide whether a complaint reflects an abnormality; and if so, where this abnormality is located and the nature of the underlying functional and structural disturbance. The student will find it to his advantage to commit these seven headings to memory, for they constitute the basis for the questions he will need to ask about each symptom.

Bodily Location. Most symptoms are localized by the patient to some region of the body. Where and how the patient localizes a symptom must be described accurately. Thus, the localization of a pain may be very precise or vague; it may spread or it may radiate; it may cover a large or small area; it may be superficial or deep.

Quality. Patients usually communicate quality by analogy. A symptom is described as being "like" something else. Either the patient selects a familiar experience, (e.g., "like whirling on a merry-go-round" to designate vertigo); or one which is based on his imagination, (e.g., "like being squeezed in a vise" to describe the chest pain of myocardial infarction). Some descriptions reflect underlying physiological or psychologic processes. For example, the expiratory wheeze of asthma clearly reflects the difficulty of expelling air through narrowed bronchioles. Other descriptions have been established by clinical experience and have no clear physiologic explanation, such as the crushing or squeezing chest pain of acute myocardial ischemia.

Quantity.   The quantitative aspect of symptoms refers to (1) the intensity of the symptom itself (e.g., mild, moderate, severe, unbearable); (2) the degree of impairment of function, often estimated by changes in the person's everyday activities; (3) the frequency, (e.g., of urination, cough, bowel movements); (4) the volume, (e.g., of vomitus, sputum, hemorrhage); (5) the number, (e.g., of convulsions, ecchymoses, attacks of pain); (6) the size or extent, (e.g., of a rash, ankle edema, abdominal swelling).

Chronology.   A precise reconstruction of the sequence of development of symptoms and events provides the best opportunity to understand the development of the underlying pathological processes. There are four major components to chronology:

1. *The time of onset of symptoms.*   The exact time of the first symptom and of each subsequent symptom must be established as precisely as possible. The intervals between symptoms and their order of development also have important diagnostic significance. For example, mild malaise, followed over the next three months by weakness, weight loss, night sweats, and cough, culminating in hemoptysis, suggests lung cancer or pulmonary tuberculosis; in contrast, a day of malaise and slight cough, followed in the next 24 hours by a shaking chill, high fever, pain in the chest, and blood-flecked sputum, is more in keeping with an acute bacterial pneumonia.

2. *The duration of symptoms.*   The duration of individual symptoms conveys important information about the underlying pathological processes. It must be established exactly whether a symptom extends over minutes, hours, days, weeks, or months. The duration of unconsciousness in syncope due to cardiac arrest, for example, is a matter of seconds or minutes at the most, since asystole longer than a few minutes would be incompatible with life. On the other hand, the weakness and fatigue of such disorders as pernicious anemia or hypothyroidism may develop slowly over months or even years.

3. *Periodicity and frequency of symptoms.*   Symptoms usually are not constant, and their pattern of variation often reflects the rhythms or periodicity of the underlying pathologic processes. Thus, obstruction of a hollow viscus is associated with the rhythmic increase and decrease of pain (colic); the chills and fever of malaria are correlated with the life cycle of the parasite. Not only may the pathologic processes cause periodic symptoms, but they also may be affected in turn by periodic

phenomena, such as times of eating, sleeping, exercise, menstruation, work, or the regular weekend visits of in-laws. The pain of peptic ulcer, for instance, characteristically occurs during periods when gastric acid is unbuffered by food.

4. *The course of the symptoms.* The time course of a symptom also reflects the nature of the underlying process and must be explored with care. Does the symptom stay the same? Does it get better or grow worse over time? Does it remain the same for a long time and then progress rapidly? Or does it run a remitting or relapsing course? For example, a pain which builds up, reaches a peak, and then slowly subsides over the course of a minute or two, thereafter recurring every three or four minutes, is characteristic of the peristaltic contractions of a hollow viscus attempting to overcome an obstruction; a steadily increasing difficulty in swallowing is indicative of a developing organic obstruction of the esophagus, such as cancer, while intermittent difficulty in swallowing which does not progress suggests spasm.

Setting. At the time an illness or a symptom is experienced, the patient is always (1) somewhere (e.g., he may be at home, in bed, in his car, on the job, or on vacation); (2) doing something (e.g., he may be sleeping, eating, bending over, shoveling snow, or watching TV); or (3) in relation to some person (e.g., he may be with, or wish to be with, someone; or he may wish to get away from someone, such as his wife, his mother, his boss, or a police officer). In the very recent past he may have suffered a serious personal loss or a job frustration. He may have been exposed to a toxic substance or an infectious agent. Exploration of these factors helps the physician to understand symptoms as well as to characterize the patient. He learns how symptoms are embedded in the matrix of the patient's life; that is, how life activities influence the symptom, and how the symptom influences the patient's life.

Aggravating or Alleviating Factors. Understanding how a symptom may be influenced by certain activities or physiological processes helps to clarify the nature of the underlying problem. For example, straining, physical exertion, eating, or coughing may respectively aggravate the pain of peritonitis, coronary insufficiency, esophageal neoplasm, or pleurisy. On the other hand, lying still, resting, avoiding food, or breathing quietly are activities that may relieve the pain of each condition. The student can best think of aggravating factors as imposing a burden beyond the functional capacity of the affected organ system, while alleviating factors reduce the demand.

Associated Manifestations. It is rare to have only one symptom associated with a disease process. Not only will the malfunction of a given organ express itself in several ways, but also there are often systemic symptoms of general bodily dysfunction. For example, a patient with an infectious disease, such as pneumonia, often has the systemic symptoms of fever, sweating, and anorexia, as well as the localizing symptoms of cough and chest pain. With experience, one becomes familiar with *symptom complexes*, which are associations and combinations of symptoms characteristic for specific disease processes. Thus, it is important to know whether vomiting occurs without nausea, or nausea without vomiting, or whether the two occur together; or whether loss of weight is associated with increased appetite, with decreased appetite, with vomiting, with diarrhea, with pain, with feelings of depression, or with no other symptoms at all. Knowledge of anatomic and physiologic principles provides a guide to the association of symptoms. For example, loss of weight in spite of increased food consumption suggests the inefficient carbohydrate utilization of diabetes or the hypermetabolism of hyperthyroidism; whereas, gain in weight despite decreased food intake suggests the possibility of fluid retention.

All seven dimensions also have relevance to the characterization of symptoms caused by psychological and behavioral disturbances. Even bodily location is pertinent, as when a psychological symptom is expressed in physical terms, such as a conversion symptom, a hypochondriacal symptom, or a somatic delusion. In contrast to organically based symptoms, the other dimensions are more likely to be elaborated in psychological, interpersonal, or social terms rather than in physiological terms.

THE IMPORTANCE OF FOLLOWING THE PATIENT'S ASSOCIATIONS WHILE DIRECTING THE INTERVIEW

The necessity to delineate the illness and to characterize symptoms in the seven dimensions requires that the student provide direction in the interview. Encouraging the patient to speak freely continues to be the basic requirement for a productive interview, since only the patient can describe what he has been experiencing. On the other hand, he usually does not appreciate all that the interviewer needs to learn from him. In order to accomplish his task of diagnosis, the student must subtly direct the course of the interview. Far from being merely a passive listener, he indicates to the patient by his responses and questions the need for certain organization and content. The patient soon comes to appreciate that events must be dated, sequences established, and symptoms described precisely. At the same time, such direction must not be achieved at the expense of prejudicing the patient's responses or of blocking the free flow of his associations. The amount of direction needed in the interview varies with the patient. Some will wander and discuss unproductive areas in minute detail; others will gloss over important historical points, and still other patients will present a coherent story where little intervention is needed. It is most important that the student be flexible in his interview technique, learn to adapt to the patient's style of reporting, and still remain in control of the situation. The student should neither passively listen to volumes of irrelevant detail, nor should he conduct the interview in the manner of a courtroom lawyer by firing repeated questions. Obviously, much practice and experience are needed to achieve the proper balance.

The two objectives, to encourage the patient's spontaneous associations and to provide direction, are best achieved by always initiating the inquiry into each new area with open-ended (nondirective) questions and by following with progressively more specific (directive) questions until the subject is fully clarified. This means that the interviewer must have clearly in his mind what details are necessary to understand the illness yet not prematurely impose his ideas on the patient. For example, he may begin the investigation of a symptom with the request, "Tell me more about it" or "What was it like?" This allows the patient to say whatever he wishes about the symptom and to bring up his own associations, unprejudiced by the interviewer. The student, as he listens to the patient's account, is alert to omissions and ambiguities, and periodically indicates what needs to be clarified; e.g., "That was when?" "What was the feeling?" "Which came first?" As the patient completes his more spontaneous account, the interviewer then follows with whatever specific questions are necessary to complete the picture. *In so doing, he always tries to formulate each successive question on the basis of what the patient has just said.* In essence, just as is done in sustaining a conversation, the student picks up where the patient leaves off. By following the patient's lead, he avoids the disruption of the patient's train of thought and important associations emerge naturally under such conditions. When a series of direct questions are posed early in the interview, the patient may respond simply by waiting passively for the next question. Only when the interviewer is satisfied that he has obtained all the information that he needs by following the patient's associations, does he again take the initiative to change the subject and introduce a new topic. Each new area is pursued in the same manner. Thus, the interview typically consists of a series of interconnected sequences, each one of which begins with open-ended questions and progresses to increasingly more specific questions until the issues are fully defined.

Throughout the interview, the student remains attentive to the patient's spontaneous associations, even when at first they may seem to be irrelevant. The patient is allowed to digress long enough to establish whether the information is pertinent to the history. If so, he is encouraged to continue. *All the while, however, the student must keep in mind what information the patient has not yet clarified, so that he can return later to ask the necessary questions at an appropriate time.*

The value of pursuing the patient's associations is illustrated in the following example.

> A 34-year-old man, complaining of headaches, mentioned that they seemed to get worse toward the end of a day's work. When asked at that point what his work was, the patient described a job in a poorly-ventilated auto repair shop. Spontaneously, he began to wonder whether exhaust fumes could be responsible for the headaches. This was a plausible suggestion, since headaches are a symptom of carbon monoxide poisoning. Inquiry about working conditions, however, revealed this cause to be improbable. Asked what he did after leaving work, he said that he often procrastinated about going home, stopping at a bar to visit with his cronies. He went on to explain that he and his wife were not getting along well, so that often he was reluctant to go home. As he mentioned this, he began to wonder whether tension could have anything to do with the headaches. Further questioning about his marital situation, however, left no doubt that the headaches preceded the difficulty with his wife by several months. Asked about other circumstances when headaches occurred, he mentioned playing golf, working in his basement workshop, and romping with the children. Exploration now revealed that repeated bending over was the common denominator for all the situations in which the headache developed. This discovery suggested that a mechanical factor was important; and indeed, it turned out that the headache was due to a brain tumor.

In this example, each of the associations had to be examined in its own right. Some proved to be blind alleys in respect to the final diagnosis of brain tumor, but all yielded information important for a better understanding of the patient.

THE TECHNIQUES USED IN OBTAINING THE PRESENT ILLNESS

Initiating the Detailed Exploration of the Illness. The detailed inquiry about the current illness begins after the patient has given a general but brief account of his difficulties (*Step 3*). The student now must decide which aspect of the illness should be inquired into first. In general, one begins with the problems which are most recent and most urgent:

1. If the illness appears to be a circumscribed incident of recent origin, the student may start with such questions as, "Exactly when did this all begin?" or "What was the very first thing you noticed?"

2. When the patient has reported several episodes of illness or a series of attacks, it is usually best to begin with the most recent one. This is freshest in the patient's mind and usually most germane to his seeking medical attention. After the details of the most recent episode have been clarified, one explores the preceding episodes and the intervals between them. In this manner, all the earlier incidents are considered until the entire complex has been reviewed.

3. Sometimes the symptoms presented in the initial phase of the interview fall into no obvious pattern. Under such circumstances, the

best approach is to begin with whatever the patient has emphasized as most important. If it is unclear what this is, he may be asked "What has been the main difficulty?" The same approach is used when the patient indicates the existence of several problems simultaneously. For example, a patient might report several weeks of malaise, poor appetite, weight loss, diarrhea, and abdominal pain. He also may mention that his "sugar diabetes" has been out of control and that he has been "down in the dumps." Beginning with what appears to be the most urgent matter, all symptoms will have to be considered in turn and their interrelationship explored.

Using the Seven Dimensions as a Framework to Clarify the Illness. The seven dimensions, *Bodily location, Quality, Quantity, Chronology, Setting, Aggravating or alleviating factors,* and *Associated manifestations,* provide a frame of reference around which the interviewer proceeds to organize his inquiry. Because of many years of practice, the experienced physician is able to pursue these dimensions with little conscious effort as he listens to the patient's report of symptoms and is aware of any omissions or ambiguities. On the other hand, the beginning student must actively concentrate to keep all the dimensions in mind and to be sure that each symptom is fully clarified in terms of the seven dimensions.

The dimension which contributes most to the organization and clarity of the history is *Chronology.* Dates and times serve to anchor the history in such a way that relationships between symptoms and events can be more clearly seen. Hence it is good practice to inquire as early and frequently as necessary "When was that?" "When did that occur?" "What year (month, day, time) was that?" "Then what happened?" or "And then?" Such reminders serve to impress upon the patient the importance of times and sequences, encouraging him to pay more attention to chronology in his spontaneous account.

The techniques of exploring each dimension are discussed in the following paragraphs. There is no fixed order of exploration, and the student must keep in mind that he is trying to reconstruct the picture of the entire illness rather than merely a succession of isolated symptoms.

Bodily location.   Generally, patients refer to bodily location in rather broad terms, such as "arm," "head," "stomach," or "back." The appropriate first question is "Where in your _____?" or "What part of your _____?" Many patients proceed to demonstrate the location; those who do not should be asked to do so. With such symptoms as weakness, dizziness, or gas, the patient may be asked "Where do you feel the _____?" Whatever the patient's response to these first questions, the matter should be pursued further by first asking more open-ended questions as "Do you feel it anywhere else?"

"Does it go (radiate) anywhere?" and finally, if the information is not yet forthcoming, more explicit questions as "Did it involve this part of your hand?" (pointing) or "Did you feel it on the surface or deep?" or "Did it go through to the back?"

Quality.   Inquiry as to the quality of the symptoms is usually best initiated by asking "What was (is) it like?" The patient is then encouraged to elaborate further. If he has difficulty or uses vague terms, like "hurts," "sick," or "dizzy," the interviewer helps him by asking, "What do you mean by _____?" or "Was it like anything you have ever felt before?" If these questions are unproductive, he offers him a choice of terms: "By 'hurting' do you mean a pain, an ache, or what?" "Do you mean sick to your stomach, sick all over, or what?" If the symptom is a pain, he might ask, "Well, was it sharp, or sticking, or dull, or aching, or what?" without emphasizing one more than another. This encourages the patient to provide a suitable term of his own, or he may respond with strong agreement to one of the terms offered him.

Quantity.   Questions concerning frequency, volume, number, or size may be approached quite directly, as "How many times did you vomit that night?" or "How much blood did you spit up?" Vague answers, as "A lot" or "Not much," are not adequate, and the patient must be encouraged to be more exact. "What do you mean by 'A lot'?" If the patient still is vague, he may be asked, "Was it two or three times or six or eight times?" "Did you bring up a few streaks of blood, a teaspoonful, or more than that?"

The intensity of a symptom and the degree of impairment of function are best estimated in more personal terms. "How bad (severe, serious) was it?" will encourage the patient to elaborate. He may then be asked to compare it to a previous experience: "Have you ever been this anxious before?" or "How does it compare to the worst pain you ever had?" Asking the patient to compare a pain to a toothache, to an injury, or to childbirth is a good way to estimate severity.

Functional impairment is best evaluated in terms of the extent to which the patient's pattern of living has changed as the result of the symptom or the illness. With a specific symptom, like dyspnea, dizziness, or stiffness of a limb, he may be asked what he is not able to do now that he could do before. Specific questions follow, such as "How many flights of stairs can you climb?" (dyspnea) or, "Can you button your jacket?" (paresis of the hand). With poorly localized symptoms, such as fatigue or anxiety, or when evaluating the overall impact of the illness, a useful approach is to have the patient describe in detail his activities on a recent day. A specific day, such as the day before hospitalization, is chosen rather than just a "typical" day. The latter often yields only a stylized report, lacking the small details that are so informative. For example, the patient may be asked, "Tell me what your day was like on Monday, from the time you got up until you went to bed." He may then be asked, "If you were well, what would your day have been like?" Obviously, such accounts also yield useful information about the patient and his current life situation, data which can be expanded further at that time or later on in the interview.

Chronology. *Every effort must be made to establish chronology in terms of calendar dates and clock times.* This requires a deliberate effort on the part of the interviewer, since people tend to keep track of time through events and circumstances that are important to them, rather than by calendar dates. Only through such associations do they establish the day or hour. Thus, a man will be sure that his pain began around 3 P.M. because it was shortly after his 2:30 P.M. coffee break; or he will recall that his first attack was at least 14 years ago because it was before his oldest son was born. The interviewer should use the same approach. Each time he asks "What date or time was this?" he should note the patient's reference points. He then uses the same points to guide him in clarifying time relationships. For example, "You began to feel sick to your stomach around 4 o'clock, while you were doing the laundry; did you vomit before you finished, or afterwards?"

On occasion, patients will spontaneously provide exact dates or times. It is always well to inquire how they remember the time so exactly, for not uncommonly it proves to be associated with some important event. For example, a patient may say without hesitation that his first episode of chest pain occurred at 7:15 P.M., March 3, 1967. He remembers the date exactly because that was the day he received word that his son was injured in an auto accident, and he remembers the time because the pain began while he was watching the evening news on TV.

Usually, patients have difficulty in accurately recalling dates. In the great majority of cases, the interviewer can resolve the uncertainty by reference to important landmarks. For example, the patient who can date the onset of illness no more accurately than, "a few months ago," may be asked how he was feeling during the Christmas holidays, during his summer vacation, or on his birthday. Familiarity with details of the patient's life is particularly helpful, for then one can refer to important specific events. For example, how was he before he moved, before he started his new job, after the baby was born, or while his father was in the hospital? Indeed, it is far easier for both the patient and the interviewer to establish the date of onset of symptoms and to keep accurate track of their sequence if they are related to concurrent events in the patient's life. Contradictions and discrepancies are more readily detected and corrected when the interviewer is able to make such comments as, "Earlier you said the pain began in January, but now you say everything was fine until a week after the baby was born. Wasn't she born on February 10th?"

By careful attention to such details, one will find that it is mainly the delirious, demented, psychotic, or mentally defective patient who is totally incapable of providing reasonably consistent dates and time relationships; indeed, their failure to do so with such an inquiry should suggest one of these diagnoses.

The date of onset of the illness must be accurately established and its entire course accounted for, right up to the time of the examination. This means that the student must investigate with great care the time of onset of the illness, and no subsequent time interval should be left unaccounted for during the course of the illness. Regardless of the point in time selected by the patient as marking the beginning of his first symptom, the student should always inquire how the patient was before that time. He must be explicit; if the patient reports the first symptom as beginning at noon, the student must inquire about that morning and the night before; if the patient dates the onset to January, he should be asked how he was during the Christmas holidays or on New Year's Day. Such questions are pursued until the patient clearly identifies a point or period in time when he definitely was feeling well. Some patients, by discounting earlier difficulties, are inclined to date the onset of the illness to the time when they first became concerned about symptoms. This tendency can be checked by inquiring whether the patient had in any way been previously restricted in his activities, or by asking, "Have there been times when you felt better?" He may then acknowledge that he had not really felt well for several months.

Having identified the time of onset, the interviewer then encourages the patient to give a sequential account of the illness and of each symptom. The frequent inquiries, "When was that?" and "Then what?" serve to reinforce for the patient the importance of accuracy of times and sequences. As the student listens to the patient's account, he makes mental note of time gaps, all of which must be accounted for in the history. With a long and complex illness, he will find it useful to jot down the sequence of dates covered so that he can check omissions before bringing the interview to a close.

At times it is important to establish as precisely as possible the duration of a symptom, for example, unconsciousness, where a difference between seconds and minutes may be crucial for the diagnosis. This is best done by having the patient reconstruct the surrounding events and estimating the probable time involved. For example, the patient may remember feeling dizzy, calling out to his wife, and then blacking out. He may next recall his wife coming toward him or someone carrying him into an ambulance. By establishing how long it would take for his wife to get to him, or for the ambulance to come, a fairly reasonable estimate of the duration of unconsciousness is possible.

Setting.   It is easy to clarify the setting if the student uses events in the patient's life as guides to evaluate functional impairment and to time the sequence of symptoms. Some patients will spontaneously interrelate their symptoms and concurrent events. Others, assuming that the doctor is not interested in personal issues, will give an impersonal account of symptoms. Patients can easily be induced to provide information about the setting if the student interposes such questions as "Where were you when this happened?" "Who was there?" "Who helped?" "What were you doing at the time?" The patient is then asked to elaborate. For example, a patient who reports an acute onset of shortness of breath and weight gain may at first answer the question "Where were you?" with "Home, asleep." In response to further questioning, he may reveal that he has been upset since his wife left him a month earlier; and because he has had to eat his meals at a nearby restaurant, he has not been able to follow his salt-free diet. From such a response, important information is obtained which bears not only on the illness itself, but also on the personal and social background of the patient. Later in the interview, these can be the starting points for further investigation of the Family Health as well as the Personal and Social History.

Finally, as diagnostic possibilities occur to the student, questions bearing on etiologic factors should be asked. For example, had the man with recurring chills and fever been in a malaria-infested region; had the farmer with acute respiratory distress been cleaning out a silo; or had anyone else at work been jaundiced? Direct questioning, on the other hand, is rarely informative in acute psychological disorders, such as an anxiety reaction or a paranoid panic. In these instances, the relevant precipitating circumstance is much more likely to emerge in the course of the patient's spontaneous account of events immediately preceding the episode.

Aggravating or alleviating factors. The first clues to aggravating or alleviating factors generally come from the patient's own account of what was going on when the symptom became better or worse. This again emphasizes the value of encouraging the patient to describe the circumstances as well as the symptoms of an illness. He may tell of awakening intensely short of breath and feeling better after sitting up; he may describe how the pain in his back suddenly increased when he tried to pick up his grandchild; or that his chest pain lessened after he stopped walking. Each such association is then examined further. The patient may be asked, "Is there anything else you found that helped, (made it worse)?" "What did you do to try to help it?"

Knowledge of clinical syndromes leads to more specific questions. Thus, the physician knows that the pain of angina pectoris develops while walking and subsides within a few minutes with rest, or that the vertigo and nausea of labyrinthitis are brought on by slight movements of the head. Questions should be worded so as not to influence the answer. Thus, when inquiring about angina, one asks, "What effect does walking have?" "Standing still or sitting down?"; or when asking about vertigo, "What happens if you move your head?" "How much movement will bring on the symptoms?"

Associated manifestations. The relationships between symptoms logically emerge in the course of developing their chronology. Nonetheless, it is still necessary to inquire directly into the nature of such associations, especially when the patient describes symptoms occurring in the past. For example, he may tell of dyspnea, orthopnea, and ankle swelling occurring "3 or 4 months ago"; and later speak of anorexia, nausea, and abdominal distress "2 or 3 months ago." In order to establish whether the gastrointestinal symptoms are related to those of heart failure (e.g., congestion of the liver and gut), a complication of treatment (e.g., digitalis toxicity), or an independent illness (e.g., conversion or gastroenteritis), it will be necessary to reconstruct the exact sequence of events.

Knowledge of clinical syndromes enables one to anticipate symptoms that the patient does not mention. If diabetes is suspected, for example, the student should inquire about polyuria and polydipsia; or if a pain is thought to represent conversion, he should ask about other symptoms of conversion, such as globus, hyperventilation, or episodes of paralysis and anesthesia.

The technique of characterizing symptoms may be summarized as follows: *The student keeps the seven dimensions in mind as the patient is allowed to tell his story in his own words. Incomplete information about any of the seven dimensions is noted, and the patient's attention is directed to these gaps, starting with nondirective questions, and following with specific questions, as necessary, until all the information is obtained. Throughout the interview, the student encourages the patient's associations, pursuing those which seem informative.*

The Wording of Questions. The basic principles determining the wording of questions are as follows: (1) the patient should have no difficulty understanding what is being asked; (2) the form of the question, while indicating what type of information is of interest to the interviewer, should in no way prejudice the patient's responses; and (3) the question should be so worded as to induce the patient to speak freely. To meet these requirements the following are essential:

1. Questions should be brief and simple. Whenever the student finds himself having to explain a question, he should stop and think through exactly what it is he wants to find out. The examples in the preceding text and in Appendix A illustrate the proper construction of questions.

2. The student should use language that is understandable to the patient. This will require taking into account the patient's level of edu-

cation and his background. It is particularly important to avoid the use of medical terms that may be unknown to the patient, such as pleurisy, jaundice, or paralysis. Instead, a brief description of the symptoms may be offered: "Did it hurt when you took a breath" "Did your skin ever turn yellow" or "Did your hand ever become so weak you couldn't use it?"

3. Only one question should be asked at a time. To string several questions together or to ask about more than one item leaves the patient uncertain as to what he should answer.

4. In exploring any issue, the inquiry should always start with nondirective questions, reserving more direct questions to fill in gaps, clarify ambiguities, or verify facts. Questions which can be answered with a simple "yes" or "no" should be used sparingly; otherwise, the patient may assume that little more is expected of him and fall into a pattern of silently waiting for the next question.

5. One should use the patient's own terms, at least until there is mutual agreement as to what the term means. Failure to do so may lead to confusion for both the patient and the interviewer. For example, a patient may refer to a sensation in the chest as a "pressure." The proper question is "Tell me more about the pressure sensation." For the interviewer to substitute some other word, such as "pain," may be a distortion of the patient's intent. It is especially confusing when the patient has reserved the word, "pain," for some other sensation.

Clarifying the Patient's Responses. It is often necessary to intervene and clarify what the patient is describing. Such expressions as "nervousness," "sick to the stomach," or "a funny feeling," usually have a quite personal meaning, and the student must inquire promptly what the patient means. Thus, it is misleading to the point of diagnostic confusion to assume that the patient's term, "sick to the stomach," means nausea, when clarification would have revealed that he really is referring to a sensation of fullness. Once the term has been clarified, it avoids confusion for the interviewer to actually use the patient's term in his further questioning: "Tell me more about being 'sick to the stomach'."

Medical or quasi-medical terms, such as "pneumonia," "tumor," "sciatica," or "nervous breakdown," must always be clarified, both with respect to the patient's understanding of the term and with respect to the details of the illness so designated. One is never justified in assuming that a name diagnosis, even if ascribed to another physician, is necessarily correct. The patient must always be asked to describe the symptoms and course of the illness in his own words. When a patient says he had an "appendectomy," for instance, the operation may indeed have been performed; but further inquiry may reveal that the history was more compatible with a conversion symptom or with regional enteritis than with appendicitis.

Some patients, when asked to tell about their illness, may omit symptoms altogether and persist instead in reporting what their doctor said and did. A patient with anemia, for instance, may give a detailed description of the medications that his doctor had given him or explain that the x-rays showed he had something wrong with his stomach, and so on. The interviewer should lose no time in making it clear that he is more interested in learning about the patient's symptoms. "Yes, I would like to know what Dr. Smith said, but first I want to hear in your own words how you have been." Occasionally, it is necessary to repeat this several times to remind the patient.

Should the thread of the story be lost, whether because the student was momentarily inattentive or because the account was disorganized, the patient must be interrupted. The interviewer should not hesitate to say "I didn't follow that" or "I'm not clear about this" and ask the patient to repeat or clarify his account. When he is consistently unable to present a coherent story, a diagnosis of delirium, dementia, psychosis, or mental deficiency is suggested.

Obtaining Essential Factual Data. Certain types of information must always be obtained and recorded as precisely as possible. The patient's account may have to be interrupted to complete such data. These include (1) the age and birth date of the patient; (2) the dates relevant to the illness; (3) the full name and location of previous physicians; (4) the dates of previous hospitalizations and the names of hospitals; (5) the name (or description) of medications, including the dosage and by whom prescribed; (6) the details of medical treatment; (7) the current ages of relevant family members or other important persons; (8) the dates of significant life events, such as births, marriages, divorce, job changes, or military service.

Pursuing the Course of the Interview. Although it is virtually impossible to predict how any interview will proceed, the student must appreciate that the process is by no means haphazard. Usually he tries to complete the investigation of a symptom or an event at the time the patient mentions it. He allows the patient to continue his spontaneous account as long as he seems to be bringing up information relevant to that symptom, and then he asks such questions as are necessary to fully characterize the symptom in its seven dimensions. Should the patient, in the context of describing the present illness, refer to a more remote illness or event, this should be followed up at the time, at least briefly. A patient may say, for instance, that he experienced similar symptoms several years ago when he had infectious mononucleosis. Then, he recalls that his father, who died of cancer of the stomach, had similar symptoms during his terminal illness. Not uncommonly, students will fail to obtain the necessary details of important information at the time the patient speaks of it. It may only take a minute or two to learn the essential facts of the patient's infectious mononucleosis or the father's age, date of death, and prior state of health before the terminal illness. The practice of briefly completing information as the patient mentions it not only takes advantage of the patient's willingness at the moment to go into more detail, but also indicates the student's interest in the material. Judgment must be used as to when one should round out the finer points of historical data so as not to interrupt the patient's train of thought. Failure to do so will necessitate the student's having to return and question the patient again in order to obtain a complete history. This not only lengthens the interview, but also may aggravate the patient who feels he has told all of this before.

After the essential information has been obtained, one returns to complete the material that has been interrupted. Sometimes patients will bring up two, three, or more items of importance in rapid succession. Here one has no choice but to select one topic first, but not without indicating interest in the other topics and informing the patient that he will want to know about them later. In all cases, the guiding principle is to invite the patient to tell the story in his own words and then progressively to direct him in such a way that the history is revealed with the least distortion.

Completing the Main Body of the Interview. This phase of the interview comes to a close when the interviewer feels that he has learned as much as he can about the present illness. With some complaints, such as an injury, a hernia, or an attack of renal colic, only a few minutes will be required. Most illnesses, however, will usually take the student 30 to 60 minutes to learn the necessary details. An experienced physician will need half the time. At this juncture, the following information usually has been obtained: a reasonably complete account of the presenting complaints and the events leading up to admission; namely, the Present Illness; some information about concurrent illnesses and illnesses in the past; and some information about the patient's personal history, including the important persons in his life.

Usually, at this point the interviewer is aware of a certain lull. The patient no longer is reporting spontaneously, and the student has run out of questions with respect to the current problems. Before he moves to the remaining sections of the history and performs a systems review, he must be sure that he has the following information which is appropriate to most present illnesses:

Pertinent positive and negative information. In considering various disease entities that might explain the patient's illness, the student should inquire about expected symptoms the patient may not have mentioned. For example, if lupus erythematosis is a consideration, the student may need to ask whether or not the patient has had a facial rash, convulsions, or pleurisy. The influence of environmental factors is also included in such questioning. If pertinent to the present illness, the possibility of infectious or chemical exposure must be considered. Has the patient traveled recently? Is there a similar illness in the family or at work?

Medications and treatment. What treatment has the patient received for his present illness? This includes physical restrictions, physiotherapy, prescribed exercises, and all medications that he is taking for this or for concomitant illnesses. The name and dosage of each drug, if not known to the patient, may be learned later from the referring physician or pharmacist. In particular, it should be remembered that patients may be taking analgesics, tranquilizers, sleeping pills, or oral contraceptives on a long-term basis. Finally, it is important to know who prescribed the particular treatment or medication, including whether it was the patient himself.

Weight. The patient should always be asked what his present weight is and whether there has been any recent gain or loss. The maximum and minimum weight in the past should also be determined.

Degree of disability. If not already known, the student should learn what limitations the patient's illness has imposed on him and his family. Such information is particularly important in chronic illnesses.

After the student has obtained what he considers a reasonably complete description of the illness, he shifts his attention to filling in the missing information relevant to the other parts of the patient's history.

Step 5: Investigating the Past Health

The inquiry into past health may be introduced by asking "How has your health been in the past?" Here, one is interested to learn about periods of good health as well as about episodes of illness. Since health is a relative experience, it is always necessary to clarify the patient's response to this question. Even "good" or "excellent" may hide significant symptoms or disability in the person who needs to see himself as strong and in control. Answers such as "pretty good" or "fairly good" should always be taken to indicate that there have been health problems. If the patient does not spontaneously elaborate, he should be asked "What does 'excellent' (or 'pretty good') mean for you?" One should inquire not only about the symptom, but also about what the patient's range of activity was like when well. "What were you able to do (or what was your life like) before you got sick?" is an effective way to evoke such a description.

An occasional patient counters the general question about his health with "Do you mean physical health?" This is his way of revealing the existence of emotional problems and is best answered with "I mean any kind of health problem."

Whatever the patient brings up as the result of this inquiry is then explored in more detail. It is important to have an adequate description to be able to accurately identify the illness, even though fewer details are needed than for the present illness. The student should learn the date of onset, the symptoms, the course, the treatment, and any sequelae. Names of physicians, the nature of diagnostic studies or of surgery, and the dates and location of hospital admissions are also noted. The student should investigate each past illness to be able to reach his own conclusion regarding diagnosis. The patient is asked to describe the illness in his own words; then specific questions may be needed to check the reliability of the diagnosis. For example, the patient who reports "gallbladder trouble" should be asked specifically about those manifestations of gallbladder disease that he failed to mention, such as jaundice, dark urine, or fatty food intolerance. *No diagnosis claimed by the patient, even when attributed to a reliable physician or medical center, should ever be accepted at face value.* There is always the possibility that the patient has misinterpreted information, or that even the most definite diagnosis may prove incomplete or wrong in the light of new information.

Sometimes the exploration of past health reveals that the present illness actually began earlier than the patient had previously indicated. For example, a patient may have described the symptoms of an acute myocardial infarction coming on in a period of "excellent" health. Later in the review of past health, he may mention a "muscle strain" that occurred six months earlier, consisting of aching pain in his anterior chest and left arm, and mild dyspnea during exertion, relieved promptly by rest. Without consulting a physician, he cut down on his physical exertion and the symptoms disappeared. He did not spontaneously associate these earlier symptoms with his present illness even though they were identical in location and character. Actually, these symptoms, angina pectoris, were the first manifestations of coronary heart disease and appeared six months earlier than the initial account of the present illness had suggested.

After the patient has been given an opportunity to tell about all the illnesses he can remember, the student completes the information in the following categories:

1. General health
2. Childhood health
3. Adult health
   a. Medical illnesses
   b. Surgical procedures
   c. Psychiatric illnesses
   d. Obstetrical history
4. Accidents and injuries
5. Allergies and immunizations

The inquiry is first a general one, beginning with questions such as "What childhood illnesses did you have?" "Have you had any other illnesses?" "Any emotional problems?" "Have you had any (other) operations?" "Injuries?" "Any problems during pregnancy or childbirth?" "Any allergies?" "Are you sensitive to any medicines or drugs?" More specific questions about each category of illness will need to be directed to the patient. For example, when he is asked "What childhood illnesses did you have?" one is not satisfied with the answer "The usual ones" but must inquire about important childhood illnesses by name. The question may need to be amplified to refresh the patient's memory. For instance, the student may need to clarify "rheumatic fever" by saying "Did you ever miss school for weeks or months because of illness?" "Did you ever have a prolonged fever that kept you in bed for several weeks?" "Did you ever have swelling or aching of your joints, frequent nose bleeds, growing pains, or St. Vitus' dance?"

Finally, one inquires specifically about illnesses which may have a bearing on the patient's current problem. For instance, inquiry about previous nephritis, urinary tract infection, or renal trauma would be important in a patient with hypertension or renal failure. In a patient with femoral artery insufficiency and intermittent claudication, one should ask about diabetes, previous foot infections, and other complications of atherosclerosis, such as coronary heart disease.

Step 6: Investigating the Family Health and Family Relationships

The student now shifts his attention to the family, asking about the health of each member and his role, past and present, in the life of the patient. In a well conducted interview, many of the family members will already have been mentioned, and a good deal learned about them and their relationship to the patient. One initiates inquiry into the family health by referring to one of these family members: "You mentioned that your wife is 43 and is working in a factory. How has she been?" If she has not been well, one should determine the nature of the illness, the degree of disability, and how the patient has been affected by his wife's illness. When asking about relationships, it is helpful to elicit the patient's feelings: "How did your wife's illness affect you?" or "How has the marriage been?" One then may inquire as to the length of the marriage and the wife's childbearing experience. This logically brings one to the children, each of whom should be identified by name, age, sex, state of health (present and past), present whereabouts, occupation, marital status, and children. When the patient's children are widely separated in age, one should always keep in mind the possibility that a parent may have remarried. In this manner, one progresses through the family, accounting for husband or wife, children, grandchildren, parents, grandparents, and siblings. One should also inquire whether any siblings or children have died, whom the patient may have forgotten to mention. Common-law partners or foster parents should be included. It is also pertinent to inquire about uncles and aunts where hereditary diseases are being considered. One should identify which family members are most important to the patient, since they are the ones whose health and activities will have the most bearing on the patient's status. At some point it is always well to inquire "Who is at home?" or "With whom do you live?" for this may reveal other persons of importance to the patient, such as in-laws, distant relatives, a common-law husband or wife, foster children, or friends. One may also learn from such a question that the patient is separated from his spouse or even living with someone else, a fact that the patient may have hesitated to volunteer.

Whenever changes in relationships with important persons are encountered, such as separations, illnesses, deaths, or retirement, dates should always be ascertained and the impact on the patient of such changes established. "How did this affect you?" or, if it is obviously distressing, "That must have been a difficult experience for you" usually suffices to bring out the feelings of the patient. In terms of understanding him and the possible implications for his illness, *how the patient reacted to the event is of far more importance than the event itself. It is not adequate merely to note the event without learning something of its effect on the patient.*

With respect to illnesses and deaths of family members, one should learn the diagnosis, the manifestations of each illness, and the age and date of death. There are at least two reasons why it is important to know the details of the family member's illness: First, it provides a check on the validity of the diagnosis reported by the patient. As an example, adequate questioning about the grandfather's "asthma" may make it evident that it was more likely congestive heart failure. Second, the manifestations of a family member's illness may have direct bearing on the patient's own symptoms. For example, if cough were a major symptom of carcinoma of the lung in the father, the fact that the patient's cough began on the anniversary of the father's death might suggest that it was a conversion symptom. Similarly, a patient with bronchitis, who knew his father died of carcinoma of the lung, may anxiously exaggerate how much he has been coughing or he may avoid mentioning it altogether, lest he discover that he too has carcinoma of the lung.

In bringing to a close the inquiry about family health, the student specifically questions the patient about diseases that might be related to his own illness through contagion, as in tuberculosis, or through a genetic factor, as in diabetes or epilepsy. It is well to remember that some inherited diseases may not be directly manifest in parents or grandparents. Hemophilia, for instance, which is attributed to a sex-linked recessive gene, may be clinically evident only in an uncle or male cousin. A good final question with which to conclude is "Has anyone in your family ever had an illness like yours?"

Step 7: Completing the Personal and Social History

By this point in the interview the student should have learned a good deal about the setting of the illness, the current life situation, and the family. If he has not, it is likely that he has conducted the interview in such a way as to neglect relating the illness to the patient's life. To introduce for the first time an inquiry into the personal and social background at this point in the interview is not likely to be productive, for it will be artificial and out of context. On the other hand, if the student has been following the course of the patient's illness in the context of his pattern of life and his family relationships, there will now remain only the task of filling in areas left unfinished earlier in the interview. Commonly, the patient's trust in the student has by this time matured to the point that he is quite willing, sometimes eager, to discuss personal concerns which he may have been hesitant to reveal earlier in the interview. These concerns may be of considerable importance for subsequent judgments about management and prognosis.

How fully each aspect of the personal and social history must be covered depends on the individual case. *In all instances, full information about the patient's current life situation is mandatory.* Beyond that, the patient himself generally indicates what is pertinent if the interviewer shows interest and follows the patient's leads. His age and the nature of the present problem give some indication as to what should be more fully explored. For example, information about early childhood is much more relevant in an adolescent or a young adult than in an elderly person. When emotional problems are prominent, a fuller exploration of the early life history is indicated, regardless of the patient's age.

The personal and social history aims to provide an overall perspective of the patient's adjustment and functioning over the years. The best way to assay this is to sample how the patient has dealt with developmental and other crises of life. Accordingly, one inquires into his performance and reactions under such circumstances as leaving school and home, military service, marriage, illness or death of important persons, or changes in his economic or social status. As already stressed, *emphasis is always on the patient's reactions and method of coping with these events, not simply on the event itself.* The interviewer's preconception of how stressful or significant an event is does not necessarily correspond with how it is perceived by the patient. Retirement, for example, may be a blessing to one person and an intolerable burden to another. Good general questions to ask whenever the patient reports some such change in his life are "How did this affect you?" or "How did you feel?" Dates and sequences are important to clarify the temporal relationship to past and present illnesses.

The details of important points in the Personal and Social History may be found in Chapter 5. The major subdivisions of the Personal and Social History are organized as follows:

CURRENT LIFE SITUATION

This covers information about *present* living arrangements and relationships to family and friends. Included are descriptions of the home and family, present occupation and economic status, social and community commitments, leisure activities, and the patient's personal characteristics and pattern of living. One emphasizes whatever may be current sources of concern to the patient and whatever may be important for his future care. Information from family or friends is also helpful in evaluating the current life situation.

PAST DEVELOPMENT

This category considers the patient's *past* personal and social history and is organized into three major subdivisions: childhood and adolescence, educational and occupational history, and marital and family history.

With respect to the interview itself, these personal issues are not dealt with in a categorical fashion. The attentive interviewer will learn a good deal just from what the patient chooses to discuss. For purposes of elaboration, the best technique is to begin with a general question referring to a major area of life experience. For example, "Tell me about your childhood" and "When did you first leave home?" are good questions to begin a discussion of childhood or adolescence. While much of the information concerning persons important to the patient, such as parents, children, husband or wife, will have already been obtained, additional details concerning relationships may emerge as the patient discusses his development. When one wishes to encourage the patient's responses, the best technique usually is to pursue information that is already known. For example, "You say you work in a bank. What do you do?" "Who is your boss?" "What was your job before that?" and so on, keeping in mind that one always follows the patient's lead and not a prepared set of questions. It is relatively easy to move from such a beginning and progress to related areas, such as schooling, military service, or outside activities, until a general outline of the patient's development and way of life has been obtained.

Obviously, new information about the present illness, past health, or family health may appear in this phase of the interview and should be pursued in detail.

Step 8: Reviewing Symptoms by Systems

The Systems Review serves to organize symptoms and signs in terms of the major systems of the body. It has two purposes:

First, it is used by the interviewer as a guide in elaborating symptoms of the patient's present illness. A complaint of chest pain, for example, should immediately suggest the need for a full review of the items covered under the Cardiovascular and Respiratory Systems. It is usually appropriate to do this at the time the presenting complaints are being investigated.

Second, the Review of Systems is used to inquire about symptoms and signs in the patient's past history that may have been overlooked in the interview. Specifically checking each system may uncover further symptoms of an illness already discussed or of an illness not yet mentioned. One may also encounter miscellaneous symptoms which do not fit into any particular diagnostic category or those which represent minor responses to psychological stress.

It is relatively easy to commit to memory the order and content of the Systems Review if one keeps in mind the several general headings and what symptoms result from specific organ dysfunction. The review proceeds systematically: Beginning with the skin and hematopoietic system one proceeds to the head and neck and down the trunk to the extremities, covering each of the major systems. Below are listed the general categories of the Systems Review. The specific items are found in Chapter 5.

Skin	Cardiovascular system
Hematopoietic system	Gastrointestinal system
Head and face	Urinary tract
Ears	Genital tract (male)
Eyes	Genital tract (female)
Nose and sinuses	Skeletal system
Mouth, pharynx, and larynx	Nervous system
Breasts	Endocrine system
Respiratory tract	Psychological status

Except when elaborating a symptom of the present illness, it is important that the direct questioning of the Systems Review be reserved for the very end of the interview. An inexperienced student may be tempted to shift to the Systems Review early when there is silence on the part of the patient or when the student feels he is running out of questions. Premature introduction of such a direct question-answer approach can serve to block the unfolding of the history by the patient, with consequent loss of important data. Whenever the student is at an impasse how to proceed, he may ask himself if he has thoroughly covered the course of the illness and evaluated the symptoms in terms of the seven major dimensions.

It is manifestly impossible to establish the occurrence of each and every symptom experienced by the patient in the course of his life. Although the Systems Review contains a great number of items, in practice, the interviewer asks a general question under each major heading and follows this with a rapid and brief query about those items that seem most relevant for the particular patient. In this fashion, he proceeds in an orderly manner through the whole sequence. Each positive response should be developed fully and its relationship to previously noted illnesses should be clarified.

An example of questioning in the Systems Review with respect to the respiratory tract would be "Have you ever had any trouble with your lungs?" "Breathing?" "Asthma?" "Wheezing?" "Cough?" "Do you cough up anything when you wake in the mornings?" "Have you ever coughed up blood?" "Ever have pleurisy, or a pain on breathing?" "Night sweats?" "When was your last chest film?" If the patient does not know what pleurisy means, an explanation must be given or a more colloquial term used. It is helpful, as the student progresses through the review of systems, to mention the names of common illnesses that the patient may have forgotten to mention; for instance, "Have you ever had pneumonia?" under the respiratory tract; "ulcer?" or "gallbladder trouble?" under the gastrointestinal system.

When a patient responds affirmatively, it is necessary to clarify whether the symptom reported represents an occasional and inconsequential manifestation (e.g., everyone coughs at some time), a normal physiological phenomenon (e.g., becoming winded after running), or whether it constitutes a significant change for him (e.g., dyspnea on climbing one flight). If the latter, the symptom should be evaluated briefly in terms of the seven dimensions.

Occasional patients respond positively to virtually every question. This is an important finding, especially in a patient who earlier described his general health as "pretty good." It may indicate a psychological illness (conversion or hypochondriasis), or be a clue to multisystem disease not heretofore recognized. Other patients minimize complaints and need to be pressed to bring out the information. Thus, a 55-year-old woman may simply state that she went through the menopause at age 45, not mentioning subsequent vaginal bleeding unless specifically asked.

Step 9: Bringing the Interview to a Close

When the student has finished the Systems Review, he should have a reasonably complete history from most patients. It must be recognized, however, that the history will not necessarily be completed in one interview. All the details of the patient's illnesses cannot be obtained in a single session. Additional questions may also be raised in the course of the physical examination, as when the physician discovers the scar of an operation not previously mentioned. If the story is long and complicated, or if the patient is quite ill, the student should be alert to fatigue or discomfort. The interview may need to be interrupted and the patient asked if he would like a brief rest. Again, such sensitivity to the patient's well-being contributes positively to the student-patient relationship and the patient's willingness to cooperate.

As an interview is brought to a close, whether the history is complete or not, it is well to give the patient an opportunity to mention anything else he may have on his mind. This is done by saying "Is there anything else you would like to bring up?" Also, if the student is not clear about a particular area of the history, it may be helpful to recapitulate briefly some of the essential features of the story. In so doing, the interviewer should ask the patient to verify the accuracy of the account: "Now as I understand it, Mr. Jones, your first experience with this pain was early in June, etc." or, one may inquire about a symptom that is still vague: "Now before we finish, let me check to be sure that I am clear about your pain." He then proceeds to relate his understanding of the symptom, inviting the patient to make corrections as he proceeds. Occasionally just as the interview is coming to a close, the patient may introduce some new piece of information as if it were a mere afterthought. The student should be aware that this may reflect concern or embarrassment and that it is important to follow up such information with interest. For instance, at the very end of an interview a patient with a rash may ask "By the way, do you think penicillin could cause this?" Up to this point he had not mentioned that he had recently taken penicillin for the treatment of a urethral discharge.

If in the course of the interview the patient has bared intimate details of a distressing nature or has exposed unpleasant feelings toward family, friends, or doctors, he may later regret that he has said too much. Commonly, he is concerned about the interviewer's opinion of him or that the confidentiality of his communication will be violated. The student may avert such a reaction by reassuring the patient that he understands his feelings and that the information will be handled with professional confidence. In all cases where the patient has been obviously upset during the interview, it is well to return later in the day to see how he is getting along.

When the interview is finished, the patient should be told what is planned next and when. Usually, it is the physical examination.

THE INTERVIEW OF INFORMANTS OTHER THAN THE PATIENT

A physician rarely deals exclusively with the patient. Interested family or friends are almost always present. *It is the student's obligation to meet these persons and to interview, at least briefly, the more important relative or friend.* The reasons for such a meeting are as follows:

1. The student should learn something of the impact of the patient's illness on the family, as well as the influence of the family on the patient's illness.

2. He must learn how to relate to family members so as to be of help to them, as well as enlist their aid for the patient.

3. The visitor serves as a valuable source of additional information and as a check on the reliability of the patient's report of his illness.

4. It gives the student an opportunity to observe directly some aspects of the relationship between the family and the patient.

Arranging the Interview with the Visitor

In general, it is best to interview the patient first before turning to others for information, even when he is limited in his ability to give a history. Only the patient can express his own feelings. His responses in the interview, although incomplete, are most important in understanding him and in diagnosing his problem. Also, unless the situation is urgent or the patient is a young child, it is wiser to interview the patient alone. This affords him privacy and prevents breaks in his flow of thought by a relative who may interrupt in an effort to be helpful. When the patient is interviewed first, the student is also able to learn which visitor is the most appropriate one to interview. To discuss the patient's problems with someone with whom he is on bad terms might jeopardize the student's relationship with his patient. In every case, however, the student should ask the patient's approval to speak with the relative or friend. "I would also like to speak with your wife. Is that all right with you?" If he seems hesitant, the interviewer gives him the opportunity to explain by saying in a questioning tone "If you would rather I'd not. . .?"

Should the patient still remain reluctant, his wish should be respected. Rarely, there are overriding instances when a relative should be seen despite the patient's objection. If so, the matter should be discussed with a staff member.

Most patients readily agree, and indeed, are pleased that the student will meet with the relative. They usually will take it upon themselves to inform the family member. Visitors are also eager to have the opportunity to speak with the staff who are concerned with the patient's care, so usually there is no difficulty in arranging such a meeting.

Conducting the Interview with a Relative or Friend

The meeting should always be in private, although the opportunity should not be overlooked to speak briefly with the patient and visitor together, since this gives some insight into how they interact. To make it quite clear that the meeting is to be more than a hurried casual encounter, both student and visitor should be seated comfortably in a private place before the interview begins.

The student must appreciate that it is an emotionally upsetting experience to have a close relative or friend sick in the hospital. The relative will often need support himself. He welcomes the opportunity to become acquainted with someone involved in the patient's care and appreciates the chance to unburden himself. Indeed, the visitor's distress constitutes an important motivation for his willingness to meet with the student, who should immediately indicate that he is aware of the relative's feelings by asking such questions as "How are *you*?" or "This must be a difficult time for you." These questions allow the visitor to tell about his own distress or ill health as well as about his concerns for the patient or for other members of the family, such as the children. The student must also be alert to the occasions when the relative is not well and is now further troubled by the illness of the patient. This is an especially common situation among elderly couples. The student's willingness to devote some time to listening to the relative's problems not only is helpful to the relative, but also may prevent the visitor from burdening the patient with his own complaints.

Sometimes the visitor begins by asking questions about the patient's condition or about plans for study and treatment. These are best handled by saying that before such questions can be answered, more must be known about the patient; in fact, this is one of the reasons for the meeting. The student may then move to a general question about the patient, such as "Tell me about your husband's illness." *He does not reveal what he has already learned from the patient*, for this may inhibit the informant from giving his own account. Instead, the relative is encouraged to elaborate details, especially in those areas where the patient was vague or where independent corroboration is needed. Often, new perspectives or different facts emerge that require further investigation.

Though usually less detailed, the interview with the visitor follows the same pattern as that with the patient. One identifies the main complaints; delineates the current illness; and explores past illnesses, family health, and relationships, as well as the personal and social history. Since the student already has the bulk of the information, he can more easily follow associations; and with a few well-chosen specific questions, he can verify or round out details already obtained from the patient.

One can sometimes get more information from an informed visitor than from the patient himself, particularly when there are details about which the patient either is unaware or is reluctant to discuss. For example, the patient may not know that his behavior was irrational or that he suffered a convulsion. Or he may minimize, distort, or deny symptoms to completely mislead the student, who may be surprised to learn from the relative how ill the patient has really been. The family member's description of the patient's behavior is especially helpful in the diagnosis of psychosis or depression; indeed, such a diagnosis can be overlooked when information from outside sources is not solicited. The relative's viewpoint is also useful in evaluating how the patient reacts to illness or to hospital procedures, especially when the relative is familiar with how the patient has handled such situations in the past. One may encourage the family members to speak about the patient by asking such questions as "How do you think your wife has been getting along?" "How disabled has she been?" "How has this affected *her*?" or "What sort of a person is your wife?"

Sometimes it is necessary to secure the entire history from a relative. This is particularly important when the patient is critically ill, delirious, demented, or psychotic. Under such conditions, the student carries out the interview in the same manner and detail as he would with the patient himself.

At the end of the interview, the visitor may have more questions. Those that have to do with the patient's condition or plans for treatment are best referred to the physician in charge.

Respecting Confidences When Interviewing Relatives

The confidential nature of some of the communications of the patient, as well as of those of the family, must always be of prime concern. Personal information is not transmitted from one to the other. Above all, the patient is never confronted with conflicting data obtained from another source, unless there is some overriding medical necessity to do so. An example of this would be when the patient withholds an important fact, such as the occurrence of bleeding or a previous venereal infection. If the patient has confided highly personal information concerning the visitor in question, it is especially important to ask his permission before interviewing that particular person and to take special pains to reassure the patient that his confidence will be respected.

The Value of Repeated Contacts with Visitors

Repeated brief contacts with visitors provide an excellent means of following the course of the patient's progress and learning which persons are most concerned about him. Sometimes the visitors will be other than the ones the student expected. For example, a wife's glowing account of her devoted husband may be cast in doubt when it is discovered that he rarely visits, stays briefly, or shows her little attention when visiting. Hence, it is valuable to know who visits and who does not and to observe how the patient relates to his visitor. Significant fluctuations in the patient's hospital course may follow the visits (or the absences) of certain persons. Such observations may prove enlightening in understanding the course of the illness and are important in planning for the patient's care after he leaves the hospital.

Occasionally it is informative to meet together with the patient and with one or more members of the family. This may reveal something of the interactions between family members. Such an interview is usually carried out after the patient has been in the hospital for some time, although very occasionally, an upset patient will insist that the family remain during the initial interview. In this situation, the best approach is to begin with a broad question as "How have things been going?" This is posed in such a way that it is not obviously directed to either the patient or the relative. One can then observe who becomes the spokesman, who contradicts, what exchange develops among the participants, and how they communicate with each other.

Other Sources of Information: Physicians and Hospital Records

On every possible occasion, a student should try to speak with the referring physician or with other staff involved in the care of the patient, such as the social worker or the psychologist. This may be done in person or by telephone. It is particularly important when accurate information is needed about medication, physical findings, and laboratory data. Generally, this is done after the student has interviewed and examined the patient; but in an emergency, or when the patient is incapable of giving a history, the information will be needed promptly. One should always check first with the resident before proceeding.

Bottles of unknown medicines can be identified by a call to the pharmacy that dispensed the drug. From the prescription number, the pharmacist will be able to give the name of the drug, its dose, and directions.

The records of previous admissions to the same hospital or to others should always be carefully reviewed but only after the student has collected his own data. *Reviewing the recorded history in the hospital chart before one interviews the patient usually hinders rather than facilitates the interview.* Only after he has finished his interview and physical examination, and after he has reasoned out his initial diagnostic impression, should the student review the old record. By completing his own study before reviewing the chart, bias is avoided; indeed, the student may come up with a finding or diagnosis unsuspected by others. After reviewing the record, however, he may wish to explore with the patient issues that were raised by previously recorded findings.

SPECIAL TECHNICAL PROBLEMS OF THE INTERVIEW

A number of technical problems may be encountered during the interview. The simplest reflect the insecurity of the student in his newly assigned role, as when the patient consults him about his medical condition or asks personal questions. Others, such as silences, crying, or hostile behavior on the part of the patient, usually stem from the patient's own problems. Clinical experience helps resolve many of the technical difficulties of the interview; however, the student will benefit from a consideration of the following common problems that may occur in any interview:

Questions about the Illness, Procedures, or Treatment

Questions by the patient concerning diagnosis, prognosis, and treatment are best referred to the physician in charge. When such questions are posed early in the interview, the student may point out that not enough is yet known about the patient's problems, which is a reason for his performing an interview and physical examination. If the patient questions him again later, the student should refer him to the physician in charge. "I think it best that you ask Dr. _____." Sometimes it may even be necessary to ask the patient who he considers his doctor to be. When more than one physician is caring for him, even though all are in complete agreement, it is still best for the physician responsible to do the counseling. Any differences of opinion between doctors may be misinterpreted by patients and lead to anxiety and a breakdown in confidence. On the other hand, the student need not hesitate to answer questions about such matters as ward routine, procedures, or scheduled tests.

Personal Questions

Occasionally, patients will ask the student personal questions. Some may inquire whether a student is married or has children. There is no reason to avoid such questions as long as one does not go beyond the factual data. Other patients will ask questions in a challenging or aggressive manner, often in response to a personal question directed to them. For example, when one inquires about a patient's reaction to a death, he may retort "How would *you* feel?" or "Did *you* ever lose a child, doctor?" Such questions can be answered honestly by saying "I would be very upset" or "No, I haven't." Sometimes the patient asks such a question because he is ashamed or because he feels the interviewer is implying that something was abnormal or unnatural about his reaction. The student's response should emphasize the upsetting nature of such an experience, that people respond differently, and that it will be helpful to know how the patient handled it.

A student may be challenged in a similar way with regard to smoking or drinking, usually because the patient feels accused. "Do *you* smoke, doctor?" is a common rejoinder. A brief honest answer is best, followed by the statement that people's behavior differ and the major concern is with the patient and his health.

Occasionally patients, notably hysterics, manic patients, and a few psychotics, make seductive or even sexual advances. Such behavior must be met in a firm professional manner, and one must avoid getting involved in any type of personal exchange.

Silences

Brief silence on the part of the patient in response to a question should not cause the student to feel uneasy, even though 20 or 30 seconds of silence may seem interminable to the beginner. The pause may reflect the patient's attempt to recall a fact or his indecision as to how he should respond. One can usually tell which is the case from the patient's expression, and the proper behavior is simply to wait expectantly. The student's manner and facial expression should indicate that he expects the patient to continue. If the patient's manner communicates some distress, a response may be facilitated by indicating awareness of his discomfort. This may be done with some remark as "You seem to be troubled," but only after one has waited long enough to see if the patient will resume spontaneously.

A common reason for prolonged or repeated silences is faulty technique on the part of the interviewer. Often, it results from failure to establish a relationship, perhaps because of clumsy handling of the introductory phase, as when some discomfort of the patient is overlooked or ignored. For instance, a patient whose pain or nausea has been passed over is likely to become preoccupied with his distress and may volunteer little information during the interview. Too many specific questions asked too early, especially those permitting only "yes" and "no" answers, or too many interruptions on the part of the interviewer, may give the patient an impression that he is only to answer questions and not to bring up other information. He therefore lapses into the pattern of answering briefly and waiting for the next question. Questions which are too complex may provoke silence simply because the patient does not know how to respond.

Some patients become silent because they have been offended by tactless remarks or a lack of consideration on the part of the student. For example, rushing ahead with a new question before the patient has finished his response may provoke silence; or interrupting when the patient obviously wants to speak of a matter of immediate concern may frustrate him and cause him to become quiet.

When the silences are not due to such technical errors, one may help the patient to resume by such nonspecific comments as "You were telling me about_____" or "Was there anything else?" or "Can you tell me more?" or "Then what?" The interviewer may also simply pick up where he left off and rephrase his last question.

Lack of communication, marked by prolonged silence, may also be a manifestation of organic brain disease, depression, or psychosis.

Crying

It is natural for a student to feel uncomfortable the first few times a patient begins to cry during an interview. Yet, crying is not only a useful clinical sign, it may also afford relief to the patient. Crying usually occurs when the patient is thinking of something that is very distressing to him. This may be the illness or death of a loved one, a threatened loss, or an extremely frustrating situation in his own life. Sometimes, crying is brought on by the patient's concern about his illness and its possible consequence. Whatever the reason, crying is a valuable clinical sign, for it informs the interviewer that the matter under discussion is of grave importance to the patient. The student should wait patiently, allowing the patient to cry and providing a tissue if necessary. By his facial expression, a sympathetic nod, or a kindly remark ("I understand how you feel"), he lets the patient know that he accepts and understands the crying. This enables the patient to relieve his feelings and unburden himself of problems that he may have long wanted to discuss with someone. One does not introduce a new subject until the patient has fully expressed himself and regained control. Such understanding behavior on the student's part goes a long way toward establishing an effective relationship.

At times, it is desirable to invite crying when the patient appears on the verge of tears and is obviously trying to suppress them. A comment, such as "It still makes you feel sad, doesn't it?" lets the patient know that his crying will not meet with disapproval. A student need not worry that he will induce a flood of uncontrollable tears. Usually, the crying subsides in a few minutes and a relieved, often grateful patient is able to resume the thread of his story; and the student will have gained insight into some of the patient's most serious concerns.

Hostility

One may encounter various degrees of hostility from patients during the interview. Some are blatantly hostile, sarcastic, demeaning, or challenging. They may refuse to answer questions, abruptly terminate the interview, or even order the student out of the room. Less overt hostility may be manifested by a curt "I have told all this before" or "My doctor knows all about me; I don't know why I have to tell you." The challenge for the student is to overcome his own natural tendency to become angry. He must try instead to understand why the patient is behaving in such a disagreeable manner. These are always trying situations, especially for a beginning student, but they can be handled appropriately if one is aware of the different situations which may provoke patient anger:

> The inconsiderate or angry student.
> The patient who is already angry.
> The aggressive, pseudoindependent patient.
> The demanding, dependent patient.
> The paranoid patient.

THE INCONSIDERATE OR ANGRY STUDENT

The first thought should always be whether the student himself has provoked the patient's reaction. Some students always assume that it is the patient's fault and give no consideration to the possibility that their own behavior is responsible. Among the possible ways the student may cause anger are the following:

1. The student may not have adequately introduced himself and made his role clear. The patient may already have been interviewed more than once and may resent being questioned again by someone he believes is not directly concerned with his care. Such a misapprehension on the patient's part is usually corrected when the student explains more fully what his responsibilities are.

2. Interruption of the patient's plan to rest or to visit with family and friends may bring about anger. Also, neglect at the outset to assure his comfort may cause the patient to become increasingly irritated until he explodes in anger at the student, whom he sees as callous and self-centered. The patient uses this means to express himself and bring an unpleasant situation to an end. This predicament may be resolved, even at this point, if the student recognizes the patient's problem and attempts to alleviate it. Sometimes the student has no alternative but to interrupt the interview and start over again at a later time when he can be more attentive to the patient's condition.

3. By failing to pay attention to what the patient has been saying or to keep track of details, the student may repeat the same question or refer to incorrect facts when asking further questions. The patient then finds himself becoming annoyed at the repetition of questions, and may eventually lose patience. Taking adequate notes and allowing more time to formulate the next question usually averts this problem.

4. Questions which are accusatory in tone or inappropriately intrusive may provoke anger. This is most likely to happen when the student fails to follow the patient's associations and asks too many direct questions, such as "Is your marriage happy?" "Were you doing anything that might have caused this?" or "Why didn't you take your medicine like your doctor told you?" The patient may then ask angrily "What does that have to do with my illness?" or refuse to answer. Under such circumstances, the only solution is for the student to recognize his error and adopt a different approach.

5. Failure to appreciate the educational or cultural level of the patient may cause resentment. This is just as likely to occur when a student talks down to an intelligent, well-educated person as when he fails to appreciate the limitations of an uneducated or culturally deprived patient. In both situations the patient feels depreciated. Sometimes such behavior on the part of the student reflects a prejudice; more often it

results from a failure to evaluate the patient's intellectual capability in the introductory phase of the interview.

6. Some patient's reactions reflect the student's personal antipathy, which may be more apparent than he realizes. Everyone has biases, although they are not always acknowledged. The student who finds his patient getting angry will do well to examine his own attitude toward the patient. He may discover that the patient belongs to a category of people whom he dislikes and that he has unwittingly communicated his feeling to the patient, who reacts to his prejudice.

7. Finally, for reasons that have nothing to do with the patient, the student may have approached the interview in an angry frame of mind. He may have been annoyed by a demand of an intern, a criticism by a senior physician, or a letter from home. The patient quickly senses his mood and responds in kind. If the student can recognize his own role in provoking the patient, he should be able to bring himself under control and avoid further difficulty. Sometimes an apology or explanation is indicated.

THE PATIENT WHO IS ALREADY ANGRY

The student may happen to begin the interview at a moment when the patient is still angry about something that has occurred in the hospital or elsewhere. Such anger is readily displaced toward the student, who is a representative of the hospital. The proper response is to hear the patient out, avoid taking sides, and try to be helpful, whether the complaint seems justified or not. It is well to appreciate that the patient can not participate effectively in the interview as long as he is preoccupied with his anger.

THE AGGRESSIVE, PSEUDOINDEPENDENT PATIENT

Some patients act aggressively as a means of dealing with their anxiety or feelings of helplessness. These are people who ordinarily handle their deep-seated fears of passivity by being perpetually active and by vigilantly trying to be in control. To be sick, immobilized, and obliged to submit to the hospital routine is very upsetting. The staff are seen as more threatening than helpful, and hospital procedures which call for passive submission are feared. Such patients struggle to maintain control and overcome these fears, often by acting aggressively toward the staff.

A number of behavioral characteristics forewarn the student that he is dealing with this kind of person. Even when quite ill, the patient is noted to be restless and overactive. He is likely to minimize or deny symptoms, at times passing off major problems as inconsequential. He is quick to tell of his past vigor and to boast of accomplishments. In small but obvious ways, he quickly tries to take control of the situation; for instance, by directing the student where to sit or informing him that he has only a few moments to talk.

The angry outburst may come at any point in the interview, especially when the patient feels his control of the situation is in jeopardy. For example, he may be provoked if the student does not allow him to take the lead or if the student interrupts him or interferes with his way of telling the story. He may become angry when he is pressed for details of symptoms which betray a greater degree of illness than he had heretofore acknowledged. He may cut off the interview when it touches on failures in his work or inadequacies in family relationships.

If the student understands that such outbursts reflect anxiety and the patient's need for control, he will handle such situations in a rational manner. The display of anger should be accepted without retaliation, and the student should attempt to help the patient regain his feeling of being in control of the situation. To accomplish this, the student moves away from the subject matter which provoked the outburst, and he becomes more passive in the interview situation. It may help to explain in very general terms that he needs certain information to be able to understand the problem and do his job. At the same time, the patient is assured that he is not obliged to speak of anything he does not wish to discuss. Such subtle emphasis on how the patient is helping the student in the performance of his duties may serve to reestablish for the patient his much-needed feeling of superiority; for example, one might say "It would help me to understand this if you could spell out what the pain was like." If the patient still demurs, the subject is dropped and the student moves to another area that is more neutral or more conducive to bolstering the patient's self-esteem; for example, one may inquire about a period when he was enjoying good health or having success in his work. If the student succeeds in supporting him in this manner, the patient will often take the initiative by coming back to the subject which led to the outburst.

THE DEMANDING, DEPENDENT PATIENT

An occasional patient voices a never-ending series of angry complaints and demands, making it very difficult to pursue the interview. He sees himself as abused and neglected. These patients are extremely dependent people who feel chronically deprived and are angrily trying to force others to take care of them. They make demands on the student from the moment he arrives; for instance, by asking to have the bed lowered, the shade drawn, or the breakfast tray removed. They may become irritable, angry, and uncooperative when they feel their needs are not being recognized. The student will find that attending to such requests at the beginning of the interview, and even periodically thereafter, will often mitigate the patient's angry demands and lead to a much more productive interview.

THE PARANOID PATIENT

The student may discover that the interview is being interrupted by angry, accusatory questions: "Why do you want to know that?" "Who told you to ask about that?" "Who wants to know that?" "Did my wife put you up to that?" Such questions carry the implication of some devious plan or design that is characteristic of the paranoid patient. The observant student will readily note an underlying quality of suspiciousness in the patient's behavior and an accusatory flavor to his account of the illness. The patient imagines that others are responsible for his plight or have designs against him. The student may be regarded by the patient as someone having a link with these outside forces. Such anger is delusional in origin and is usually beyond appeal to reason. It is wise not to dispute the patient's false ideas, and one should abandon further questioning about the subject which aroused the patient's suspicions.

*****

As with crying, anger does not last indefinitely. The problem may be resolved merely by sitting it out or by coming back to see the patient on some more propitious occasion. It should also be remembered that the patient who does react with anger may later feel sorry. He should be given an opportunity, at that time, to express his feelings of remorse and be reassured that his behavior was understood and accepted as part of the stress of illness. Such a sequence often is the medium whereby an effective relationship becomes possible.

Denial or Withholding

Some patients minimize or completely deny symptoms. This tendency may be a way of averting anxiety, or it may represent a character trait which is the patient's typical manner of dealing with any difficulty. Such patients are not aware of the degree to which they are distorting the facts. Other patients deliberately withhold or distort information about which they are ashamed or afraid. Denial or withholding usually is betrayed by the obvious disparity between the patient's condition and how he reports it. There may be the too hearty, smiling insistence that all is well or that a symptom does not exist. He may dismiss all symptoms by categorizing them as familiar minor disorders, such as "gas," "a little indigestion," "a touch of rheumatism," or "just a virus." Or the patient who is consciously withholding information may respond with repeated flushing, hesitation, revealing gestures, or inappropriate smiling when a sensitive topic is under consideration. As the interviewer recognizes this tendency, he must modify his approach in order to obtain the needed information without provoking anxiety by undermining the patient's defences. This is best done by coming back to the sensitive subject in an indirect manner at a later point in the interview. For example, a patient, fearful of the possibility of heart disease, might refer to his attack of chest pain and shortness of breath as, "just a little gas" or "indigestion." When questioned directly, he may emphatically deny cardiac symptoms. Following the patient's lead, the interviewer should then shift the inquiry to a consideration of digestive symptoms. He asks the patient to tell more about his previous experiences with "gas" or "indigestion" and the circumstances under which they have occurred. Approached from this perspective, the patient may now reveal that in more recent attacks the "gas" sometimes "cuts off my breath" or "squeezes me here" (pointing to his sternum); or that it has come on while playing golf and when he is under emotional pressure. By having the patient describe his daily activities, perhaps later in the interview, one may discover that, over a period of time, he has gradually restricted or eliminated activities because of his symptoms. In this manner, the interviewer succeeds in eliciting the essential details of the history without forcing the patient prematurely to face the possibility of heart disease.

When confronted with this type of patient, it is essential to interview a reliable informant as well. Usually such a person is quite familiar with the patient's propensity to deny or withhold. But with rare exceptions, the patient should not be confronted with the information obtained from an outside source. Occasionally, however, the information is vital and its reliability must be ascertained directly from the patient; for instance, the history of tuberculosis, epilepsy, a psychiatric illness, or of alcohol ingestion. When this is the case, the student will have to explain that the information is necessary if proper treatment is to be instituted, and he must insist on an answer. The probable alcoholic, who admits only to "an occasional beer now and then," may be enticed into a more accurate response when the interviewer suggests a specific amount that might be consumed daily or on weekends. Information which may initially be withheld is often revealed later on a second or third contact, after a relationship of trust has been established.

It should not be forgotten that sometimes the presence of other patients within hearing may be responsible for the patient's withholding information. A later interview in privacy may easily solve this problem.

THE INTERVIEW MODIFIED BY THE PATIENT'S ILLNESS

The student will encounter patients who will be limited in their ability to relate a history because of their underlying illness. In some instances, the acute nature or severity of the patient's illness necessitates an abbreviated interview; in other instances, because of the disease, the patient will be handicapped in telling his story.

The basic outline of the interview is applicable to all situations. There is always an initial introduction, a quick evaluation of the patient's present state, and a series of more detailed inquiries, each proceeding from the more general to the specific. Where it is necessary to modify the interview because of the patient's illness, information must be derived from other sources in order to complete the history. These sources include family, friends, or previous hospital records, as well as the student's subsequent interview of the patient at a more opportune time.

The Acutely Ill Patient

In an acute emergency, the patient's condition demands prompt action. He may be bleeding, in shock, severely dyspneic, in intense pain, or in a psychotic crisis. In such situations, the student must combine the techniques of both the interview and physical examination. Observation of the obvious physical or psychological disturbance is made on approaching the bedside. The student introduces himself and inquires as to the problem. By taking the patient's hand or feeling his pulse, he communicates at once an intent to help as quickly as possible. Except for an occasional psychotic patient, physical contact provides considerable reassurance. At times, it is appropriate to start with a quick examination before questioning him further. Such an approach may reduce the anxiety of a seriously sick person sufficiently enough so that, although previously uncommunicative, he may now be able to respond. As soon as the main area of distress is identified, the student moves quickly by direct questioning to gain the information necessary to determine a course of action. It should be emphasized that, even with the abbreviated work-up of patients in an emergency situation, adherence to the general order of the interview first, followed by the physical examination, will lead to more accuracy; and in the long run will take less time.

The Seriously Ill Patient

In some cases, because of the severity of the illness, the patient cannot be completely interviewed. He may be too weak, too dyspneic, too disorganized, or in too much pain. One must give priority to those aspects of the history which appear most relevant to the immediate situation. Which information is important is not always obvious to the beginner; but in general, the best approach is to explore the first complaints reported by the patient in response to the opening question. If he is having difficulty speaking at any length, more specific questions should be asked sooner than is ordinarily done. It may be necessary to limit oneself to a series of brief interviews for 10 or 15 minutes, distributed over a period of time, rather than to try to get a full history in one or two sessions. For instance, the patient may need more time between bouts of pain or nausea to respond to the questions. In general, by being attentive to the comfort of the patient, the student will succeed ultimately in obtaining an adequate history.

The Delirious or Demented Patient (Organic Brain Disease)[3]

The inability of a patient to report his history in a logical or coherent fashion poses special problems. The interviewer must judge the extent of the patient's deficit, as well as evaluate the reliability of the report. If the patient is capable of providing some of the history, the student adapts his technique so as to make the effort as productive as possible. When the patient appears incapable of giving a reliable history, then a relative or friend must be utilized as the primary source of information. Such serious interference is found in two major groups of disorders: organic brain disease (delirium or dementia) and the functional psychoses, such as schizophrenia, mania and hypomania, or psychotic depression. In practical terms, the student must recognize at the outset that the patient is having difficulty in presenting a coherent story, and an abbreviated mental status examination is carried out to evaluate the nature of the problem. This can easily be done in the framework of the interview.

Patients with organic brain disease have defects in attention, memory, and abstract thinking which make it difficult, if not impossible, to obtain an accurate history. In delirium, the defect is based on a reversible disorder of cerebral metabolism secondary to an inadequate metabolic supply (deficiency of oxygen or glucose), an electrolyte imbalance, or a blocking of the metabolic pathways by endogenous or exogenous toxic substances. In dementia, the defect results from the irreversible

---

[3]Engel, G. L.: Delirium. *In* Freedman, A. M., and Kaplan, H. I., Eds.: Comprehensive Textbook of Psychiatry. Williams & Wilkins Co., Baltimore, 1967, pp. 711-716.

destruction of brain substance, which may develop gradually, as in cerebral atherosclerosis; or abruptly, as with head trauma. Hence, the student should have a high index of suspicion of delirium when he approaches any seriously ill patient, and of dementia when he sees any elderly patient who is sick. Demented patients are especially vulnerable to further metabolic insult, as from hypoxia or drugs; and they will commonly have superimposed the reversible defect of delirium as well.

For practical purposes, the basic psychologic abnormalities are in the cognitive sphere and are the same in delirium and dementia: reduced attention and awareness, defects in recall and recent memory, and reduced ability to think abstractly, as evidenced by difficulty in orientation or in the performance of calculations. Some patients may also exhibit psychotic behavior, with hallucinations, sense deceptions, delusions, or panic. But it is the underlying, usually readily demonstrable, cognitive defect which establishes the diagnosis of delirium or dementia in such patients and differentiates them from those patients with only functional psychoses.

Organic brain disease is first suggested when the patient is noted to be inattentive, unsure of his responses, vague, and inconsistent. Even when answering relatively simple questions, he may appear to be puzzled and to exert an unusual effort. Such a patient responds slowly, hesitantly, with a furrowed brow, and often searches the room as if the answer literally is to be found by looking around for it. He may attempt to deflect the inquiry by humor, sarcasm, or an irritable denial of knowledge. Some patients frankly acknowledge that they are having difficulty in remembering.

When the patient behaves in this way it is wise to interrupt the sequence of the interview and examine the patient's cognitive performance. This is best done by remaining within the general framework of the interview and concentrating on known factual data. Using information in the hospital chart, the student may test the patient's ability to report accurately such items as his home address, his telephone number, the names of relatives, the date of hospital admission, the number of days he has been in the hospital, the present date, and the name of the hospital. One is particularly concerned with the patient's attention, memory, orientation, and ability to calculate. The questions are best posed in the guise of seeking information needed for the record, not in the form of a test. For example, "Which day was it you came here?" "And, let's see, today is the. . .?" "So you have been here how long now?" *The interviewer inquires as though he is the one who is unsure,* and the questions are designed to test orientation for time as well as the ability to perform simple calculations. The latter can easily be evaluated further by having the patient check the ages of relatives against their birth dates. "Your daughter is how old?" "When was she born?" To respond correctly the patient not only must know the current year and remember the birth year, but must also be aware of whether the age reported is consistent with the dates given. By repeating some of the same questions after an interval, one can check on inconsistencies. In so doing, it is often better to behave as if the interviewer himself does not remember, rather than suggesting that it is the patient who does not. "Let's see, how old did you say your daughter is?" In this way, the person with a milder defect is less likely to be offended.

If the patient makes errors in responding to such questions, delirium or dementia is suggested, and a more formal examination of cognitive performance may then be indicated. One may start by asking "Have you been having difficulty in remembering?" coupled with the reassuring comment that this is not uncommon when someone is sick. The patient may then be questioned about his level of education and the type of his employment to give some guide as to his optimal level of intellectual performance. Commensurate with his estimated ability, he may be asked to perform some familiar calculations. A housewife with a grade school education, for example, may be asked to add in her head a small grocery list or to make change. Serial subtractions of 3 or 7 from 100 is a simple and informative technique, but this requires at least a sixth grade education to be reliable. The patient is asked to subtract 3 or 7 from 100 and to continue subtracting until he reaches zero. This tests not only the ability to calculate, but also how well he is able to keep figures in mind without sensory guidance. In the presence of delirium or dementia, the patient exhibits increased effort, takes more time, and makes errors. He may count on his fingers; repeat all the numbers, (e.g., three from 100 is 97, three from 97 is 94, etc.); repeat errors, (e.g., 100, 97, 94, 91, *87*, 84, 81, 77. . .); perseverate, (e.g., 100, 93, 93, 93); lose his place (100, 93, 86, 79, 82, 75); or give some reason not to continue. The student records the length of time taken, the number and kind of errors made, and any pertinent description (e.g., perseveration, concreteness, appeal for outside guidance).

Usually more detailed testing for information, vocabulary, reasoning, and judgment is not needed to establish the diagnosis of organic brain disease, but these procedures are useful when following the course of a delirium.

Patients with defects due to delirium or dementia are not likely to provide a reliable history. The extent of mental limitation should be established early, since it is a waste of time to attempt to pursue a complete interview with such patients. However, the patient who is able to correct errors by exerting more effort can be successfully interviewed. With such a person, the student should word his questions as simply and clearly as possible, give the patient plenty of time to respond, and repeat questions to check the consistency of the responses. Too demanding tasks will increase confusion and provoke fatigue, so it is wise to keep the interview sessions brief. Also, one should not attempt to pursue an interview with a patient who is extremely anxious, hallucinating, experiencing sense deceptions, or who is highly distractible, since this may only serve to upset him further.

The Psychotic Patient

Some patients with psychoses are difficult to interview because they are inarticulate, unresponsive, or silently preoccupied with fantasies, hallucinations, or bodily sensations. Others are difficult because their capacity to relate to others is seriously impaired by disorganized thinking and language, or by behavior which is uncontrolled and bizarre. Yet many clearly psychotic people may give a reasonably reliable and complete history, whether it be of the psychiatric illness or of a concurrent physical illness. As soon as the interviewer suspects that the patient may be psychotic, his approach to the interview is altered in order to incorporate an abbreviated mental status examination. While collecting such factual material as he can, he pays particular attention to the *behavior* of the patient. Is it appropriate and acceptable? Does he display unusual postures, gestures, mannerisms, or inappropriate facial expressions? The *mood* of the patient is noted. Is he in excessively good spirits, profoundly dejected, inappropriately angry, or seductive? His *speech* is evaluated with respect to quality (e. g., tone, loudness, blocking), quantity (e.g., poverty of speech, pressure of speech), and organization (e.g., coherent, circumstantial, flight of ideas, punning). One is alert to *illusions*, where the patient misinterprets sensory data; *delusions*, where he expresses false beliefs; *feelings of persecution, influence, or reference*, where he believes outside forces are affecting him; *hallucinations*, where he sees visions, hears voices, or experiences other false sensations. The patient may have peculiar ideas about his body; for example, that his brain has shriveled up, his nose is deformed, or that one hand is smaller than the other. One also observes how *distractible* the patient is, whether he wanders from the subject or becomes preoccupied and silent.

The patient with a functional psychotic disorder is likely to display abnormalities in many of these areas, yet in contrast to the patient with organic brain disease, he is quite likely to be oriented to date and place, to have intact memory with retention and recall of factual details, and to be capable of performing calculations appropriate to his educational level. Indeed, when discussing matters which are remote from the underlying emotional problems, the patient may be entirely lucid. In practice, this means that the main problem is to deal with the patient's distractibility. The interviewer must repeatedly draw him back to the subject under discussion. With some effort and patience, it will eventually be possible to secure a reasonably complete and reliable account of an organic illness in a psychotic patient.

Psychotic patients who are extremely withdrawn are very difficult to interview. Such patients usually are severely disturbed schizophrenics (catatonic) or are psychotically depressed (retarded). They have great difficulty in making contact with other persons since they are intensely preoccupied with their own morbid thoughts. These patients may be curled up in bed or seated in a slumped position; they may wander distractedly about the room; or may be gesturing, posturing, muttering, and actively hallucinating. Obviously, if such behavior persists for any length of time, a productive interview is out of the question. But some seemingly withdrawn patients will begin to take note of the student and even direct remarks to him if he remains patiently in the room or at the bedside. Very occasionally a patient, who at the outset seemed quite out of contact, may become progressively more responsive; and an interview can proceed, although it is likely to be fragmentary and incomplete. In general, when questions are posed to the more disorganized psychotic patient, he is very likely to stray in his response long before a satisfactory answer can be obtained. Hence, time and persistence are required to piece together the fragments of factual information, and much of the historical information must be gathered from family or friends.

The Depressed Patient

It is important to recognize that many patients with any type of illness may be mildly depressed. This is evident not only from the pessimistic content of their speech, but also is indicated by a lack of spontaneity and a downcast facial expression. The seriously depressed patient, whether psychotic or not, may find it difficult to respond in an interview. He is slowed down and feels burdened or preoccupied. He volunteers little, his responses may be brief, and he does not elaborate. He may complain that he cannot remember or think clearly, although when pressed he is found not to have any significant memory defect. He may express the feeling that it is not worthwhile to report his story, that others are sicker or more in need of attention, and that his own condition is not of sufficient interest to waste the doctor's time. More ominous are expressions of futility, extreme pessimism, self-accusation, and preoccupation with alleged past misdeeds. Thoughts of suicide may be elicited on direct questioning. Psychotically depressed patients ordinarily also complain of poor appetite, constipation, weight loss, and inability to sleep. The presence of depression interferes with interviewing mainly because of the patient's reduced spontaneity and his preoccupation with his own pessimistic thoughts. However, firm but kindly persistence will enable the interviewer to overcome these barriers and to secure an adequate, if not a full account.

Recognition that depression is the cause of difficulty in obtaining a history is of great importance because a suicide risk can exist, and psychiatric consultation may be indicated.

The Mentally Defective Patient

The adult who is mentally defective, unless to an extreme degree, does not manifest a reduced level of awareness or attention. Since he is limited in the ability to learn and perform simple mental operations, he gives the appearance of stupidity or ignorance. This is in contrast to patients with delirium and dementia, whose superficial appearance of stupidity actually is based on a reduced level of attention and a memory deficit. The degree of intellectual retardation of the mentally defective person may be judged by his vocabulary, literacy, and age at the highest grade of schooling. If one is careful to keep inquiry at a level commensurate with the patient's abilities and level of completed education, mental deficiency, unless of extreme degree, usually does not preclude obtaining an adequate history.

The Dysphasic Patient

When a patient has had cerebral injury, such as in a cerebral vascular accident, he may have an expressive aphasia preventing an adequate interview. He may appear totally unresponsive or seem mentally incompetent, but at the same time *can be acutely aware of all conversation around him.* The student must be particularly careful of injudicious comments within the patient's hearing. Such patients may be taught simple signs for "Yes" or "No," enabling some degree of communication. It is also important to recognize that some patients who cannot speak are able to respond in writing.

The Patient Who Is Hard of Hearing

If a patient appears to be hard of hearing, one should always check whether he has a hearing aid available and help him make use of it. If he does not have his hearing aid with him, the assistance of the family or friends should be sought to have it brought to the hospital. The patient who is totally deaf may respond to written questions, or, if able to use sign language, may be able to communicate through an interpreter.

Reference

Engel, G. L.: Delirium. *In* Freedman, A. M., and Kaplan, H. I., Eds.: Comprehensive Textbook of Psychiatry. Williams and Wilkins Co., Baltimore, 1967, pp. 711-716.

Chapter 4

THE APPROACH TO THE PHYSICAL EXAMINATION

This chapter describes the basic physical examination common to physicians of all specialties, and emphasizes the following three principles: (1) How to relate to the patient during the physical examination. (2) How to apply the general techniques of physical diagnosis. (3) How to do an efficient and orderly examination.

The student should clearly recognize that the order of doing the physical examination differs from the order in which it is recorded. The actual examination is best done by regions, whereas the write-up is organized by organ systems (see Chapter 5). The present chapter helps the student to prepare for and organize his examination by regions. For a more detailed description of techniques, examples of abnormal physical findings, and the interpretation of findings, he should consult the conventional physical diagnosis texts.

GENERAL PRINCIPLES

Observing the Patient

The physical examination begins the moment the student first sees his patient. In the initial few minutes, the patient's dress, his speech, gait, and relationship to accompanying relatives will yield important information. How he walks down the hall or undresses himself will tell far more about his neurologic status, for example, than manipulating the patient's limbs on an examining bench. The student should also train himself to study the patient's facial expression, his posture, and gestures, which may yield important information regarding his psychologic status. Observation continues even as the interview proceeds. For example, the patient may have the pallor of anemia; the pigmentation of adrenal insufficiency; cyanosis of pulmonary disease; jaundice; the pale, sweaty brow of shock; or the downcast facies and slumping shoulders of depression. Only if something is looked for will it be found.

Just as the patient's appearance and behavior may yield important clues, so may his surroundings. The hospital bedside table is his link with the outside world. It should be carefully scrutinized. The choice of reading matter, be it a comic book, the Bible, or Shakespeare, gives an insight into his intellectual achievement and interests. Are there flowers and get-well cards, or is he bereft of attention? Does the diabetic have a gift of chocolates; or the cardiac, salted nuts? Does the patient have his own pills that he may be taking in addition to what is ordered? Is there a sputum cup on the table? If so, its contents should be examined for the color, consistency, and volume of the sputum.

Observation of the patient must be practiced in a deliberate but discreet manner. The patient is greeted in a friendly way and the interview begins as outlined in Chapter 3. While the patient is talking, the student systematically but unobtrusively studies him and his surroundings. When the general physical examination begins and as he starts to study each new region, the student should pause to carefully observe. The patient understands and accepts this brief delay.

Relating to the Patient During the Examination

It is important that the interview precede the physical examination. Not only does the patient's history indicate where physical abnormalities are likely to be found, but the interview also serves to establish a relationship with the patient. By means of the interview, the student may become aware of the patient's concerns about being examined, and therefore is better prepared to cope with them. Patients may be fearful as to what the examination will reveal, may be anxious about the discomfort it may provoke, or may be sensitive about having their bodies looked at and manipulated. Special concerns are likely to surround the examination of the eyes, the pharynx, the breasts, the heart rate, the blood pressure, the rectum, and the genitals. Some patients are afraid that they will be subjected to pain or other unpleasant sensations, as indeed they may have been in the past. Other patients are ashamed of defects or deformities and find it humiliating to display them. Still others are ashamed of their condition, that they are unkempt, have involuntarily soiled themselves, or simply are not able to perform up to their own standards. Most patients will demonstrate increased anxiety as the physician begins his examination, a reaction which may also affect such physical findings as heart rate, blood pressure, skin color, and sweating.

The guiding principle for the student during the physical examination is to respect the patient and his body. The observant student will know from the interview what are likely to be the patient's concerns about the examination — perhaps from the patient's questions (e.g., "Do you think it's my heart, doctor?"), or from his preoccupation with the illness of some other person (e.g., the heart attack or stroke suffered by a parent). The patient's remarks about previous examinations or the findings of other physicians often will give a clue. Apologies and excuses for his appearance or behavior identify the patient who is prone to shame; for example, "I look a mess, doctor," "If I had known you were coming, I would have tried to fix myself up a little" or "I'm sorry I can't move my arm any better." As the student gets ready for the examination, the patient may reveal his anxiety by saying "I gag easily, doctor" or "Don't blow up that blood pressure thing too tight." He may watch apprehensively as the student prepares his instruments and may inquire as to their use.

Accordingly, the student takes special pains to respect the patient's sensitivities. He is gentle and considerate as he approaches the parts of the body that cause the patient concern. He lets the patient know what he is about to do and encourages him to relax. When a procedure may cause discomfort, such as the examination of the pharynx or the rectum, the patient is prepared in advance. He is told "This may be a little uncomfortable. I will be gentle; be sure to let me know if it hurts." Sometimes it may help to defer a painful procedure to the end of the examination.

When shame or embarrassment are prominent features, the student is especially attentive to the privacy of the patient during the examination. He makes sure that the patient is properly draped, and he does not linger unduly in his examination of sensitive areas. The air of brisk, professional competence, which the student will soon acquire, goes a long way to mitigate such feelings on the part of the patient.

By and large, the examination is carried out in silence, except for the necessary instructions to the patient, as well as for a few brief questions should symptoms be evoked during the examination. The student must have all of his powers of concentration acutely attuned. Talking hinders him from concentrating fully on his techniques of physical diagnosis as well as from the mental visualization of possible underlying abnormalities. However, the examination is not done in complete silence. It is necessary to instruct the patient how to cooperate; for example, to fix his vision on a particular point when his fundus is being studied, to breathe slowly through his mouth to facilitate listening to his lungs, and to put his hands to the side and draw up his knees in order to relax his muscles during the abdominal examination. Sometimes it is also important to divert the patient's attention by a question or two while taking the blood pressure or checking his reflexes. Should patients bring up new information which they neglected to report during the interview, the examination is interrupted long enough to establish the relevance of such data. On the other hand, the student will need to ask some patients to remain quiet: "I am going to ask you not to talk for a few minutes because I want to listen to your chest."

The student must be alert to his own conduct. As he carries out his task, he avoids comments, facial expressions, or gestures which can be misinterpreted by the patient as indicating alarm or puzzlement. He should be cautious, too, about ill-founded reassuring comments. It is difficult for a beginning student to reassure a patient convincingly, since his statements are not likely to be based on firm experience. The best reassurance he can give the patient is to carry out his examination with meticulous care and with sensitive attention. The student should be serious and business-like, not somber and detached.

How should he handle the patient who repeatedly and anxiously demands reassurance? "Will I be all right, doctor?" "Will the bleeding stop?" "Will I be able to move my arm?" Such questions obviously represent serious concerns that cannot be ignored. The most effective approach for the student is to invoke the prestige of the institution and the staff. "Well, you've got the best doctors and nurses in the hospital, and we are all going to do everything we can to help you." At the same time, the student demonstrates by his behavior that he takes seriously what concerns the patient and indicates that he will be in close contact with the staff about his problem.

The full physical examination may be very tiring for the patient, especially when conducted by an inexperienced student. One must be attentive to signs of fatigue or discomfort, and if necessary, give the patient a rest between parts of the examination. The seriously ill patient, in particular, should be told at the outset "Let me know if you get too tired, so that we can give you a rest."

The Physical Examination in Diagnostic Perspective

What is the role of physical diagnosis in the modern era of highly accurate and abundant laboratory tests? At first glance, one may suspect that physical diagnosis has become obsolete. On the contrary, the great advances in laboratory technology have served to refine the techniques of physical diagnosis and to complement the physical examination as the latter complements the interview. The student who halfheartedly feels for the cardiac apex or superficially examines the lung fields, with the conviction that the chest film will pick up the abnormality, is cheating not only himself but the patient as well. It is clearly recognized, for example, that early obstructive emphysema is better detected on physical examination than on the chest film; or that a small bronchogenic carcinoma in the hilum may be missed on roentgenographic studies, yet be revealed to the clinician by the presence of a unilateral wheeze. It is true that the chest film is more accurate in measuring cardiac size, but it will not discriminate dilatation from hypertrophy. The experienced clinician can diagnose left ventricular hypertrophy by feeling a discrete apical thrust. Laboratory tests extend the techniques of physical diagnosis and are selected to *confirm* a suspected diagnosis, not to *make* that diagnosis.

In the physical examination, it is not only important for the student to become skilled in applying his techniques, but he must also understand the reasoning behind the physical signs. If he knows the theoretical basis for the mitral opening snap, he will understand why its absence in mitral stenosis means a rigid or calcified valve; and he will realize that vertical nystagmus means a brain stem lesion rather than labyrinthitis, or that right upper quadrant abdominal muscle spasm does not necessarily point to an abdominal problem, but may well mean pneumonia in the right lower lobe. Even the most experienced physician will benefit from reviewing the mechanisms of physical signs and from studying his own techniques. As in any field of knowledge, advances proceed as technology develops. Witness the present emphasis on listening for bruits over arterial vessels: The development of angiography has led to auscultation of the carotid bruit in suspected cerebrovascular disease, the bruit of renal vascular disease in hypertension, and the bruit of partial femoral artery occlusion in peripheral vascular insufficiency.

The Systematic Approach

There are two major principles underlying an efficient yet comprehensive physical examination. First, the student must study the patient by regions; and second, there must be a well organized order of examination.

THE REGIONAL EXAMINATION

Not only is a regional examination more efficient, but it also takes into account the comfort of the patient by eliminating the need for frequent shifts in position. All organs in a given region, such as the neck, are examined together: the lymph nodes, salivary glands, muscles, bones and joints, trachea, carotid arteries, jugular veins, and thyroid. This approach is far more efficient than tracing out all the lymph nodes in the body, then checking all the pulses, and perhaps returning again to study the nose, trachea, and lungs.

While doing the physical examination, the student must constantly be thinking: *What is the underlying anatomy? What abnormality may be present?* When examining the thyroid, for instance, he must mentally visualize its anatomic location. As he palpates, he asks himself what abnormalities might be present. Is the gland diffusely enlarged? Is one lobe larger? Is there a nodule? Is the nodule hard and fixed? Are adjacent lymph nodes enlarged? By keeping in mind these possible abnormalities, he will direct his techniques appropriately. In every region examined, the student must constantly search for possible hidden disease: Is there a small carcinoma in the breast? Are apical lesions of tuberculosis present? Or is there an asymptomatic abdominal aneurysm?

THE ORDER OF EXAMINATION

An overall order of examination by regions is outlined in Tables 4-1 and 4-2 on pages 90 and 92. Just as the student should develop a systematic approach in the general examination, so must he have a logical order of examination for each region. He begins with a *general survey* of an area and then focuses on its component parts. If no abnormality is found, the examination is brief but comprehensive. If an abnormality is present, it is studied meticulously, using special maneuvers as needed. Some beginning students will examine each region superficially without concentrating on the abnormality, while others will lose perspective in an overly detailed examination of each region. With experience, the student will strike the proper balance. A student cannot and should not use all techniques available in every part of the physical examination. He must learn to spend more time and apply all available techniques on the region where there is a suspected abnormality.

In general, the order of examination in a given region progresses through *observation, palpation, percussion,* and *auscultation.* The great importance of observation cannot be overemphasized. The value of the other three techniques varies with the particular region of the body. All four are important in the examination of the heart and lungs. However, auscultation is only rarely employed during the examination of the extremities, for example, when listening for joint crepitus or when an arteriovenous fistula is suspected. Percussion is not useful in the joint examination and is of limited help during the study of the abdomen.

Since the human body is bilaterally symmetrical, one takes advantage of the fact that there is a symmetrical area for comparison. This means that more subtle changes can be appreciated. The student should never be satisfied to measure hearing or vision on only one side but must always compare it with the other. Pulses, sensory changes, muscle strength, joint abnormalities, reflexes, pulmonary and abdominal findings should always be cross-checked, comparing the right to the left side.

Finally, a prescribed order of examination does not imply a lack of flexibility. The examination varies with the condition of the patient and the type of problem present. If an abnormality is found in one area, the student may wish to return to examine other regions in the light of the new finding. For example, he may wish to recheck neck veins or hepatic tenderness when he finds a gallop rhythm pointing to early congestive heart failure, or to reexamine the fingernails for clubbing when there is a suspicious pulmonary finding. Likewise, if the initial physical examination has not been entirely satisfactory, the student should not hesitate to return at a later time to check his findings. Through his medical reading, he may learn new maneuvers to help detect the abnormality. Circumstances when reexamining the patient may be more favorable; both the student and patient may be less fatigued or the room better illuminated and quieter.

THE GENERAL PHYSICAL EXAMINATION

Preparing for the Examination

THE STUDENT'S PREPARATION

The student should allow himself adequate time to do an unhurried physical examination. If possible, he should choose a time in the ward routine when he will not be interrupted frequently. He begins and ends every examination by washing his hands. Any instruments that will be needed should be present and properly cleaned. The following items are usually necessary in the general physical examination and may be kept in a small physician's bag:

> Stethoscope
> Aneroid blood pressure cuff
> Ophthalmoscope with attachable otoscope
> Pocket flashlight
> Reflex hammer
> Tuning fork (128 cycles per second)
> Centimeter ruler and tape measure
> Wooden tongue depressors
> Two large straight or safety pins and a wisp of cotton
> Rectal glove, lubricant, and filter paper
> Clean paper towels and tissues

Before the patient is examined, the instruments are removed from the doctor's bag and are placed in an orderly fashion on the bedside table to be easily accessible. Tongue depressors may be kept uncontaminated by placing them on a clean towel or tissue. Cluttered furniture about the bed is removed and, if so equipped, the bed should be elevated electrically to a comfortable examining height. Adequate lighting is of special importance. Daylight is generally better than artificial light. When shining obliquely across the patient's bed, daylight may bring out subtle shadows or early jaundice. The student as well as the patient must be comfortable during the examination. A proper examination cannot be carried out from an awkward and uncomfortable position.

PREPARING THE PATIENT

The patient's comfort must be assured before one begins the physical examination. If he is in pain and anxiously awaiting medication, this should be given. He may want a glass of water or need to go to the bathroom. Should he be anxious to talk with a waiting relative, it is better to let him do so and return after the brief visit.

When the patient stands, one makes sure that he is wearing slippers or that paper toweling is put on the floor. The examiner's hands and instruments should not be uncomfortably cold. The student may warm his hands at the sink in warm water or rub both palms briskly together. The cold stethoscope is also warmed in one's hand before placing it on the patient's chest.

During the examination the patient is properly draped to keep him warm and to protect his modesty. In the office, he may wear an examining gown or be covered with a large sheet. A small hand towel may be used to cover the female breasts when examining her anterior lung fields while she is on her back. When the examination is done in the hospital bed, sheets or blankets may be manipulated to keep the patient warm yet adequately exposed. For example, the student may study the full length of the legs of a patient who is lying flat by keeping him covered with a sheet and bringing his legs out on either side while the sheet is drawn together across the perineum. In this way, the legs are fully exposed while the rest of the torso remains covered. One must make sure that the region to be studied is always adequately exposed at the time of examination. Palpating the abdomen with a girdle pulled down, not off; examining the leg with socks left in place; or observing the breast partially hidden is poor technique. To insure the patient's privacy on a ward, it is also important to close tightly the curtains that may surround the bed. The curtains are easily kept together by the simple device of a safety pin.

Proper positioning of the patient during the physical examination is of considerable importance. Thought must be given to his comfort. He should not be required to move excessively or to hold a given position for too long a time. Should the patient be very ill and need support, a nurse, a ward aide, or a fellow student should be asked to help raise and hold him. In addition, it is important to obtain the optimal patient position for each region examined. For example, the patient's head must be raised and lowered to study the jugular venous pulse; he must be in the sitting position to properly study the posterior lung fields; and the deep tendon reflexes may be easier to obtain when the patient is sitting than when he is on his back.

When the examination is completed, it is appropriate to inquire whether there is anything else the patient cares to mention. Occasionally, he may express some concern or raise a new issue that justifies further study. If not, the student assists the hospitalized patient to put on his gown, helps rearrange the bed clothes, turns off the spotlight, replaces the bedside table, sees that the side rails are in place, lowers the bed, and in general, restores conditions to their former state. In the office, the patient is afforded the necessary privacy to get dressed. Following the examination, the student should not forget to indicate his interest in the patient by asking if he has any immediate needs and by telling him when he will be seen again.

THE INITIATION OF THE EXAMINATION

First, the patient is placed in the proper position. It is ideal to have him sit on the side of the bed or examining bench and face the examiner. If he is too ill, the bulk of the examination will need to be done with the patient supine. When not squarely in front or in back of the patient, the examiner always examines from the patient's right side. Students who are left handed should decide which side is more effective.

One of the more reassuring ways to begin the physical examination is to take hold of the patient's hand and palpate it or feel the pulse. To begin the examination by abruptly reaching to feel the patient's head, or by staring at him for a protracted time, may be disconcerting. As already stressed, the physician must be constantly aware of his own facial expression and attitude during every part of the examination. If he repeatedly returns to study an area with a frown, for instance, the patient may become fearful that something is wrong.

The Order in Which to Examine Regions

Each physician will develop his own order of examination, which is designed to cover all areas thoroughly and to maintain the patient's comfort with a minimum number of position changes. With experience, the complete physical examination will take 30 to 45 minutes. Any time longer than one hour may tire the patient unduly, not to mention the examiner.

Two outlines for the order of examination are given in Tables 4-1 and 4-2, the first for the ambulatory patient and the second for the bed-bound patient. The latter differs in that the major part of the examination is carried out with the patient supine. These outlines can serve only as a guide. The student must adapt his approach to the needs of each individual patient. Some cannot sit up for any length of time because of fatigue, weakness, paralysis, or pain. Others, such as those with congestive heart failure, may not be able to lie flat without becoming severely short of breath.

GENERAL INSPECTION AND VITAL SIGNS

Ambulatory

THE EXAMINER. *Standing before the patient and moving as needed.*

THE PATIENT. *Sitting or lying on the bed or examining table.*

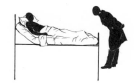

Bed-bound

THE EXAMINER. *Standing at the foot of the bed.*

THE PATIENT. *Lying on his back with the head of the bed slightly elevated.*

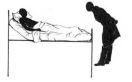

The importance of inspection has been emphasized in the section, "Observing the Patient," at the beginning of this chapter. One first begins by studying the patient's general characteristics, which include awareness, gait, speech, posture, and behavior.* One then focuses on specific regions of the body, looking for abnormalities. The student must train himself to observe the subtle details of disease as he progresses through the physical examination: the slight pill-rolling tremor of Parkinson's disease, the stare of thyrotoxicosis, the unilateral decreased chest wall motion of pneumonia, or the flank fullness of early ascites.

Vital signs include respiratory rate, pulse rate, arterial blood pressure, and temperature, which usually are taken at the beginning of the physical examination. Some examiners prefer to measure vital signs at the time of the chest and cardiac examination. There is an advantage to repeating the pulse and blood pressure determinations later, since patient apprehension may cause the initial measurements to be abnormally elevated. Temperature will usually have been taken by the nurse

---

*Also part of the neurologic examination. The various components of the neurologic examination will be indicated by an asterisk in this chapter.

(Text continued on page 94.)

TABLE 4-1. A SUMMARY OF THE EXAMINER'S AND PATIENT'S POSITIONS
DURING THE PHYSICAL EXAMINATION

REGION	THE AMBULATORY PATIENT THE EXAMINER'S POSITION	THE PATIENT'S POSITION
1. *General inspection and vital signs*	Standing before the patient and moving as needed.	Sitting, or lying on the bed or examining table.
2. *The head*	Standing, facing the patient.	Sitting on the side of the bed or examining table.
3. *The neck*	Standing, facing the patient, then moving behind him.	Sitting on the side of the bed or examining table.
4. *The back; posterior thorax and lungs*	Standing behind the patient.	Sitting on the side of the bed or examining table.
5. *The anterior thorax and lungs*	Standing, facing the patient.	Sitting on the side of the bed or examining table.
6. *The breasts and axillary regions*	Initially facing the patient, then examining from the patient's right side.	Sitting, facing the examiner, then lying supine.
7. *The heart*	Standing at the patient's right.	In three positions: sitting, lying on his back, and on his left side.
8. *The abdomen*	Standing at the patient's right.	Lying on his back.
9. *The extremities*	Standing, facing the patient, and moving to the patient's right.	Lying flat, then sitting on the side of the bed, and finally standing.
10. *The male external genitalia*	Standing before the patient and slightly to his right.	Standing, facing the examiner.
11. *The female genital tract*	Sitting on a stool facing the perineum, and standing for part of the examination.	Lying on her back on an examining table with both knees flexed and her feet in stirrups.
12. *The rectum*	Standing, facing the buttocks.	Bending at the hips over the bed or examining table. The female retains the same position used in the examination of the genital tract.

Fig. 4-1 The Ambulatory Patient.

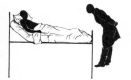

General
inspection and vital
signs

Head
Neck

Back, posterior
thorax and lungs

Anterior thorax
and lungs
Breasts, axilla
Heart, sitting

Breasts,
axilla
Heart,
recumbent

Heart,
left lateral

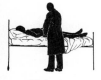

Abdomen

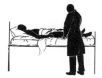

Extremities

Extremities

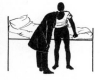

Extremities
Male
genitalia

Female
genital tract

Rectum

TABLE 4-2. A SUMMARY OF THE EXAMINER'S AND PATIENT'S POSITIONS DURING THE PHYSICAL EXAMINATION

REGION	THE BED-BOUND PATIENT THE EXAMINER'S POSITION	THE PATIENT'S POSITION
1. *General inspection and vital signs*	Standing at the foot of the bed.	Lying on his back with the head of the bed slightly elevated.
2. *The head*	Standing at the right side of the bed, then moving to the left side.	Lying on his back with the head of the bed slightly elevated.
3. *The neck*	Standing at the right side of the bed.	Lying on his back with the head of the bed slightly elevated.
4. *The back; posterior thorax and lungs*	Standing at the right side of the bed, examining across the bed, *or* from the right posterior oblique side of the chest.	Sitting on the left side of the bed with his back to the examiner *or* sitting up in bed with assistance.
5. *The anterior thorax and lungs*	Standing at the right side of the bed,	Lying on his back.
6. *The breasts and axillary regions*	Standing at the right side of the bed.	Lying on his back.
7. *The heart*	Standing at the right side of the bed.	In three positions: lying on his back, on his left side, and sitting.
8. *The abdomen*	Standing at the right side of the bed.	Lying on his back.
9. *The extremities*	Standing at the right side of the bed.	Lying flat on his back, then on his abdomen; if able, sitting on the side of the bed facing the examiner.
10. *The male external genitalia*	Standing at the right side of the bed.	Lying on his back.
11. *The female genital tract*	Sitting on a stool facing the perineum, and standing for part of the examination.	Lying on her back obliquely across the bed, with both legs flexed.
12. *The rectum*	Standing at the right side of the bed.	Lying on his left side with both legs flexed at the hip.

Fig. 4-2 The Bed-Bound Patient.

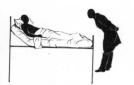

General
inspection and
vital signs

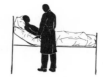

Head, right

Head, left

Neck

Back,
posterior
thorax and lungs

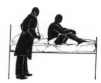

Back,
posterior
thorax and lungs

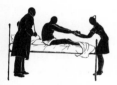

Back,
posterior
thorax and lungs

Anterior
thorax and lungs
Breasts, axilla
Heart, recumbent

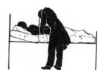

Heart, left
lateral

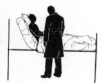

Heart, sitting

Abdomen

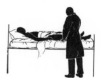

Extremities
Male
genitalia

Female
genital tract

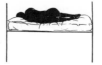

Rectum

but may be repeated if one suspects that it may have changed at the time of examination. Although not a vital sign, weight is important and should be obtained, noting the time relationship to meals and how the patient is dressed.

Respiration. The student observes the rate, depth, and regularity of breathing. Any respiratory "noise," such as audible wheezes, rhonchi, or rales, is noted. Since he may consciously alter his breathing pattern, it is best for the patient to be unaware that his respirations are being observed. At least a minute of observation is necessary if such phenomena as Cheyne-Stokes breathing or frequent sighing are not to be overlooked.

Pulse. To feel the pulse, one places his index and middle fingers over the radial artery. The pulse is counted for 15 seconds and multiplied by 4 to give the pulse rate per minute. If an arrhythmia is suspected, a count for 1 to 2 minutes is indicated. Not only the rate, but also the pulse regularity, contour, and amplitude are carefully studied. These findings may be more readily appreciated by feeling the larger brachial or carotid arteries. It is also worthwhile to feel both radial pulses simultaneously for differences, such as a delayed or softer pulse on one side, indicating proximal partial arterial occlusion.

Blood Pressure. The cuff is snugly wrapped around the upper part of the arm, and the diaphragm of the stethoscope is placed on the medial antecubital fossa over the brachial artery. With experience, the student may estimate the exact anatomic area without feeling for the brachial pulse. While taking the blood pressure, the student may wish to distract the patient's attention by conversation. The recording scale should also be turned away from his line of sight. The cuff pressure is increased to a level in the neighborhood of 200 mm. Hg, so as not to miss expected systole. The first sound heard on slowly deflating the cuff indicates the level of systole. Diastole usually lies at a point between the sudden muffling and the total disappearance of sounds. The American Heart Association recommends that both levels be recorded.[1] The cuff should not be inflated for a protracted time because of the discomfort to the patient. It should also be completely deflated before rechecking the pressure. Blood pressure recordings in both arms are occasionally indicated, as with suspected occlusion of the subclavian artery. A blood pressure determination in the leg is rarely needed and requires a special broad cuff which is wrapped around the thigh. Such a cuff may also be required to measure the arm pressure of a very obese person.

The position of the patient at the time of the blood pressure determination should always be noted, since in conditions such as mild shock

---

[1]Kirkendall, W. M., Burton, A. C., Epstein, F. H., and Freis, E. D.: Recommendations for Human Blood Pressure Determination by Sphygmomanometers. Circulation, 36:980, 1967.

or postural hypotension the blood pressure may be normal in the supine position but low when seated or standing. If these conditions are suspected, the blood pressure should be determined with the patient first supine, then seated, and finally standing for 2 to 3 minutes.

THE HEAD

Ambulatory

THE EXAMINER. *Standing, facing the patient.*
THE PATIENT. *Sitting on the side of the bed or examining table.*

Bed-bound

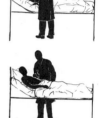

THE EXAMINER. *Standing at the right side of the bed; then moving to the left side.*
THE PATIENT. *Lying on his back with the head of the bed slightly elevated.*

The techniques used are inspection and palpation.

  Initial inspection and palpation
  Ear and hearing
  Eye
  The use of the otoscope and ophthalmoscope
  Nose
  Mouth and pharynx
  Completion of the cranial nerve examination

Initial Inspection and Palpation.   The face is inspected for abnormal movements, edema, and asymmetry. The *skin* is closely examined for color, texture, sweating; for lesions, such as a small basal cell carcinoma in the muzzle area; telangiectasia; or abnormal pigmentation. The student indicates to the patient the reason for studying his face by asking him whether or not he has noted any sores there. One then checks the scalp for scars, contusions, tenderness, or masses. The texture and distribution of the *hair* of the head and face, including eyebrows, are observed. Any suspected *lesion* is palpated: the parotid gland and auricular nodes for enlargement and tenderness, or the temporal artery and facial sinuses for tenderness. The odor of the *breath* is noted.

Ear and Hearing.* The *pinnae* and *periauricular tissues* are studied for deformity, masses, and tenderness. A quiet room is necessary when one tests hearing. Each ear is tested separately. The examiner masks sound in one ear by moving the tip of his index finger in the outer canal of that ear. Hearing in the opposite ear is then tested by asking the patient to repeat a whispered phrase with his eyes closed. If he cannot hear, the intensity of the examiner's voice is increased. The procedure is repeated as sound is masked in the opposite ear. Another method for testing hearing is to face the patient directly and bring a ticking watch (or two fingers rubbed together) progressively closer to his ear from a distance of 2 to 3 feet. The watch should be moved toward the patient along a line that is equidistant from both the patient's and examiner's ear. The student will then know if the patient can hear the ticking at the same time he does. The distance that the patient first hears the sound is noted for each ear.

Eye.* The palpebral and bulbar *conjunctivae, sclera, cornea*, and *iris* of each eye are carefully inspected, using a flashlight when necessary. The conjunctivae of the lower lids are studied by depressing each lid with a finger placed just proximal to the eyelashes. To examine the conjunctivae and *lacrimal glands* of the upper lids, the examiner asks the patient to maintain a downward gaze as he gently places his thumb proximal to the eyelashes, raises the lid, and moves his thumb slightly sideways to roll the lid off the globe. *Ptosis of the lids* is looked for by noting the width of the palpebral fissures at rest and with upward gaze.

The size of the pupil, its *regularity*, and its *reaction to light* are observed and compared with the opposite eye. In order to check the light reflex, the flashlight is held lateral to each eye, and its beam is directed on the pupil.

The range of ocular motion is tested in six directions with the patient holding his gaze long enough to permit detection of nystagmus. These directions are in the horizontal and two oblique planes to the right and left. The examiner holds the chin of the patient with his left hand to keep the head still and directs the patient to look at the finger of his right hand as it is moved in the six cardinal directions. *Accommodation* is checked by asking the patient to observe the tip of the index finger as it is brought from a distance close to his eyes at the level of the bridge of his nose. Alternatively, the examiner observes the change in pupil size, as the patient is asked to read the time on a watch that is brought 2 or 3 inches in front of his eyes.

In the absence of a Snellen chart, the patient's *visual acuity* is tested by asking him to hold his hand over one eye and to read with the other

---

*Part of the neurologic examination.

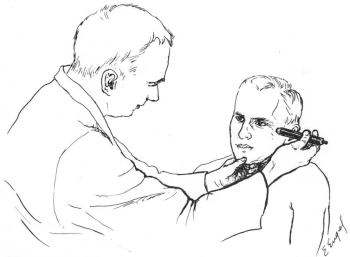

Fig. 4-3 The light reflex of the left pupil is demonstrated by casting a beam of light on the left eye from its lateral aspect. The examiner holds the patient's chin to keep him from moving his head.

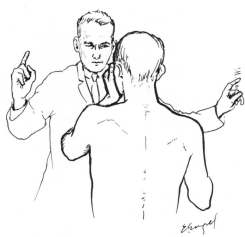

Fig. 4-4 Gross testing of visual fields by confrontation. Using his own visual field as a guide, the examiner stands directly in front of the patient and closes one eye. The patient covers the eye opposite to the examiner's closed eye and is asked to fix his gaze on the examiner's nose. As he holds both hands at the periphery of the field of vision, the examiner asks the patient to point to the wiggling finger with his free hand.

eye the smallest print on a readily available newspaper or tissue box held at a distance of about 2 feet. In a similar way, visual acuity is tested for the opposite eye. The size of the print and distance are noted. If used, glasses should be worn by the patient during the examination.

Testing of *visual fields* by confrontation is part of the general physical examination if a neurologic deficit is suspected. Here, the examiner squarely faces the patient, who is approximately 1½ to 2 feet distant and who is asked to cover one eye as he fixes his gaze with the other on the tip of the examiner's nose. Holding his hands in a plane equidistant between the patient's and his own face, the examiner extends both arms so that his index fingers are held at the nasal and temporal periphery of the patient's field of vision. As the examiner keeps his arms in this position, he wiggles either index finger. The patient is instructed to point to the moving finger with his free hand without shifting his gaze from the examiner's nose. By closing the eye opposite to the patient's occluded one, the examiner superimposes his visual field upon the patient's, which enables him to see if his finger motion is at the periphery of vision. The four quadrants can be tested by wiggling each index finger when the examiner's hands are held in different positions about the circumference and within the field of vision. Each eye is tested separately.

The Use of the Otoscope and Ophthalmoscope.   The examiner tells the patient in advance that he is going to darken the room in order to check his eyes and ears. The lights are turned off, the blinds drawn, and the patient is asked to face away from the window. The otoscope head is attached, introduced into the ear, and directed in line with the external auditory canal in a slightly anterior direction. Moderate traction up and posteriorly on the external helix will help to open the canal. With the bed-bound patient, the examiner moves from the right to the left side of the bed to examine the left ear. Wax, inflammation, discharge, and masses are looked for in each canal as the instrument is introduced. Landmarks on the drum are identified; and one observes the color of the drum and the mobility with swallowing, as well as any abnormalities, such as scars, opacities, or perforations. The speculum is then withdrawn from the canal and is wrapped in a tissue. Following completion of the physical examination, it is carefully cleaned.

While the room is still darkened, the ophthalmoscopic examination is done.* The instrument should have sufficiently strong batteries to provide the best possible light. The patient is instructed to fix his vision on a designated point straight ahead and slightly above eye level. The ophthalmoscope is held firmly. The examiner's free hand is placed on the patient's forehead with his thumb over the patient's lateral eyebrow, in order to elevate the upper lid. The examiner must be quite close to the patient, even to the point that his forehead touches the knuckle of

---

*Part of the neurologic examination.

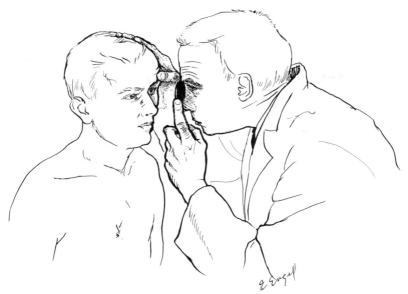

Fig. 4-5 Ophthalmoscopic examination. The examiner looks into the patient's left eye with his own left eye as he holds the ophthalmoscope in his left hand. The patient's left lateral lid is elevated slightly with the right thumb.

the thumb that supports the patient's lid. The right hand and right eye are used when examining the patient's right eye, and the left hand and left eye, as one looks into the patient's left eye. When the patient is bed-bound, the right eye is examined from the right side of the bed and the left eye from the left side. By putting the beam of light onto the pupil at about 15 degrees lateral to the patient's line of vision, the light will be directed into the eye and on the disc. The dial to adjust diopter readings may be turned with the forefinger. By beginning at a reading of +8 or +10, the *iris, pupil, lens,* and *media* may be studied before focusing on the disc. Opacities in the lens and media, as well as irregularities of the pupil, are detected in this way.

If the *optic disc* is not immediately seen, a major vessel may be traced proximally until it is found. The color, sharpness of the margin, degree of elevation, and cupping of the disc are studied; and the *arterioles* and *veins* are followed out peripherally in each quadrant. The retina between the vessels is then carefully inspected, ending with the *macula.* In general, it is easier to have the patient continue to fix his vision on a single point as the fundus is examined, but the fundus also can be studied by having the patient fix his gaze at the extreme periphery in each of the six cardinal directions.

Nose.   The external appearance of the nose is observed for scars, deformities, and asymmetry. By tilting the patient's head back slightly with one hand and gently pushing up the tip of the nose with the thumb, the examiner may directly inspect with a flashlight the nasal canal, turbinates, septum, and superior nasal cavity for color, secretion, and masses. If the nasal septum is perforated, light directed into the nostril on one side may be seen shining through the septum on the other side. Relative patency of the airways is determined by occluding first one nostril, then the other as the patient breathes through his nose. In order to adequately visualize the airways, the examiner should also use a nasal speculum, the handles of which are held comfortably in the palm of his hand and the blades are opened gently so as not to scrape the sensitive septum. An otoscope speculum should not be used because it is too small to allow an adequate study of the interior of the nose.

Mouth and Pharynx.   The *lips* are first observed for color, moisture, pigment, masses, ulceration, or fissures. The mobility of the *temporomandibular joint* is observed as the patient is instructed to open his mouth. If there is any abnormality, the joint is palpated on each side as the patient opens and closes his jaws. A wooden tongue depressor is used to study the *oral cavity*, which is illuminated with a flashlight. The cheeks and lips are carefully retracted to observe the *teeth, gums, mucous membranes,* and *orifices of the salivary ducts.* If false teeth are present; the patient is given a tissue so that he may remove and hold them, while the underlying membranes are studied. One notes abnormal lesions, such as petechiae, ulcerations, pigmentation, scars, and masses. If a mass is seen, it should be palpated with a gloved finger. Any lateral *tongue* deviation is noted when the patient is asked to stick it straight out. After the tongue is withdrawn, the tongue depressor is firmly pressed on the posterior surface as the patient says "Aaah." The uvula should rise in the midline. The *posterior pharynx* and *tonsillar areas* are then inspected. The gag reflex is tested by forewarning the patient and gently touching each side of the pharynx.

The Completion of the Cranial Nerve Examination.*   Cranial nerves I, V, VII, and XI remain to be tested. The first cranial nerve is not checked unless there is a neurologic abnormality. The *corneal reflex* of the fifth cranial nerve (trigeminal) is tested with a wisp of cotton or tissue. The left lower lid is pulled down with the thumb as the patient looks up to the right. Slowly and gently, the tip of cotton is brought to the lateral edge of the left cornea (not the conjunctiva). This normally causes a blink and a feeling of slight irritation. The right cornea is similarly tested with the patient looking up to the left. The *three sensory divisions of V* are tested for light touch and pain; first checking one side of the face, then comparing symmetrical sides. The patient is asked to close his eyes and to say "sharp" or "dull," when he feels the point or head of

---

*Part of the neurologic examination.

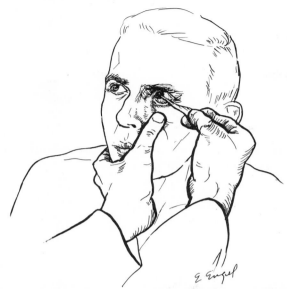

Fig. 4-6 The corneal reflex of the left eye is tested by touching a wisp of cotton to the lateral edge of the cornea as the patient looks up to the right and his lower lid is depressed with the left thumb.

the pin; and "yes," when he feels the light touch of cotton. After identifying the sensation, the patient is asked to compare the intensity of the stimulus applied to symmetrical sides of the face. The *motor division of V* is tested by having the patient open his mouth. The student then observes if the jaw deviates to either side.

Cranial nerve VII (facial) is examined by watching facial symmetry as the patient spontaneously smiles and frowns; and when he is asked to show his teeth, close his eyes tightly, and wrinkle his brow. *Cranial nerve XI* (spinal accessory) is tested by having the patient turn his head to each side against the student's resisting hand or shrug his shoulders against resistance.

THE NECK

Ambulatory

THE EXAMINER. *Standing, facing the patient, then moving behind him.*

THE PATIENT. *Sitting on the side of the bed or examining table.*

Bed-bound

THE EXAMINER. *Standing at the right side of the bed. (Inspection of posterior neck and palpation of the thyroid from behind are done when the patient sits up for the next step of the examination.)*

THE PATIENT. *Lying on his back with the head of the bed slightly elevated.*

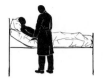

The techniques used in examination of the neck are inspection, palpation, and auscultation for bruits.

> Skin and musculoskeletal structures
> Lymph nodes and salivary glands
> Jugular veins
> Carotid arteries
> Trachea
> Thyroid

Skin and Musculoskeletal Structures.   The skin is observed for its color, texture, scars, and underlying masses or pulsations. The patient is then asked to move his head its full range to test mobility of the neck: flexion, extension, rotation to each side, and lateral bending. Passive motion of the neck is done with the patient relaxed and his head held by the examiner's two hands. Limitation of motion, stiffness, or pain is noted; and if weakness is suspected, the patient is asked to move his head against resistance or, while supine, to bring his chin to his chest. It is also important to test full anterior flexion of the neck when meningeal irritation is suspected.*

Lymph Nodes and Salivary Glands.   By palpating one side of the neck at a time with the index and third finger (using a firm rotary motion), the student may study the salivary glands under the jaw as well as the lymph nodes in their respective chains. The distribution, size, mobility, tenderness, and consistency of palpable glands are noted. If the patient is sitting and bracing himself with both hands on the examining bench, it may be necessary to ask him to rest his hands on his lap in order to relax the muscles in the supraclavicular area and to permit more accurate palpation.

Jugular Veins.   One examines the neck veins with the patient *in two positions:* when semirecumbent, to note pulsations, and when the head is elevated, to determine the degree of venous distention. Neck veins may be studied at the time of the neck examination or later during the heart examination.

---

*Part of the neurologic examination.

The gentle transmitted *pulsations of the deep jugular veins* may be seen through the muscles at the base of the neck, with the patient flat or with his head elevated slightly. The neck musculature should not be taut and the head should be turned slightly to one side. The pulse waves transmitted through the muscles are best seen by creating shadows with a beam of light directed tangentially across the lower neck. It may be necessary to turn the patient's head or to change the elevation of the head in order to enhance venous pulsation. The carotid pulse behind the anterior aspect of the sternocleidomastoid muscle is distinguished by being more discrete; it is palpable, and it is not obliterated by gentle pressure of a finger over the clavicular end of the sternocleidomastoid muscle. To properly time the *a, c,* and *v* waves (see the schematic diagram of the simultaneous events in the cardiac cycle on p. 126), the student should feel simultaneously the carotid pulse high in the neck or identify the first heart sound with the stethoscope, both of which immediately follow the *a* wave.

The patient's head and shoulders are next raised to 45 degrees to look for *external jugular distention.* This and the uppermost point of pulsation of the *internal jugular veins* are measures of increased central venous pressure. The location of the external jugular vein may be established by gently occluding it with firm finger pressure over the clavicular end of the sternocleidomastoid muscle and observing it fill. Any distention of the external jugular veins when the patient's head is elevated to 45 degrees or more, indicates an abnormal elevation of venous

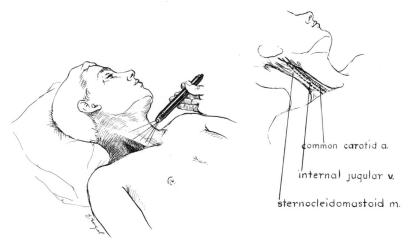

common carotid a.

internal jugular v.

sternocleidomastoid m.

Fig. 4-7 When the patient is flat, the pulsations of the deep jugular vein are visible through the sternocleidomastoid muscle as moving shadows in a tangential light. Note that the beam of light creates on the surface of the lower sternocleidomastoid muscle a sharp border of shadow which reflects the pulsations of the underlying deep jugular vein.

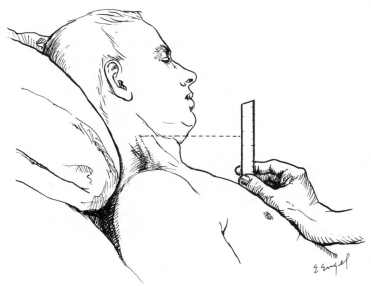

Fig. 4-8 Central venous pressure is estimated by measuring the vertical distance in centimeters from the sternal angle to the upper level of distention of the right external jugular vein, with the patient's head and shoulders elevated at 45 degrees.

pressure. The degree of distention of both veins should be examined since local obstruction can cause unilateral distention. The elevation of venous pressure may be expressed in centimeters by measuring the vertical distance above the sternal angle or by measuring from the top of the clavicle to the upper level of the external jugular distention. When measuring from the clavicle, the examiner must note the angle at which the patient's head is elevated.

Carotid Arteries. The amplitude and the location of the carotid arterial pulsations are observed first. Each artery is then palpated to determine the character of the vessel wall, as well as the pulse contour, and to compare the amplitude on both sides. The student should palpate gently, approximately halfway up the neck to avoid the carotid sinus, which is located just below the angle of the jaw. Both carotids should not be palpated simultaneously because of the danger of occluding blood flow. As the patient briefly holds his breath, bruits are listened for over the carotid as well as over the subclavian arteries behind the clavicles.

Trachea. The level of the thyroid cartilage and any vertical movement with respiration are noted. To determine whether the position of the trachea is in the midline, the index finger is introduced straight into the sternal notch, as the patient faces directly ahead. The finger is then slipped off the trachea, first to one side, then to the other. Deviation of the trachea from the midline is estimated by the relative amount of room the finger finds between the trachea and the sternal manubrium on each side.

Thyroid.   When the student examines the thyroid, it is important that he visualize its anatomic location. Although somewhat variable, the isthmus usually crosses the trachea just below the cricoid cartilage, and the two lateral lobes are largely covered on their anterior lateral aspect by the sternocleidomastoid muscles. It is important to appreciate that the thyroid gland lies low in the neck, not at the level of the thyroid cartilage. Particularly in patients with short necks, the lower part of the gland may lie behind the sternal manubrium.

The thyroid should first be inspected. For the bed-bound patient, one elevates the head of the bed to the sitting position. Inspection is best done by having the patient extend his neck slightly and swallow. The entire outline of the gland may be seen to rise and fall behind its muscular covering. Its contour and symmetry are noted. The patient may need to swallow several times in order to visualize the gland. Since he may have difficulty in swallowing repeatedly, the patient should be offered water that he can hold in his mouth until he is directed to swallow.

On occasion, a subtly enlarged gland or nodule may be more clearly defined by observation than by palpation. The latter technique is generally more satisfactory, however, and may be done from two positions: with the examiner facing the patient and using one hand, or from behind the patient using both hands. Some examiners prefer one

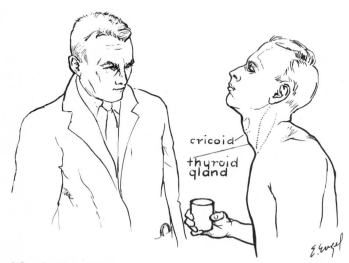

Fig. 4-9 The thyroid is inspected as the patient extends his neck and swallows, which causes the gland to rise. The thyroid isthmus crosses the trachea below the cricoid cartilage.

method over the other, although a thorough examination includes both. The student should initially run his index or third finger in a vertical direction over the trachea just below the cricoid cartilage to feel for the isthmus. The finger is then swept horizontally across the midline above the cricoid cartilage to feel for the pyramidal lobe.

When the lateral lobes are palpated, the patient's neck should be slightly extended, but not to the degree that the sternocleidomastoid muscles are taut. In palpating from an anterior position, the examiner inserts the index and third finger of his right hand behind the anterior border of the left sternocleidomastoid muscle and palpates the left thyroid lobe with a firm circular motion. Enough pressure needs to be exerted to cause slight discomfort. It is then necessary to hold one's fingers still as the patient swallows in order to feel the lobe ride up under them. The outline, consistency, size, and surface contour of the lobe are noted. In the same manner, using two fingers of the same or opposite hand, the examiner repeats the examination of the right lateral lobe. He may also attempt to feel each lobe, as the patient swallows, by inserting his thumb anterior and his second and third fingers posterior to the sternocleidomastoid muscle. The trachea is displaced toward the palpating hand by using the thumb of the opposite hand. This method is most useful when a lobe is enlarged.

Palpation of both lobes of the thyroid may be done simultaneously from the posterior position. When standing behind the patient, the examiner must first be sure he is palpating at the proper level in the neck,

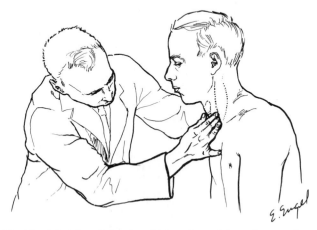

Fig. 4-10   The left lobe of the thyroid is palpated from the anterior position with the patient's neck flexed sufficiently to relax the sternocleidomastoid muscle. As the patient swallows, the gland is felt to ride up under the examiner's fingers.

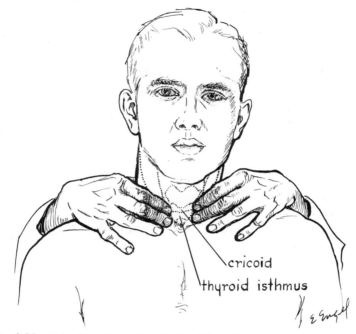

Fig. 4-11   Palpation of the thyroid gland from the posterior position, using both hands.

which is accomplished by finding the cricoid cartilage. The patient's neck should be slightly extended to the degree that the examiner can easily insert the second and third fingers of each hand medial to the anterior border of each sternocleidomastoid muscle. Palpation is then conducted as described above.

If the gland is grossly enlarged, the student should listen over it with his stethoscope for the bruit of increased vascularity. Also, if the gland is hard and fixed, not moving on swallowing, or if there is a large nodule, the regional lymph nodes should again be carefully palpated.

THE BACK, POSTERIOR THORAX, AND LUNGS

Ambulatory

THE EXAMINER.   *Standing behind the patient.*
THE PATIENT.   *Sitting on the side of the bed or examining table.*

Bed-bound

THE EXAMINER. *Standing at the right side of the bed, examining across the bed, or from the right posterior oblique side of the chest.*

THE PATIENT. *Sitting on the left side of the bed with his back to the examiner or sitting up in bed with assistance.*

For the ill, bed-bound patient, sitting up may be exhausting, painful, or conducive to a fall in blood pressure. The examiner should proceed with maximum speed and efficiency; should frequently inquire how the patient is doing; and, if necessary, should tell him how much longer he will need to sit up. The student should be alert to the development of pallor, sweating, and sighing, which are signs of falling blood pressure. If the length of time the patient can be seated clearly is limited, one restricts the examination to obtaining only the most important information.

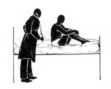

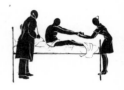

Inspection and palpation are the major techniques used in studying *the back*. The examiner first observes the skin of the back, which is fully undraped. The patient's posture, spinal curvature, strength, and symmetry of the back muscles are noted.* The mobility of the spine is tested by firmly holding both iliac crests as the patient bends forward at the waist, backward, to each side, and rotates to the right and left. If back pain is a symptom, palpation is helpful in locating tender points. The palpating fingers are pressed firmly over the vertebral spines, spinal ligaments, and paraspinal muscles, comparing both sides for tenderness and tone. The vertebral spines may also be struck successively with a quick tap of the point of a reflex hammer to elicit underlying bone tenderness.

If the patient's history suggests a specific disorder, the examiner directs his attention and techniques to the abnormal area. If, for instance, rheumatoid spondylitis were suspected, one should carefully check the full range of spinal motion, including a measurement of thoracic expansion. This is done with a tape measure, comparing the widest circumference of the thorax at the height of deep inspiration with deep expiration. If acute pyelonephritis were suspected, the examiner may test for kidney tenderness by placing the palm of one hand over the costal vertebral angle and delivering a jarring blow with the ulnar aspect of the other fist, comparing the right with the left side. The patient is

---

*Part of the neurologic examination.

forewarned, "I'm going to jar your back. Tell me what you feel." One always begins with a gentle blow and increases its strength if there is no discomfort. Or, if fluid retention were a problem, one would study the sacral area for edema. Sacral edema is brought out by pressing the point of the index finger firmly into the skin overlying the sacrum. If a pit is left in the subcutaneous tissue, edema is present.

One next proceeds to examine the *posterior thorax and lungs*. The four major techniques of physical diagnosis are used in the examination of the lungs, usually in the order listed below. However, the student should not necessarily follow such a rigid outline. For example, if he finds an area of dullness in one anterior apex, he may wish to check tactile fremitus and listen for rales before completing percussion of the entire posterior chest. Also, he may wish to reexamine other areas of the body in the light of his new findings. For instance, he may look again at the fingernails for clubbing, reexamine the eyes for Horner's syndrome, or recheck the position of the trachea. The four techniques used are:

1. Inspection
2. Palpation
3. Percussion
4. Auscultation

In examining the thorax, the student should develop a systematic order. Usually, one begins at the apex and progresses down the medial, mid, and lateral aspect of each hemithorax, not neglecting the axilla. Symmetrical areas on each side of the chest are compared, and one *always specifically searches for abnormalities which have been suggested during the interview.*

Inspection. The contour, mobility, and symmetry of the thorax are best seen by standing squarely in back of the seated patient. If the patient is on his back in bed, the examiner should first observe the chest from the foot of the bed. Respiratory motion is carefully watched for a possible lag or splinting of one side of the chest compared to the other. Abnormal respiratory movements include the use of accessory muscles, prolonged expiration, and intercostal muscle retraction or bulging as the patient breathes.

Palpation. Thoracic expansion and asymmetry may be determined by grasping the low posterolateral rib cage firmly in both hands, exerting most pressure with the fingers and keeping the arms relaxed. The examiner's thumbs are pointed toward the spine, and, as the patient takes a deep breath, the distance each thumb moves away from the midline is a measure of thoracic expansion. Such a maneuver may demonstrate an initial lag in motion, as well as a decreased expansion on one side.

Light palpation of the posterior chest wall with the finger tips of one hand is done first, looking for rib tenderness or intercostal muscle spasm and tenderness. Feeling vibrations in the chest as the patient repeats in a resonant voice the number, "99" or "1,2" (*tactile fremitus*), is also valuable in delineating underlying lesions. One is looking for areas in which the intensity of the vibration is significantly increased or decreased, even to the point of being absent. Tactile fremitus is best elicited by using the palmar surface of the fingers or the ulnar surface of the entire hand. It is more accurate to use one hand, successively comparing similar areas on each side, than to use both hands simultaneously, since sensitivity may differ in the two hands.

One tests tactile fremitus beginning at the posterior apex and progressing down the medial, mid, and lateral aspects of each hemithorax, sampling three or four places between the apex and the diaphragm. While progressing downward, the student should always compare one side with the symmetrical area of the other.

Percussion.   One of the techniques that the student must repeatedly practice is that of percussion. The plexor or striking finger is usually the third finger of the right hand, the nail of which is cut short. The pleximeter finger, or the finger receiving the blow, is usually the third finger of the left hand. One strikes the pleximeter finger briefly and sharply on its terminal phalanx. Some examiners prefer to strike just proximal to or just distal to the joint. Firm pressure is applied by the pleximeter finger to keep the underlying skin taut; the other fingers must be kept off the patient's skin to prevent damping of the percussion note. There is a

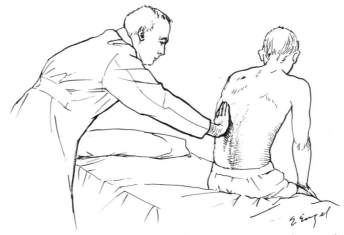

Fig. 4-12 Tactile fremitus is detected by placing the palmar surface of the fingers firmly over the chest wall as the patient repeats "99" or "1,2" in a resonant voice.

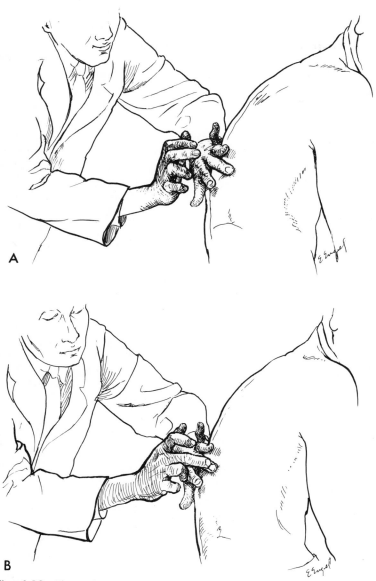

Fig. 4-13 The technique of percussion. *A,* The third finger of the examiner's left hand is pressed firmly against the skin, while the other fingers are held off the surface. *B,* As the right hand swings freely at the wrist, the tip of the third finger strikes the underlying terminal phalanx sharply to produce a percussion note.

relaxed free swing at the wrist of the percussing hand with no significant motion of the forearm. One will gradually learn to percuss with a flexible wrist so that the plexor finger strikes like a piano hammer; and it is important that each stroke be as uniform as possible with regard to force and rhythm. One soon appreciates that feeling the vibration is as important as listening to the sound produced. The student should practice percussion on himself to compare different notes: resonance over his upper anterior lung fields, hyperresonance over the stomach bubble, dullness over the liver, and flatness over the muscles of his anterior thigh.

Percussion is initiated by asking the patient to bend slightly forward and to rest his elbows and forearms on his thighs. This will spread the scapulae and expose more of the lung fields. The student may first check the *level and range of motion of the diaphragm.* The level of the diaphragm on one side of the chest is determined by percussing in a vertical line starting below the scapula tip and progressing downward until a level of dullness is reached (the paraspinal area of heavy musculature is avoided). This level of dullness is noted and the patient is then instructed to take and hold a deep breath. It is also helpful for the examiner to hold his own breath to let him know when the patient needs to take another breath. Percussion continues downward 4 to 6 cm. to a new level of dullness as the patient maintains full inspiration. The distance between the two levels of dullness measured in centimeters represents the degree of descent of the diaphragm. The opposite thorax is percussed in a similar manner, comparing the relative levels and excursions of diaphragmatic dullness on both sides. In the thin patient, one may determine the anatomic level of the diaphragm in relationship to the vertebral spines by counting down from the prominent seventh cervical spine; or by counting up from the third lumbar spine, which is identified by a line that connects the two iliac crests and crosses between the third and fourth lumbar spinous processes.

Following the determination of the diaphragmatic level, each hemithorax is percussed in the medial, mid, and lateral areas from top to bottom, comparing right and left sides, as was done for palpation.

Auscultation.   A proper fit of the stethoscope is particularly important in the examination of the lungs and heart. Regardless of the type of stethoscope used, the earpieces must be large enough to comfortably adapt to the external ear canals, and the curved metal tubing of these pieces must be properly directed to conform to the angle of the canals. Either the diaphragm or the bell may be used in listening to the lungs. Some examiners prefer the bell for the lower pitched vesicular breath sounds. The stethoscope head is held firmly yet comfortably between the thumb and forefinger, with the remaining three fingers resting on the chest wall to provide support. If one is listening to low pitched sounds, the bell should be held lightly against the skin of the chest wall, not firmly, since the tense skin acts as a diaphragm. If the patient is thin and his ribs are prominent, one must be sure the entire rim of the bell or the diaphragm makes contact with the chest wall.

The student should practice listening to various areas of his own chest to learn the different types of breath sounds:[2] vesicular, over the lower anterior lungs; bronchovesicular, below the medial head of the right clavicle; and bronchial breath sounds mimicked by the harsher sounds heard over the trachea. Adventitious sounds, such as rales[3] or a pleural friction rub, are not normally present. The student will learn to distinguish rales from the fainter sounds of muscular contraction in a shivering patient, for instance; or from the sound of hair moving under the stethoscope when the diaphragm is not pressed firmly against the chest.

Before beginning auscultation, the examiner will need to tell the patient how to cooperate in breathing; that is, to breathe through his open mouth, but not to hyperventilate, as this will distort breath sounds and may make him dizzy. It may help to demonstrate how the patient should breathe. The student then examines the posterior lung fields from above downward as before, always being sure to crosscheck from one side of the chest to the other and to compare sounds in symmetrical areas. The intensity, pitch, and relative duration of the inspiratory and expiratory phases of breath sounds are compared. The presence and location of extra sounds, such as rales, in the inspiratory or expiratory phase are then noted. The stethoscope must be kept in a given area for at least two or three breaths to allow adequate evaluation.

If there is an abnormal area, this should be further defined by testing *vocal fremitus*. The patient is instructed to say "99" or "1,2" repeatedly as the student listens for any distortion, comparing the abnormal to the normal area of the opposite chest. The same sounds are then whispered, which may be a more sensitive test than using the spoken voice. Whispered sounds ordinarily are poorly heard over the aerated lung but are well transmitted through solid lung tissue (*whispered pectoriloquy*). Since whispered voice is normally well heard over the trachea and major bronchi, these areas provide a good example for comparison with

---

[2]Vesicular breath sounds are low pitched, the inspiratory phase being longer and louder than the expiratory phase. Bronchial breath sounds are pathological, harsher, and usually higher pitched. The expiration sound is longer and louder than the inspiration sound. Bronchovesicular sounds are a combination resembling the vesicular inspiratory phase and the bronchial expiratory phase.

[3]Pronounced "rahls" not "rails." The classification of rales is quite variable. A simple description is to call the more musical sounds emanating from the bronchial tree, wheezes or rhonchi; those from the terminal bronchi and alveoli, coarse, medium, and fine rales.

other regions of the thorax. *Egophony* is useful in detecting a pleural effusion. The patient is asked to repeatedly say "E" and when the stethoscope crosses the upper level of the effusion, the sound is like "A."

THE ANTERIOR THORAX AND LUNGS

Ambulatory

THE EXAMINER.   *Standing, facing the patient.*
THE PATIENT.   *Sitting on the side of the bed or examining table.*

Bed-bound

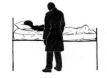

THE EXAMINER.   *Standing at the right side of the bed.*
THE PATIENT.   *Lying on his back.*

When studying the anterior lung fields, the student should remember that the right and left sides of the chest are not strictly comparable, since the heart is located on the left and the right main bronchus is directed more anteriorly, resulting in bronchovesicular sounds in the region of the right apex. The examination of the anterior lung fields may be done either with the patient sitting or lying on his back. If the patient is acutely ill, he will be more comfortable in the supine position, and it is easier to percuss the chest in this position. Some examiners may combine the inspection of the anterior thorax, breasts, and cardiac pulsations while the patient is sitting, before going on to the separate examination of each system when the patient is lying on his back.

The same order of examination is used to study the anterior chest as was followed in examining the posterior thorax. With the female as well as with the male patient, the entire chest should be exposed during the examination, with the drape covering the upper abdomen. First, the student pauses to inspect the skin, noting hair distribution, color, masses, nevi, scars, lesions, and pigmentation. The contour and symmetry of the chest are observed, including the prominence or depression of the sternum. Chest expansion is watched as the patient takes a deep breath. This is best done by facing the patient squarely when he is sitting, or by standing at the foot of the bed when he is supine. Subtle differences in the degree of expansion and the lag in motion of one hemithorax can then be compared.

Palpation, percussion, and auscultation are done in a systematic fashion from above downward in the regions of the midclavicular, anterior axillary, and midaxillary lines. Rib tenderness may be demon-

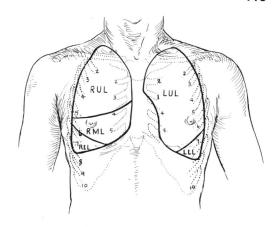

Fig. 4-14 Projections of the major lung fissures on to the anterior (*above*) and posterior (*below*) body surfaces. Note the extra fissure dividing the right middle lobe (RML) and right upper lobe (RUL). Posteriorly the right lower lobe (RLL) and left lower lobe (LLL) reach the spine of the fourth dorsal vertebra.

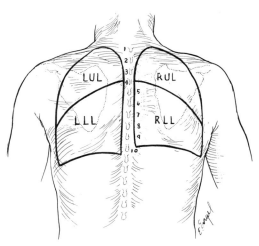

strated by compressing the sides of the thorax between two hands and further localized by pressing the finger over the costochondral articulation or the body of a rib. It is particularly important that the apical regions be studied carefully, including the region above the clavicles, and that both axillary lung fields be examined, since these sites may contain significant abnormalities which cannot be detected from the examination of the posterior thorax. Abnormalities in the right middle lobe, for example, can only be detected in the anterior thorax and the right axilla. (See Figure 4-15.)

When an area of abnormality is detected, the student should reapply all his techniques to clearly define it. He again uses inspection and palpation to compare contour and expansion with the opposite hemithorax. He determines whether the lesion has affected the contour and space between the ribs and whether there is tenderness or muscle

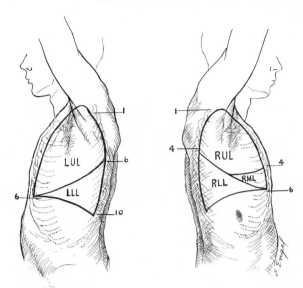

Fig. 4-15 Projections of the major lung fissures on to the left and right lateral body surfaces. Note that the right middle lobe (RML) and the lower portions of both lower lobes project anteriorly, as seen in Figure 4-14.

spasm. If the abnormality is a large one, he checks for mediastinal shift by looking for displacement of the trachea or the cardiac apical impulse. Percussion is then used to help define further the limits of the abnormality. One percusses from an area of normal resonance to dullness. Breath sounds, as well as spoken and whispered voice, are listened for over the suspicious area, noting the variations from the adjacent normal and opposite symmetrical lung field. Special techniques should also be applied to further define the lesion, and the patient will need to be instructed how to cooperate. For example, he should be asked to cough at the end of an expiration in order to establish whether posttussive rales appear on the next inspiration.

THE BREASTS AND AXILLARY REGIONS
Ambulatory

THE EXAMINER.   *Initially facing the patient, then examining from the patient's right side.*

THE PATIENT.   *Sitting facing the examiner, then lying supine.*

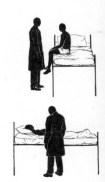

Bed-bound

THE EXAMINER. *Standing at the right side of the bed.*

THE PATIENT. *Lying on his back (when the patient sits up for examination of the heart, the breast examination is completed).*

The techniques used are inspection and palpation. A helpful reference on the breast examination is that of Haagensen.[4]

The patient sits with her arms relaxed at her sides with the anterior chest undraped. The contour, size, level, and symmetry of each breast are systematically studied. In particular, one looks for any surface irregularity that might point to an underlying mass. The nipples and areolae are inspected for nipple inversion, discharge, ulceration, or a mass. The arms are raised above the patient's head to determine if there is asymmetry and localized skin retraction caused by an underlying tumor. If there are suspicious lesions, other maneuvers are done, such as asking the patient to press her hands to the sides of her hips, which contracts the pectoral muscles and may bring out local skin retraction.

Palpation of the breasts can be done with the patient seated by gently feeling the dependent tissue between the thumb and fingers of one hand or by using two hands; however, *palpation is more accurate when the patient lies on her back and should preferably be done in this position.* The breast is gently felt by pressing downward with a slight rotary motion against the chest wall, using the palmar surface of the fingers of one hand. Each quadrant in succession is systematically studied by palpating repeatedly from the periphery to the areola to cover the entire breast. If the breast is large, it may be helpful to place a small pillow behind the patient's scapula on the side being palpated, which will cause the breast to lie more evenly on the chest wall. Normally, breast tissue is slightly lobular, and one is searching in particular for a hard, fixed mass hidden in the glandular tissue. Palpation of the subareolar tissue and the axillary region of the upper outer quadrant should not be overlooked. The entire examination is done gently; the student should avoid excessive palpation. While one breast is being palpated, the other is draped.

In the male patient, inspection and palpation of both breasts should not be forgotten, with attention especially directed to gynecomastia or neoplasm.

---

[4]Haagensen, C. D.: Carcinoma of the Breast. American Cancer Society, Inc., New York, 1958.

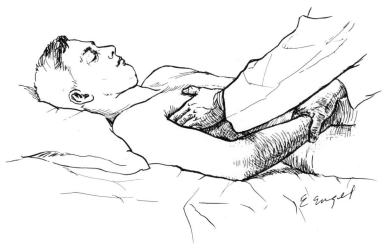

Fig. 4-16 The right axilla is palpated with the finger tips of the examiner's left hand. The patient's arm is closed against the palpating hand in order to relax the axillary musculature and allow palpation high in the axilla. The left axilla is palpated with the right hand.

Both axillary regions are next inspected with the patient's arms elevated. One looks for skin lesions, such as furuncles and rashes. The patient's upper arm is then partially closed against the examiner's palpating hand, enabling him to reach higher into the axilla, as the axillary musculature is relaxed. The right axilla is easily felt with the left hand; the left axilla with the right hand. Lymph nodes, in particular, are felt for by using a rotary motion with two or three finger tips.

THE HEART
Ambulatory

THE EXAMINER.   *Standing at the patient's right.*
THE PATIENT.   *In three positions: sitting, lying on his back, and lying on his left side.*

 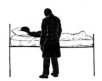 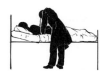

Bed-bound

THE EXAMINER. *Standing at the right side of the bed.*

THE PATIENT. *In three positions: lying on his back, lying on his left side, and sitting.*

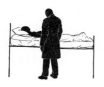 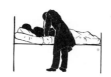 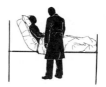

The techniques of inspection, palpation, percussion, and auscultation are important in the examination of the heart. The student should systematically apply the four techniques in the order given above. However, if an abnormality is found, he may wish to focus all of these techniques briefly on the problem before going on to complete the cardiac examination. For example, if he visualizes a prominent apical impulse, he may wish to check his finding by palpating the apex and percussing the left cardiac border. Also, other parts of the cardiovascular examination may be combined with the study of the heart, particularly if an abnormality is found. These include the blood pressure, arterial pulses of the upper extremities and neck, and the jugular venous pulse. The majority of the examination of the heart is best done with the patient on his back, where it is easiest for the examiner to apply his techniques and most comfortable for the patient. However, the student *must always examine the patient in the left lateral and sitting positions as well;* in particular, searching for the murmurs of mitral stenosis and aortic regurgitation. Following the breast examination, the patient will be in the supine position. The examination of the heart may proceed with the patient remaining in this position and includes inspection, palpation, percussion, and auscultation. After a complete study with the patient on his back, he is turned on his left side as one palpates and listens over the apical area. The cardiac examination may then conclude with the patient sitting in order to recheck the apical impulse, if necessary; to feel for other pulsations of the heart or great vessels; and to listen for the murmurs of semilunar valve insufficiency. One avoids having the patient sit up and down repeatedly; however, the student should not hesitate to change the patient's position at any time during the cardiac examination to clarify findings or detect abnormalities. For example, if there is difficulty finding the cardiac apex in the supine position, the location of the impulse, as well as its character, may often be brought out by palpation when the patient is turned in the left lateral position, even though the apex will be displaced laterally. The lateral position forces the heart closer to the chest wall, and the location of the apex with respect to the intercostal space can be better defined. When the patient is again on his back, the exact location of the apical impulse may now be recognized by palpation and percussion.

Inspection. The student is chiefly looking for pulsations, but he should not forget other abnormalities, such as a subcutaneous pattern of venous distention or the bulging contour of the left anterior hemithorax, which may be prominent because of long standing cardiac enlargement. At some point in the examination of the anterior thorax or heart, inspection for pulsations should be carried out with the patient sitting and bending slightly forward, since the heart tends to drop away from the chest wall when the patient is on his back.

It is important to look for the cardiac apical impulse. Normally, in a patient with a thin chest wall, a single systolic thrust of the heart apex may be visualized as a faint impulse in the region of the left midclavicular line and the fifth intercostal space. In other normal individuals with a thick chest wall and in women with heavy breast tissue, even though retracted upward, the apical impulse may not be seen in the sitting position.

The student next systematically looks for abnormal pulsations of the chest wall. Those originating from the heart itself are located between the apical impulse and the sternum, or beneath the lower sternum; whereas pulsations of a dilated proximal aorta or a pulmonary artery are seen in the right and left parasternal second intercostal spaces, respectively. Oblique lighting is helpful by virtue of the shadows cast; so too is holding the breath in expiration, which brings the heart and great vessels closer to the anterior chest wall. Visible pulsations should be carefully examined by palpation as well.

Palpation. The student should feel for the cardiac apical impulse that may or may not have been visible. If the patient is a woman, the right hand is placed on the chest wall underneath the left breast; if very large, the breast is retracted with the left hand. The location of the point of maximal impulse (P.M.I.) of the cardiac apex is a measure of cardiac size and should be recorded as to the level of the interspace and the number of centimeters to the left of the midsternal line or to the right or the left of the midclavicular line.[5] The distance from the midsternal line to the P.M.I. is measured tangentially to the sternum and is normally 8

---

[5]The midclavicular line is a vertical line halfway between the midsternal line and a vertical line dropped from the distal end of the clavicle. The point of maximal impulse normally lies on the left midclavicular line or slightly medially.

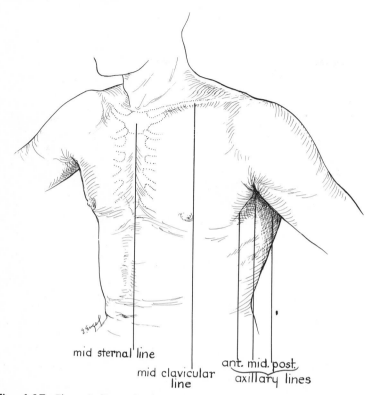

mid sternal line

mid clavicular line

ant. mid. post. axillary lines

Fig. 4-17 Thoracic lines of reference used in the examination of the heart.

to 10 cm., depending on thoracic contour. One can determine what interspace the cardiac apical impulse is in by palpating down from the left second intercostal space. The sternal angle, where the manubrium joins the body of the sternum, is used as a landmark to identify the second intercostal space, since the second rib articulates at the angle.

With practice, right and left ventricular hypertrophy can be evaluated by palpation. To determine right ventricular hypertrophy with the patient supine, the butt of the examiner's hand is placed over the low sternum or left parasternal area. If a *diffuse heave* is observed or felt, this indicates an underlying hypertrophied right ventricle. In the apical area, a *localized sustained thrust*, lifting the finger, is a sign of left ventricular hypertrophy; a more diffuse and briefer impulse is more characteristic of a hyperdynamic left ventricle.

Palpation is of special value in helping to define cardiac abnormalities. Proper patient positioning is imperative. For example, a *diastolic gallop* may be easier to feel than hear. One turns the patient halfway on

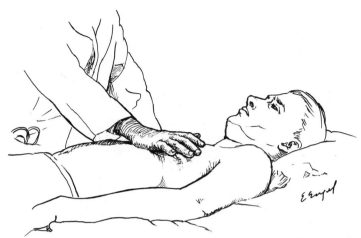

Fig. 4-18   The diffuse heave of right ventricular hypertrophy is felt for by placing the butt of the right hand over the low sternum or left parasternal area.

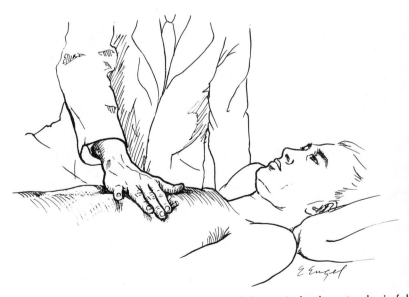

Fig. 4-19   The localized sustained thrust of left ventricular hypertrophy is felt for at the cardiac apex with the tips of the index and third fingers.

his left side and feels for a faint second apical impulse. So may the apical thrust of left ventricular hypertrophy be better defined with the patient on his left side. The *thrill* of a loud apical systolic or diastolic murmur is enhanced when the patient holds his breath in full expiration and lies in the left lateral position. One is aware of a buzzing sensation under the palmar surface of the hand pressed firmly against the chest wall. A thrill is particularly important, because the anatomic defect lies directly beneath its point of maximum intensity. The systolic thrill of a ventricular septal defect, for instance, may be felt just to the left of the midsternum when a patient is on his back. The thrill of severe aortic or pulmonic stenosis is located at the base of the heart when the patient is sitting, bends forward, and exhales fully. Finally, a loud *pericardial friction rub* may be felt as a grating to-and-fro sensation with the patient on his back, left side, or even when he lies prone on the palpating hand of the examiner.

Percussion.   This technique is used to estimate cardiac size, especially when the apical impulse is not seen or felt. The pleximeter finger is held either parallel or perpendicular to the direction of the ribs and is lightly struck as it is brought successively from lung resonance to the area of cardiac dullness. The pleximeter finger is kept within the intercostal space. The location of the left border of cardiac dullness from the third to fifth or sixth intercostal space is expressed in centimeters to the left of the midsternal line. It is very difficult to determine the right heart border because of sternal resonance unless there is considerable cardiac enlargement. However, very light percussion in the right third and fourth interspaces may show a change of note just lateral to the sternum, indicating the normal cardiac border.

Auscultation.   In learning to listen to the heart, the student should review the events of the cardiac cycle and the mechanism of heart sounds and murmurs. He must develop a logical order in listening to the heart; and in particular, learn to listen to one event at a time, screening out all other sounds. It is good practice to listen to one's own heart to become familiar with the character of each sound and to learn how heart sounds vary in the different areas of auscultation. A detailed description of heart sounds and murmurs is given in Leatham's review.[6]

Four areas of auscultation are classically described: the aortic area in the second intercostal space just to the right of the sternum, the pulmonic area in the second intercostal space to the left of the sternum, the mitral area at the cardiac apex, and the tricuspid area to the left of the low sternum. It should be recognized that sound is transmitted from the valves widely, so that the student should also listen in the general vicinity of these areas. It may be easiest to begin auscultation in the aortic area,

[6]Leatham, A.: Auscultation of the Heart. Lancet, 2:703 and 757, 1958.

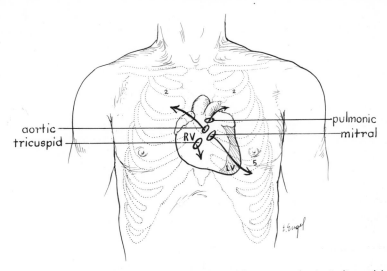

Fig. 4-20 The four areas for auscultation of heart sounds. As indicated by the arrows, each area projects a distance from the anatomic location of the corresponding valve. The sound generally follows the direction of blood flow. The *aortic area* is in the second right intercostal space, the *pulmonic area* in the second left intercostal space; the *mitral area* is at the midclavicular line in the fifth left intercostal space, and the *tricuspid area* is at the lower end of the sternum. Note that from the anterior view the right ventricle (RV) lies immediately behind the sternum, while the left ventricle (LV), which lies posteriorly, is located mainly at the cardiac apex.

where the second heart sound can be identified as being louder than the first; then, move to the pulmonic area; next, listen at the left of the midsternum, then, at the apex; and finally, in the tricuspid area.

When he listens to the heart, the student should be comfortable and the room kept as quiet as possible. Sometimes, closing his eyes will help him concentrate. Even when the patient breathes quietly, some murmurs are very difficult to hear. Hence, he should be asked to stop breathing briefly. It is better that he be instructed to stop breathing rather than to hold his breath, since a deep inspiration may distort cardiac sounds and lead to audible chest wall contraction noises. The examiner also holds his own breath, which lets him know when the patient should breathe again. For most of the cardiac examination, the student uses the diaphragm of the stethoscope, which is best for the higher pitched systolic and diastolic murmurs. One uses the bell to hear the low-pitched apical diastolic gallops and the murmur of mitral stenosis (see Table 4-3, page 125).

Heart Sounds. Before concentrating on the individual heart sounds, the examiner should listen carefully to the cardiac rhythm. Is it regular? If not, how does it vary? Is there a gradual change related to respiration; are there occasional or frequent beats that come early; do

TABLE 4-3. THE USE OF THE BELL AND DIAPHRAGM OF THE
STETHOSCOPE IN THE CARDIAC EXAMINATION

The Bell (*Low pitched sounds*)	Gallops	Diastolic murmur of mitral or tricuspid stenosis		
The Diaphragm (*High pitched sounds*)	Ejection click; opening snap	Systolic murmurs	Diastolic murmur of aortic and pulmonary regurgitation	Pericardial friction rubs

beats drop out; or is the rhythm totally irregular, as in atrial fibrillation? If there are many premature beats, it can be quite confusing because of the variation of heart sounds and increased splitting. Under such conditions, the rhythm can better be determined by feeling the arterial pulse. It is also very helpful to study the jugular venous pulse in arrhythmias, such as in complete heart block where the pulse associated with atrial contraction has no relationship to ventricular systole.

The heart sounds in each auscultatory area should be individually analyzed for the following:

1. Identification of first and second heart sounds
2. Intensity of heart sounds
3. Splitting of each heart sound
4. Extracardiac sounds

Identification of first and second heart sounds. The loudest sound in the aortic area normally is the second heart sound, occurring at the time of closure of the aortic and pulmonary valves.[7] The first heart sound may be identified in any area by gently feeling the carotid pulse which occurs simultaneously with the first sound. The radial pulse is less satisfactory for timing, being slightly delayed because of its distance from the heart. At the mitral area the first heart sound, at the time of mitral and tricuspid valve closure, is normally louder than the second.[7] With time and experience, one learns that the systolic interval between the first and second heart sounds is shorter than the diastolic pause which follows the second sound.

Intensity of heart sounds. After identifying both sounds in a given area, the student next concentrates on their relative intensities. With experience, he will learn their normal limits. He will also recognize that

---

[7]The actual cause of the first and second heart sounds is controversial and appears related to acceleration and deceleration of blood flow, causing vibration of valvular and muscular structures within the heart and of the wall of the proximal ascending aorta. For a detailed description of the genesis of heart sounds see: Delman, A. J.: Hemodynamic Correlates of Cardiovascular Sounds. *In* De Graff, A. C., Ed.: Annual Review of Medicine. Annual Reviews, Inc., California, 1967, Vol. 18, p. 139.

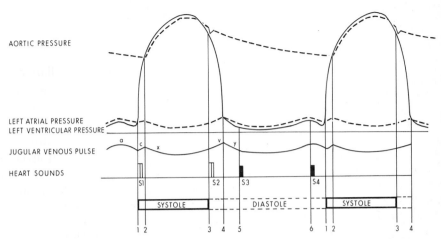

Fig. 4-21 Simultaneous events in the cardiac cycle — schematic diagram. Two cardiac contractions are diagrammed. The aortic and left atrial pressure curves, indicated by dashed lines, are superimposed on the left ventricular pressure curve (solid line).

The jugular venous pulse waves are also diagrammed to demonstrate their relationship to the cardiac cycle. However, it should be emphasized that the jugular pulse is directly related to the pressure changes in the *right* atrium, which are *not* shown here. The jugular venous pulse includes the positive *a wave*, which is caused by right atrial contraction; the inconspicuous *c wave*, which may be due to transmitted carotid pulsation or perhaps to closure of the tricuspid valve; the negative *x descent*, which is due to right atrial relaxation; the positive *v wave*, which is caused by rapid venous filling of the right atrium; and the negative *y descent*, produced by the opening of the tricuspid valve and release of blood into the right ventricle.

The numbers at the bottom of the diagram refer to mechanical events of the left heart: (1) closure of the mitral valve, (2) opening of the aortic valve, (3) closure of the aortic valve, (4) opening of the mitral valve, (5) rapid filling of the left ventricle, and (6) left atrial contraction.

Systole extends from the first to the second heart sound, and the longer *diastole* from the second to the first heart sound.

S1 represents the first heart sound, which occurs at the time of closure of the atrioventricular valves. *S2* represents the second heart sound, occurring at the time of semilunar valve closure. *S3* coincides with the phase of rapid filling of the left ventricle and *S4* with augmented left ventricular filling due to left atrial contraction. *S3* and *S4* are usually inaudible in the normal adult heart. (*S3* is audible in the child.)

Splitting of the first sound in the normal heart is due to the asynchronous closure of the atrioventricular valves, the mitral closing before the tricuspid. Splitting of the second heart sound is caused by the asynchronous closing of the aortic and pulmonary valves, the former normally preceding the latter.

the intensity of sounds, particularly those in the pulmonary area, vary with the position of the patient. Finally, it is worthwhile to compare the relative intensities of the second sounds in the aortic area and pulmonic areas (more accurately, to compare the aortic component of the second heart sound with the pulmonic component). This is done by repeatedly moving the stethoscope from the aortic to the pulmonary area. Normally in adults, the second sound in the aortic area is louder than that in the pulmonic area. Abnormal accentuation of the second sound may give a rough estimate of aortic or pulmonary artery hypertension. Valve damage, on the other hand, may decrease the intensity of the second heart sound.

Splitting of heart sounds. The student should listen in the pulmonic area for splitting of the second sound when the pulmonic valve closes after the aortic, and in the tricuspid area where splitting of the first sound occurs when the mitral valve closes before the tricuspid valve. Splitting of the second heart sound in the pulmonary area is increased in the normal heart during inspiration, because as more blood is returned to the right heart, right ventricular ejection is prolonged and pulmonary valve closure is delayed. One listens for splitting as the patient is instructed to breathe "a little deeper"; splitting of the second heart sound will normally be heard to increase towards the end of inspiration compared to end-expiration.

Extracardiac sounds. Extraheart sounds are usually not heard in the normal adult heart. The student first identifies the systolic extra sounds. Then he listens in diastole for any diastolic extra sounds. Those sounds in systole include the early ejection click, associated with the opening of the semilunar valve in the presence of a dilated aorta or pulmonary artery, and the mid or late systolic clicks, associated with mitral valve dysfunction. In diastole, the low-pitched S3 and S4 gallops are most important. One may also hear the sharp early opening snap of mitral stenosis or the early diastolic knock of constrictive pericarditis. To bring out a gallop, the examiner lightly places the bell of his stethoscope at, or medial to, the cardiac apex, with the patient in the left lateral position. A pericardial friction rub may also be heard as a coarse to-and-fro sound in systole and diastole, composed of two or three audible components.

Cardiac Murmurs. When the student has finished analyzing heart sounds, he next directs his attention to cardiac murmurs, listening first for a murmur in each area during systole, then in diastole. He should identify the following characteristics for every murmur:

1. Anatomic location
2. Location in systole or diastole
3. Intensity (grade 1 to 6, grade 4 being associated with a thrill)

4. Pitch and quality
5. Duration
6. Radiation

The practice of diagramming heart sounds and murmurs for each valve area is especially helpful for the beginning student. If he disciplines himself to record what he hears, he will train himself to separate cardiac events and to better understand timing. An example of diagramming sounds and murmurs is given on page 129.

Systolic murmurs. When the student listens in a given area, he identifies first the systolic interval and then concentrates on the characteristics of the murmur so as to be able to answer all six points mentioned above. With time and experience, he will be able to differentiate systolic from diastolic murmurs by their pitch and quality alone, and to distinguish systolic murmurs originating from the semilunar valves from those of the atrioventricular valves by their pitch, quality, and duration. For example, the typical diamond-shaped aortic systolic ejection murmur is harsh, increases in intensity in midsystole at the time of greatest flow, and ceases before the aortic component of the second sound. The typical murmur of mitral regurgitation is blowing in quality and holosystolic, maintaining the same intensity throughout systole up to the second sound. When analyzing a murmur, one mentally visualizes the characteristics of the murmur first, before interpreting its meaning.

If the murmur is loud, it will radiate in the direction of blood flow beyond the valve. For example, the systolic murmur of aortic stenosis will radiate to the carotid arteries in the low neck. One listens for the murmur in the neck as the patient briefly holds his breath.[8] Likewise, when a loud apical systolic murmur is present, the student should listen laterally to see if it radiates to the left mid or posterior axillary line.[9]

Diastolic murmurs. One carefully listens in diastole at each cardiac area. Diastolic murmurs from the aortic or pulmonic semilunar valves are typically very high pitched, decrescendo, and blowing; whereas those from the mitral valve are low pitched and rumbling, being most prominent in mid or late diastole. All six characteristics of the murmur are identified.

The position of the patient and the proper use of the stethoscope

---

[8]On occasion, especially in a young person, one may hear a venous hum in the supraclavicular fossa or upper anterior chest. This is a musical, continuous murmur that is accentuated in diastole, caused by rapid flow through the jugular veins, and can be mistaken for a patent ductus murmur. It is not abnormal; it is intensified by the upright position or by turning the head to one side, and is eliminated by compressing the veins at the base of the neck.

[9]The axillary lines may be defined as follows: The anterior axillary line is dropped perpendicularly from the anterior axillary fold, the posterior axillary line from the posterior axillary fold, and the midaxillary line is halfway between (see Fig. 4-17, page 121).

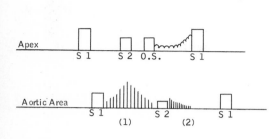

Fig. 4-22 Diagramming heart sounds and murmurs. **Upper,** Mitral stenosis. The first heart sound (S1) is increased; there is an opening snap (O.S.) close to the second heart sound (S2), and a rumbling murmur (mm) with presystolic accentuation. **Lower,** Aortic stenosis and regurgitation. The aortic component of the second heart sound (S2) is decreased. There is a diamond shaped aortic systolic murmur (1) and a decrescendo early diastolic murmur (2).

are most important to bring out diastolic murmurs. The aortic diastolic murmur is best heard when the examiner uses the diaphragm and listens to the patient in the sitting position bending slightly forward with the breath held in full expiration. One should tell the patient to breathe out fully and then stop breathing. The student should listen not only in the aortic area, but also to the left of the midsternum, where the aortic diastolic murmur may be more prominent. He must always turn the patient in the left lateral position to search for the murmur of mitral stenosis, gently placing the bell of the stethoscope just medial to the apical impulse. Since this murmur may be quite localized, he should also search for it in the general vicinity of the cardiac apex.

In conclusion, auscultation of the heart is complex and requires considerable experience to develop proficiency. The student must practice frequently and use an orderly system of examination to become adept. He will develop his own overall approach to the patient as time goes on and will learn to combine the techniques of inspection, palpation, percussion, and auscultation to do an efficient, yet thorough examination.

THE ABDOMEN

Ambulatory

THE EXAMINER. *Standing at the patient's right.*
THE PATIENT. *Lying on his back.*

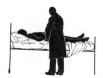

Bed-bound

THE EXAMINER.   *Standing at the right side of the bed.*
THE PATIENT.   *Lying on his back.*

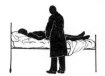

The abdominal examination begins with inspection. Palpation is the most important technique and is used to elicit tenderness, abnormal masses, or organ enlargement. Percussion and auscultation are of secondary importance.

There are two major principles that aid in the accurate examination of the abdomen: the proper patient positioning and a systematic approach.

Proper Patient Positioning.   The patient must be in a comfortable position with the head of the bed lowered, so that his abdominal muscles are relaxed. His hands should be at his side or resting on his anterior chest. If he places his hands behind his neck, this stretches the abdominal wall and interferes with the examination. Flexing the knees will also help to relax the abdominal muscles. When palpation begins, the patient is told, "Now, I'm going to examine your abdomen. Please try to relax." The abdomen should be completely exposed from above the xiphoid to the pubis, but care should be taken to protect the patient's modesty. Although the examination is done chiefly with the patient on his back, one should not hesitate to vary his position to help detect an abnormality. The electrically controlled bed is fully elevated so that the examiner's forearm is level with the patient's abdomen. This will enable him to palpate with the palmar surface rather than with the tips of his fingers.

A Systematic Approach.   Palpation of the abdomen is gentle, deliberate, and done with the flat of the hand so as not to cause muscle spasm or a tickling sensation. Being certain that the hand and stethoscope are warm will also help to avert tensing of the abdominal muscles.

One begins with light palpation and progresses to deep palpation in the four quadrants of the abdomen. *Light palpation* is done with one hand by gently moving the fingers up and down at the metacarpalphalangeal joints. *Deep palpation* involves applying a little more pressure and using a slight rotary movement. *Bimanual palpation*, after initial light and deep palpation, is indicated for those organs, such as the liver, spleen, or kidneys, that extend to the posterior part of the abdomen. Here, the palpating hand is placed on the anterior abdominal wall, while the other hand is directly behind on the flank. The posterior hand lifts upward, without assistance from the patient, and brings the organ forward toward the anterior palpating hand. The patient is then instructed to take a slow deep breath, which causes the liver, spleen, or kidney to descend and ride under the palpating anterior hand. Finally, if one has difficulty examining structures deep in the abdomen because of obesity or muscle spasm, palpation with two hands may be used. The right hand is placed on the abdomen, and the fingers of the left hand are pressed down on the dorsum of the fingers of the right hand. This allows the palpating fingers to relax and have a more sensitive sensation of touch.

Not only should the student carefully examine the four quadrants of the abdomen, but he must also be sure to identify structures successively from the anterior to the posterior wall. The examination must be orderly and thorough. One systematic method is outlined as follows:

I. Initial General Survey (abdominal wall, intestines, abnormal intraperitoneal masses)
    A. Inspection
    B. Auscultation
    C. Light palpation of the four abdominal quadrants
    D. Deep palpation of the four abdominal quadrants
II. Organs in the Anterior Abdomen
    A. Liver
        1. Inspection
        2. Light palpation
        3. Bimanual palpation
        4. Percussion
    B. Spleen
        1. Inspection
        2. Light palpation
        3. Bimanual palpation
        4. Percussion
    C. Bladder and enlarged uterus
        1. Inspection
        2. Light palpation
        3. Percussion
III. Retroperitoneal Structures
    A. Kidneys (bimanual palpation)
    B. Retroperitoneal masses
    C. Abdominal aorta
IV. Inguinal Region
V. Special Techniques

Initial General Survey

Inspection

The general shape and symmetry of the abdomen are first observed from the foot of the bed, noting particularly muscle tone, subcutaneous fat, abdominal distention, and bulging in the flanks. Tangential light is helpful in bringing out subtle contours. The student should next scan the surface systematically, observing scars, pigmentation, striae, abrasions, ecchymoses, venous pattern, and any skin lesions. The abdominal musculature is watched during respiration to compare one side with the other for evidence of splinting or guarding. By asking the patient to raise his head off the bed, one detects herniation in sites of scars, at the umbilicus, or between the rectus muscles. The deeper structures are next studied systematically for visibly enlarged organs, masses, pulsations, peristaltic waves, and dilated loops of bowel. When masses are obvious, their movement in relationship to respiration should be noted.

Auscultation

Auscultation may be done during any part of the abdominal examination. However, when the diagnosis of adynamic ileus, peritonitis, or bowel obstruction is suspected, auscultation should be performed prior to palpation, since palpation may depress or increase peristalsis of the irritated bowel and thus interfere with a helpful diagnostic sign. In the case of the ticklish or hypersensitive patient, the stethoscope may also be of help in the initial search for tenderness when one applies gentle pressure with the head of the stethoscope in each region of the abdomen.

The examiner listens for peristalsis by placing the diaphragm of the stethoscope over two or three areas of the abdomen. It is left in place long enough to determine the pitch, quality, and frequency (rate per minute) of the bowel sounds. The examiner next listens in the mid-epigastrium for bruits which may arise from a stenotic renal artery or from an abdominal aortic aneurysm, and for a venous hum should portal hypertension be suspected. One must be careful to distinguish an abdominal bruit from a cardiac murmur transmitted from the chest; the latter will increase in intensity as the stethoscope is moved closer to the heart. Each iliac region is examined for the bruit of ileofemoral artery stenosis. Rarely, one may hear a friction rub with respiration over a metastatic liver nodule or over the site of a splenic infarct.

Light palpation of the four abdominal quadrants

The student first compares symmetrical areas of the right and left sides of the abdomen. He palpates lightly with one hand, using the full palmar surface of his fingers. During such palpation, the patient's face is watched for an expression of pain or discomfort. If tenderness is suggested, this particular region is noted and the remainder of the abdominal survey completed before returning to the tender area. After the initial survey comparing two sides, the four quadrants are each examined by light palpation, looking particularly for tenderness, muscle spasm, or resistance of an underlying organ or mass. When generalized muscle spasm is felt, a further effort must be made to encourage relaxation. The patient's attention can be distracted by conversation; he may be asked to take a few deep breaths or to flex his knees and hips. The finding of localized spasm is abnormal and indicates peritoneal irritation.

Should tenderness be found, the student must decide what structure is tender and then estimate the intensity of the pain. Light stroking of the skin with cotton or a pin will detect an area of skin hyperalgesia. Pain in the abdominal wall itself may be determined by grasping the skin and subcutaneous tissue in a fold between the fingers. Peritoneal irritation may be demonstrated by slowly depressing the abdominal wall with one or two fingers and then abruptly releasing the pressure. This maneuver, which evokes quick pain as pressure is released, is called rebound tenderness. Tenderness of deeper structures is identified by deep palpation and is produced when the underlying organ or mass is touched or compressed between both hands.

Deep palpation of the four abdominal quadrants

After the abdomen has been surveyed by light palpation, the examination is repeated with gentle but deeper rotational palpation. The student should concentrate intently on the sensations of his fingers; and should constantly think of the anatomy of the underlying area, asking himself "What organs and structures are under my hand?"

The left lower quadrant is a good place to begin deep palpation, because tenderness is not common in this area. Normally one should only feel bowel. If there is a very large spleen, it can project into the left lower quadrant, as can an asymmetrically enlarged uterus or ovary. The sigmoid colon is usually easily palpable as a firm, smooth, tubular structure; if it contains hard feces, it may feel nodular, suggesting an abnormal mass.

One moves systematically across the midline to survey by deep palpation the right lower quadrant where lie the cecum, appendix, and distal ileum. Gas is usually present in the cecum, which can be felt as an easily compressible organ. The edge of an enlarged liver may descend into this region, and rarely an enlarged ovary or uterus may be felt low in the right lower quadrant.

In the right upper quadrant, one may feel the resistance of an enlarged liver. The gall bladder is not palpable unless grossly distended, as with hydrops, and one normally can not feel the underlying head of the pancreas or duodenum. The lower pole of the right kidney lies deep in the vicinity of the midclavicular line above the umbilicus. *One postpones the necessarily very deep palpation of the kidney until the later examination*

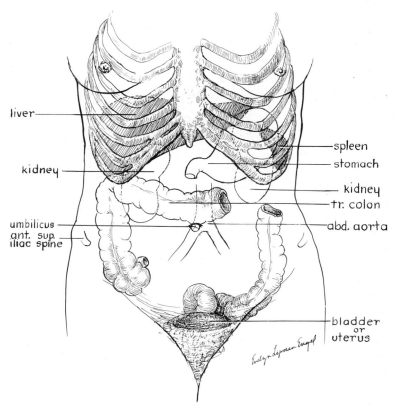

Fig. 4-23 The abdominal organs accessible by physical examination. The shaded organs represent those located in the anterior abdomen; namely, the liver, the spleen, and the bladder or uterus. The kidneys and abdominal aorta lie posteriorly in the retroperitoneal space. The aorta divides into the iliac arteries at the level of the umbilicus. The stomach is not palpable but yields a tympanitic note on percussion, as do the small and large intestines. The caecum may sometimes be felt as a compressible air-containing structure in the right lower quadrant, while the sigmoid may be felt as a firm structure in the left lower quadrant.

of retroperitoneal structures, so as not to cause patient discomfort and muscle spasm. The epigastric area is difficult to palpate because of the thick rectus muscles. One is particularly looking for tenderness in this region. Some patients may note tenderness when pressure is applied over the aorta, which is recognized by its pulsation.

The stomach, spleen, left renal pole, and colon lie in the left upper quadrant. The spleen and left kidney are not usually detected by deep palpation unless enlarged. The stomach and colon are not palpable, but sizeable masses associated with them may be.

As the student surveys the four quadrants by light and deep palpation, he is particularly alert to the possibility of discovering an abnormal mass. The mass may represent an abnormally enlarged organ, such as liver, spleen, or lymph nodes; a lesion extrinsic or intrinsic to an organ, such as a cyst of the liver or a carcinoma of the bowel; or adherent structures, such as loops of small bowel matted together around an abscess. Should such a lesion be found, it is studied for the following characteristics:

1. Location	5. Consistency
2. Size	6. Mobility
3. Tenderness	7. Pulsation
4. Contour	

One or both hands may be used to define the mass, depending on its depth in the abdomen. The regional location of the lesion should be determined, as well as its relationship to neighboring structures. The dimensions are measured in centimeters to express size. Tenderness, contour, and consistency are determined by systematic pressure over the available surface of the mass, first using gentle palpation; then firmer pressure, as is tolerated. If the lesion is near the diaphragm, it may move with deep inspiration; or if it is attached to the omentum, it may be displaced to a different region of the abdomen. Masses or organs extending to the posterior abdominal wall, such as the liver, spleen, or kidneys, may be brought forward by bimanual palpation. A large mass that extends to the posterior flank may also be displaced forward to tap the anterior palpating fingers by a series of quick thrusts of the fingers of the posterior hand (ballottement). One should not forget that changing the patient's position may help to delineate a mass. An enlarged liver or spleen may be more apparent in the semisitting position, and placing the patient on his hands and knees may make an intraabdominal mass palpable by bringing it forward. A large fecal mass in the colon will move with time and can be distinguished from a tumor, being absent when the patient is reexamined following a bowel movement or enema. Finally, the palpating hand or hands should be placed on the sides of the mass, if possible, to feel for pulsation. Expansile pulsation indicates that the lesion is an arterial aneurysm and not pulsation transmitted to a mass from a neighboring large artery.

Organs in the Anterior Abdomen

Liver

Following a systematic survey of the abdomen by light and deep palpation, the student next concentrates on specific organs. One first pauses to observe whether the edge of the liver can be visualized to descend in the right upper quadrant with deep inspiration. The examining fingers of one hand are then placed lightly but firmly on the abdominal wall below the right costal margin. The hand is parallel and lateral to the right rectus muscle with fingers pointing toward the patient's head. As the patient takes a slow deep breath through his mouth, the examiner may feel a sharp or rounded liver edge ride under his fingers. If the patient does not take a deep enough breath to cause the liver to descend, it may be necessary for the student to demonstrate how to do so. The hand is kept in the same position, and is not pushed inward as the patient inspires. Repeated efforts may be needed to determine the presence or the absence of an enlarged liver. The examiner's hand must explore for the liver edge by moving closer to and further from the costal margin, as well as medially and laterally. Bimanual palpation is then used. The student now presses the palmar surface of the fingers of the right hand gently into the anterior abdominal wall and lifts the posterior aspect of the lower rib cage and right flank with his left hand to bring the liver forward. The patient should not attempt to assist lifting his rib cage since this action will tense his muscles. The patient is instructed to "breathe slowly in and out." Inspiration must be deep enough to cause the liver to descend adequately. The right hand is kept in the same position, waiting for the liver edge to meet it. If palpable, the liver edge is then traced laterally and medially into the epigastrium by repeating the maneuver in these positions. It is more difficult to feel the liver medially under the rectus muscles, and the

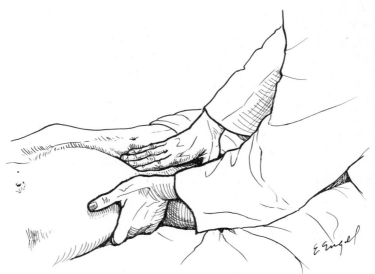

Fig. 4-24   In bimanual palpation of the liver, the posterior rib cage is lifted with the left hand as the palmar surface of the fingers of the right hand are pressed gently into the abdominal wall. The patient inspires slowly and deeply to cause the liver edge to descend and meet the tips of the palpating fingers.

tendinous inscriptions can be erroneously interpreted as the liver edge. When palpable, the characteristics of location, size, tenderness, contour, consistency, and pulsation are noted, as with any abdominal mass. The location of the lower border of the liver is estimated by measuring the number of centimeters it extends below the costal margin in the mid-clavicular line at the height of deep inspiration, and by measuring in the midsternal line, should the liver be enlarged. Normally, the lower border extends to the costal margin in the midclavicular line or 1 or 2 cm. below. One should not forget that an abnormally distended gallbladder may be palpable just below the liver edge in the midclavicular line, and it will also descend with inspiration. At times, when an organ, such as a liver, spleen, or kidney, is felt, the patient may be aware of a slight uncomfortable sensation. This can be helpful in confirming that the organ had indeed been palpated.

Percussion of the upper and lower borders of the liver is a useful method to estimate hepatic size. One method of liver percussion is to percuss continuously with the finger in just one spot just below the right costal margin. As the patient takes a slow deep breath, the resonant note may become dull, indicating the presence of the liver edge as it descends below the rib cage. When the liver is low lying, it may normally descend 2 or 3 cm. below the costal margin; so the upper hepatic border must be checked by percussion as well. To determine the extent or span of liver dullness, one percusses in the midclavicular line above from the resonant lung to liver dullness and from the tympanitic intestines below toward dullness at the costal margin. The span of liver dullness from the upper to lower border is normally not greater than 11 to 12 cm. If there is a pleural effusion or pneumonia above the liver, one will not be able to determine the upper border; and rarely, distended, air-containing bowel may obscure the dull percussion note at the lower border.

Finally, if liver tenderness is suspected, one may place the left hand, palm down, over the right lower anterior rib cage and jar the under-lying liver by striking the left hand with the ulnar aspect of the right fist. The left anterior lower costal margin is struck in a similar way for comparison, beginning with gentle blows on each side.

Spleen

If the spleen is enlarged and the abdominal wall thin, one may see the splenic contour descend below the costal margin on deep inspiration. The examiner next places the palpating fingers of the right hand just below the left costal margin with the fingers pointing toward the costal margin. Gentle pressure is applied and the hand held still, as the patient is asked to "slowly take a deep breath in and out." The spleen in the adult is felt only when it is enlarged. If the spleen is not felt initially, the palpating hand should be moved medially and laterally. Some examiners prefer to palpate with fingers parallel to the costal margin to cover a larger area. Rarely will a spleen be so large as to extend into the left lower quadrant. In this instance, the student may feel resistance in the left upper quadrant and should move his hand further down until he is below the splenic edge. The initial light palpation is followed by bimanual palpation. The left lower posterior rib cage is pulled forward with the left hand to assist in bringing the spleen forward. *If the spleen is not felt when the patient is on his back, he should be turned on his right side with the thighs flexed, and bimanual palpation should be repeated.* The palpable splenic edge is usually firm and rounded, and the splenic hilum may be felt as a notch medially. If the spleen is enlarged, one should measure the number of centimeters the lower border descends below the costal margin in the midclavicular line at the height of inspiration.

Splenic percussion can be unreliable because of the hyperresonance of an air-filled stomach or colon, or if there is dullness above caused by pneumonia or a pleural effusion. However, percussion should not be

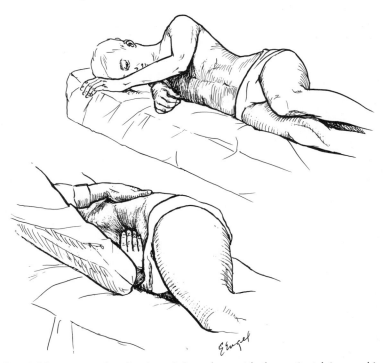

Fig. 4-25 Bimanual palpation of the spleen with the patient lying on his right side. *Upper,* Demonstrates the patient's position with his knees drawn up, and *Lower,* the position of the examiner's hands. The left hand pulls the left lower posterior rib cage forward. The palmar surface of the fingers of the examiner's right hand are pressed gently into the left upper quadrant to feel the descent of the spleen as the patient inspires deeply.

omitted and may be done by two methods. First, with the patient on his right side, one percusses continuously in one spot just under the left costal margin in the region of the anterior axillary line. The patient is then asked to take a slow deep breath. The change of the percussion note from resonant to dull suggests descent of the spleen. By repeating this in two or three locations medially and laterally, one may find a dull area, which indicates where to palpate for the splenic tip. A second method is to percuss across the anatomic location of the spleen, with the patient again lying on his right side. Beginning at the lowest area of lung resonance in the left mid or posterior axillary line, one percusses in an intercostal space, first toward the costal margin; and then from subcostal resonance to dullness across the rib margin in the same interspace. Normal splenic dullness does not exceed 6 to 8 cm.

Bladder and enlarged uterus

If either organ is enlarged, one may see a convex fullness above the symphysis pubis and may palpate a midline mass. Percussion is carried out in the midline from the umbilicus downward, and the extent of dullness above the symphysis is measured in centimeters. Pressure over the mass that gives a sensation of wanting to void and disappearance of the mass after urination confirms bladder distention. A suprapubic mass in the female always raises the possibility of pregnancy or of a uterine tumor.

Retroperitoneal Structures

Kidneys

When the student begins deeper palpation in the retroperitoneal area, the patient should be forewarned, "I am going to feel deep in your abdomen now. Please try to relax and I will be gentle." Bimanual palpation is used to feel for the kidneys. The student starts by supporting the patient's right flank behind the kidney with his left hand, while his right hand is placed on the anterior abdominal wall lateral to the right rectus muscle above the level of the umbilicus, with the fingers pointing toward the left costal margin. The patient is asked to breathe deeply, and the anterior hand is advanced steadily during successive expirations as the muscles relax. When both hands are approximated, the lower pole of the right kidney may be felt, on inspiration, as a vague mass passing between the fingers of the two hands. The fingers of the posterior left hand may give a quick thrust forward when the patient maintains deep inspiration to confirm the presence of the organ. The same procedure is repeated for the left kidney with the left hand pressing up in the left flank and the right hand in the medial left upper quadrant. However, the left kidney, being higher, is rarely felt; and when the patient has an obese abdomen or heavy musculature, it may be impossible to palpate deep enough to reach the region of either kidney.

Retroperitoneal masses

Very deep palpation is usually necessary to feel retroperitoneal masses, such as a pancreatic pseudocyst, tumor of the transverse colon, or retroperitoneal lymphadenopathy. Some retroperitoneal masses may be so large as to be confused with intraperitoneal structures. A huge ovarian cyst, for example, may even mimic ascites, except for the fact that dullness is prominent in the midabdomen with resonant flanks, in contradistinction to ascites where the reverse is the case. The technique of very deep palpation is difficult and may be virtually impossible if the abdomen is obese or if there is inadequate relaxation. The patient is told before starting that the examiner is going to feel deep in his abdomen. The fingers of one hand are pressed on the dorsum of the fingers of the other, slowly advancing during expiration as the abdominal muscles relax. When the mass is reached, a rotary motion will help delineate its outline.

Abdominal aorta

The abdominal aorta should be felt for at the conclusion of the abdominal examination. The patient is told to breathe a little deeper than usual; and the palpating hand, placed in the midline above the umbilicus and pointing toward the ensiform process, is steadily advanced toward the aorta during successive expirations. The thumb and fingers are held 4 to 5 centimeters apart so as to come down on each side of the aorta, which is recognized as a deep pulsation. The fingers are held parallel to the abdominal surface so not to cause muscle spasm. The width and degree of the pulsation of the aorta are of particular importance. In the thin patient, one may also be able to trace the iliac arteries as they branch from the aorta.

Inguinal Region

Both sides are inspected for skin lesions and are observed for a hernial bulge when the patient coughs or strains down. Palpation is then done in a rotary fashion to feel for masses and lymph nodes. The femoral artery is palpated with the patient's leg relaxed, slightly abducted, and externally rotated. One feels just below the inguinal ligament medial to the sartorius muscle with two or three fingers transverse to the longitudinal direction of the vessel. Firm pressure is needed, and additional pressure on the dorsum of the palpating hand may be needed to help relax the underlying fingers. The pulse is compared on each side; and if the patient is hypertensive, the radial pulse is felt simultaneously with the femoral. A weak and delayed femoral pulse is compatible with coarctation of the aorta.

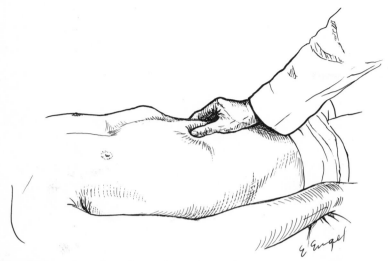

Fig. 4-26 Palpation of the abdominal aorta with the thumb and fingers 4 or 5 cm. apart and held parallel to the abdominal surface. The hand is placed in the midline above the umbilicus. As the patient's muscles relax during expiration, the hand is steadily advanced toward the aorta, which is recognized as a deep pulsation.

Special Techniques

In the presence of ascites, one may palpate an enlarged liver or spleen by ballottement or dipping. The tips of the fingers are placed over the enlarged organ and suddenly thrust downward. With the abrupt displacement of fluid, the underlying mass may be briefly felt. Even though the maneuver is quick, it should be gentle.

Percussion is used to demonstrate shifting dullness in the presence of peritoneal fluid. With the patient supine, the upper borders of flank dullness are marked by parallel lines drawn with ink on the skin. When the patient turns to one side, the level of dullness rises above the line on the dependent side and is replaced on the superior side by tympany, as the gas-containing intestines float to the top. The demonstration of a fluid wave by an abrupt tap of the lateral abdomen is less helpful, since the finding is positive only with a tensely distended abdomen when the ascites is already obvious. A progressive increase in abdominal girth may be documented by measuring the circumference at the level of the umbilicus with a tape measure.

If the patient is suspected of having a neurologic abnormality, one may wish to check the abdominal reflexes before leaving the region. The patient must be relaxed. The pointed end of a broken throat stick or the point of a pin is drawn diagonally and briskly, first across each upper quadrant, then across each of the lower quadrants. Contraction of the underlying musculature is compared on each side.*

---

*Part of the neurologic examination.

THE EXTREMITIES

Ambulatory

THE EXAMINER. *Standing, facing the patient, and moving to the patient's right.*

THE PATIENT. *Lying flat, then sitting on the side of the bed, and finally standing.*

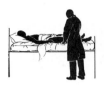 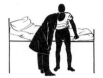

Bed-bound

THE EXAMINER. *Standing at the right side of the bed.*

THE PATIENT. *Lying flat on his back, then on his abdomen; if able, sitting on the side of the bed, facing the examiner.*

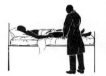

    The essential principle used in the examination of the extremities is to constantly compare structure and function of symmetrical parts. If necessary, the entire examination can be carried out with the patient in bed; however, a complete study requires that he also sit and stand. Inspection and palpation are the chief techniques used. The major systems examined are the skin, lymph nodes, muscles, bones, joints, blood vessels, and nervous system.

    By this point in the general examination, the examiner will already have observed any gross defects of the extremities, such as limitation of motion, weakness, paralysis, ataxia, or involuntary movements, which are obvious when the patient moves about or removes his clothes. These abnormalities are now studied in more detail.

    The patient is first asked to extend both arms in front of him (at an angle of 50 degrees in the recumbent patient), to pronate and supinate, and then to hold his arms steady with fingers outstretched.* This maneuver brings out gross asymmetries, limitation of the motion of the joints, weakness (seen when one arm drifts downward), ataxia, and involuntary movements. Coordination and the ability to follow directions are tested by asking the patient to touch repeatedly the tip of his nose with the index finger of the right hand; then the left, first with the eyes open, then closed.*

    The arms are lowered and first one then the other is held and

---

*Part of the neurologic examination.

turned as one inspects and palpates carefully from the fingers to the shoulder. Particular attention is paid to the skin and nails; muscle mass; limitation of joint motion, swelling, or tenderness; enlarged epitrochlear nodes; and arterial pulsations.

Finally, the biceps, triceps, and radial reflexes are tested.* *For the elicitation of the deep tendon reflexes, adequate patient relaxation is essential. A mild degree of passive tension on the muscle is also necessary.* If the patient is not completely relaxed, it is helpful to reinforce the reflex just before striking the tendon by asking him to bite down hard; or to link his fingers and pull, in the case of the knee and ankle jerks. One may use the broad head of the reflex hammer to strike accessible tendons, such as the Achilles, and the pointed end for smaller less accessible tendons, such as the biceps. The reflex hammer should be loosely held so that gravity contributes to the descent of the heavy head against the tendon, yielding a brisk and consistent blow. This, along with the symmetrical alignment

*Part of the neurologic examination.

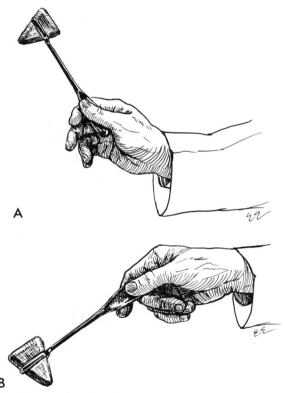

Fig. 4-27 To properly elicit deep tendon reflexes, the reflex hammer should be held loosely between the thumb and fingers *(A)* and allowed to fall by gravity against the tendon *(B)*. This yields a brisk and consistent stroke.

of the extremities, assures a comparable stimulus on the two sides, enhancing the accuracy of the comparison. *It is most important that symmetrical reflexes be immediately compared.* For example, the student compares the biceps jerk of one arm with the other; then both triceps jerks, going back and forth as necessary. He does not test all the reflexes of one arm and then all those of the other. Reflexes may be graded from 0 to 4+. 1+ is a slight detectable response, 2+ is normal, and 4+ very brisk. When there has been motor cortex or corticospinal tract damage and very brisk reflexes are present, clonus or repetitive muscle contraction can sometimes be induced. Ankle clonus may be elicited, for example, when the ankle is initially relaxed and the knee partially flexed. The distal foot is then briskly dorsiflexed and a slight degree of dorsiflexion is subsequently maintained to provide tendon stretch, yielding ankle clonus.

With the patient in the recumbent position, the best way to elicit the biceps reflex is to place both of his hands symmetrically on his abdomen to provide slight tendon stretch; the examiner strikes his own thumb or forefinger, which is pressed firmly on the tendon in the antecubital space. To elicit stretch for the triceps jerk, the patient's hands are brought up to his anterior chest, and the tendon is struck directly just above the elbow. The radial jerk is obtained by striking the brachioradialis tendon directly over the lower third of the radial aspect of the forearm. The wrist may need to be flexed slightly in an ulnar direction to provide tendon stretch. In the seated position the patient's hands are allowed to rest comfortably on his lap, while the examiner lowers or elevates the forearms to induce slight tension on the biceps or triceps tendons, respectively.

At this point, the examination of the lower extremities may begin. Since it is well to compare deep tendon reflexes in the legs with those of the arms, the reflexes should be tested first. To elicit the knee jerks in the recumbent position, the examiner supports the lower posterior thighs with his left arm to slightly flex the knees and stretch the tendons. The patient should be completely passive in this maneuver, and the knees are kept slightly apart. The broad patellar tendon is struck directly. To test ankle jerks several positions are useful: the patient's knee may be flexed slightly and the hip externally rotated; the lateral foot and ankle may be placed on the opposite shin; or the patient may lie on his abdomen, with his knees flexed to 90 degrees, which is the most reliable position. In all positions, the examiner should press gently on the ball of the foot in order to induce slight dorsiflexion and, therefore, put tension on the tendon. The Achilles tendon is struck directly. Lower extremity reflexes in the seated position are easy to obtain because the patient may be better able to relax. He should sit far enough forward so that his legs can swing freely. The knee jerk is elicited by striking the patellar

(Text continued on page 148.)

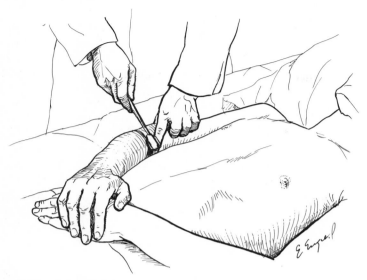

Fig. 4-28   The right biceps reflex. First the patient's hands are placed on the abdomen. The tip of the left index finger is pressed firmly on the biceps tendon and is struck briskly with the hammer.

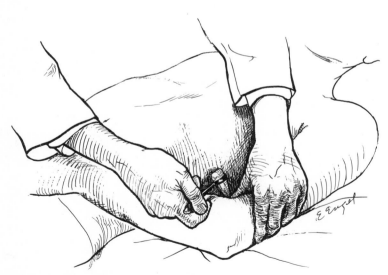

Fig. 4-29   The left biceps jerk is obtained by striking the examiner's thumb which is held firmly over the biceps tendon.

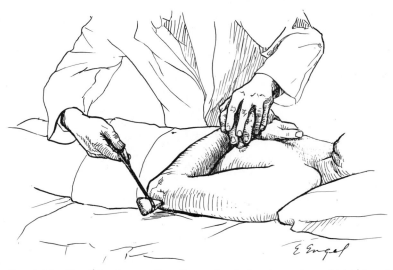

Fig. 4-30   The left triceps reflex. The patient's hands are brought to his anterior chest, and the triceps tendon is struck directly just above the elbow.

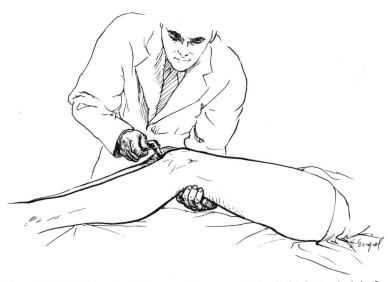

Fig. 4-31   The knee jerk. The examiner supports both thighs to slightly flex the knees and strikes the patellar tendon directly.

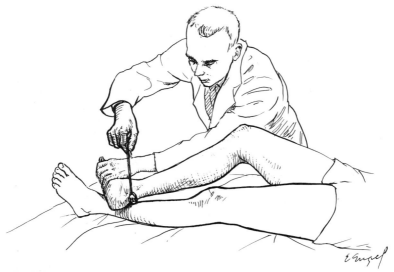

Fig. 4-32 The right ankle jerk is obtained by striking the Achilles tendon directly as the patient rests his foot on his left shin. Stretch of the tendon is provided by slightly dorsiflexing the patient's foot.

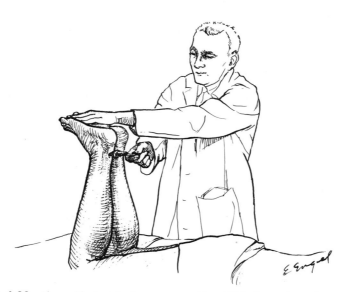

Fig. 4-33 The ankle jerk in the prone position. With the patient's knees flexed to 90 degrees, the examiner presses gently on the balls of the feet to stretch the Achilles tendon, as he briskly strikes the tendon with the reflex hammer.

tendon as both legs hang in a perpendicular position. The reflex on one side is compared to the other. For the ankle jerk, the examiner slightly elevates the distal foot with his hand. If no response is obtained, good relaxation of the Achilles tendon may be achieved by having the patient kneel on a chair.

The important plantar reflex is abnormal when there is damage to the motor cortex or the corticospinal tract. To obtain the response, one stimulates the lateral plantar surface of each foot with the teeth of a key or the irregular end of a broken tongue blade. A deliberate, but light, stroke is carried up the lateral aspect of the foot from the heel across to the ball of the great toe. The direction of the initial movement of the metatarsal-phalangeal joint of the big toe is noted. The limb should be relaxed as much as possible. Dorsiflexion of the great toe or an extensor plantar reflex is abnormal. Where the deficit is marked, there will be fanning or spreading out of the other toes. Before attempting to obtain the reflex, the student should prepare the patient for the noxious stimulus by saying "Now I am going to scratch the bottom of your foot."

One then goes on to inspect and palpate the legs from the toes to the groins. Each extremity is studied for skin lesions, bone and joint deformity, and muscle asymmetry. Points or areas of tenderness are located and evaluated in relationship to the responsible structures. Less accessible regions, such as the soles of the feet and the back of the legs, should not be overlooked. The study of the circulation of the legs is of particular importance. One first looks at the feet for visible arterial pulsations. The dorsalis pedis and posterior tibial pulses are then felt for by placing the index and following one or two fingers of the palpating hand along the longitudinal direction of the artery and pressing firmly to

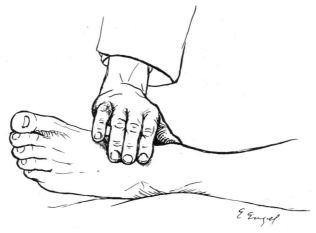

Fig. 4-34 The dorsalis pedis pulse is felt for with two or three fingers by successively shifting the fingers across the dorsum of the foot.

compress the vessel slightly. The fingers are successively shifted across the dorsum of the foot and behind each internal malleolus to find the vessels. The pulses are graded 1+ to 4+, and those of one foot compared with the other. Grade 1 is barely palpable after considerable search, and grade 4 is full and bounding.

The popliteal pulses are also felt for, as the knee is flexed about 30 degrees to relax the popliteal fascia. The artery is located deep in the popliteal space and lateral to the midline. The pulse is felt for by firmly pressing the fingers of one hand into the lateral popliteal fossa, as the fingers of the other hand press down on the dorsum of the palpating fingers. Arterial insufficiency is demonstrated by holding both legs in an elevated position for one to two minutes when the patient is on his back; then by having him sit up and dangle his legs. The return of color and the filling of the surface veins of the adequately perfused foot should take 15 seconds or less. Distention of varicose veins and cyanosis are also best seen when the legs are dependent.

Should slight swelling of one leg be suspected, caused by deep thrombophlebitis, or should slight muscle atrophy be suspected, it is helpful to measure and compare the circumferences of both legs. To obtain calf circumferences, for example, a given distance down each calf is first marked in ink, measuring from a fixed reference point, such as from the superior border of the patella. The circumference on each side at this level is then measured, using a flexible cloth tape when the muscles are relaxed. The distance from the superior patella and the dimensions of each circumference should be immediately recorded for future reference.

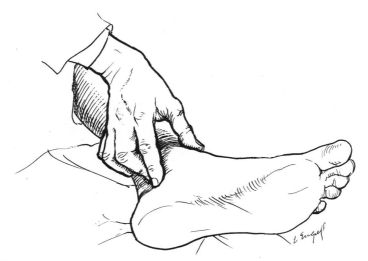

Fig. 4-35 The posterior tibial pulse is felt with the index and third fingers of the examiner's hand placed behind the internal malleolus.

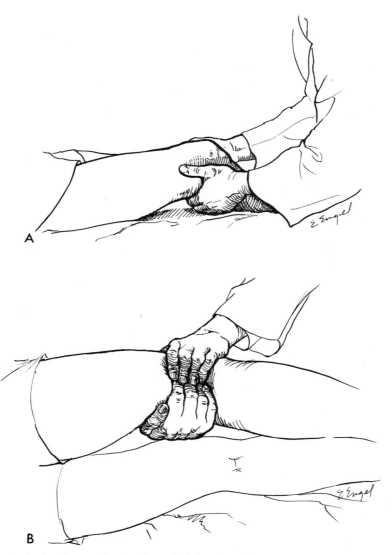

Fig. 4-36 The popliteal pulse, which lies lateral to the midline in the popliteal fossa, is palpated by flexing the knee slightly and by pressing the finger tips of the examiner's right hand firmly into the popliteal fossa with the fingers of the left hand. A, The position for the examination. B, View from behind the knee to show the position of the fingers.

To determine whether or not there is ankle edema, one presses the skin of the lower leg or ankle firmly against the bone with the tip of the index finger or thumb for about 5 seconds. A residual pit which can be both felt and seen indicates edema.

This completes the usual extremity examination, but the student should be prepared to expand his investigation when abnormalities are found. The screening examination then becomes focused and requires the application of special techniques to fully evaluate any abnormality. In the extremities, this is most pertinent to orthopedic or neurologic lesions.

When there is suspected *orthopedic disease*, all joints are carefully studied successively, with comparison of those on the right to those on the left. See Beetham et al. for a detailed description of the joint examination.[10] The muscles and joints of the hands, wrists, elbows, shoulders, feet, ankles, knees, and hips are first inspected, then palpated. The patient is next asked to move the affected joint through its full range of motion. If limitation is found, the examiner also tests passive joint movement by holding the limb above and below the given joint, and moving it through its full range of motion while the patient is asked to relax. Bony fixation, contracture, or muscle spasm may cause limitation of passive movement. The patient's face must also be observed for any indication of pain during such manipulation. Limitation of active and passive flexion, extension, abduction, adduction, or rotation are noted and are estimated in terms of the degrees of the arc of a circle. To do an adequate examination, the examiner will need to put the patient in various positions. For example, when testing for extension of the hip, one should place the patient on his side or on his abdomen. Study of gait and posture may require that the patient be fully undraped.

Further detailed inspection and palpation are required to study involuntary movements, muscle contour, fasciculations, tenderness, and tone.*

*Muscle strength** may be tested and compared by having the patient squeeze simultaneously with both hands, two or three of the fingers of the examiner's right and left hands. Rising from the lying to the sitting position tests the power of the trunk muscles. Leg and hip strength are observed as the patient stands on his toes and heels and rises from a squatting position. The in-bed patient may be asked to elevate one leg at a time, extended to about 45 degrees, and to hold the position for 15 to 20 seconds. Wobbling or drifting downward of the leg indicates weakness. At the same time, by placing his hand under the opposite heel,

---

[10]Beetham, W. P., Jr., Polley, H. F., Slocumb, C. H., and Weaver, W. F.: Physical Examination of the Joints. W. B. Saunders Co., Philadelphia and London, 1965.
*Part of the neurologic examination.

the examiner tests the extent to which the patient utilizes his other leg for leverage. When paralysis is of conversion origin, the normal leg is not used; whereas with organic paralysis, strong pressure is applied by the normal leg in an effort to raise the paralyzed limb. Patients who are weak and are unable to raise their entire leg may be asked to raise the knee while the examiner exerts counter pressure. Muscle power across each joint may be tested further by stabilizing the limb above the joint with one hand while the patient is requested to push against the other hand, which holds the limb below the joint as it is moved through its normal range of motion. Again, one limb should be compared with that on the opposite side. Strength may be graded 0 to 5.

0 No visible muscle contraction.
1 Contraction without joint movement.
2 Movement with gravity eliminated.
3 Ability to move against gravity.
4 Movement against gravity and some resistance.
5 Normal strength.

When weakness is detected, the involved muscles are carefully inspected for wasting, tenderness, tone, fasciculations, or unusual bulk.

Coordination and involuntary movements* are examined by noting how the patient moves his extremities spontaneously while he walks, takes off his clothes, buttons or unbuttons, or ties his shoelaces. The finger-to-nose test, described on p. 142 at the beginning of the examination of the upper extremities, is a good way to evaluate coordination in the upper extremities when the patient is in bed. Coordination of the legs may also be tested in the recumbent position by directing the patient to place the heel of one foot on the opposite knee and to run it slowly down the shin (heel-to-shin test).

Incoordination of the upper extremities with the patient sitting may be elicited by having him pat his thighs alternately with the palm and the back of both hands as rapidly as possible, or hold his hands in the air and rapidly pronate and supinate both forearms. Performance on the two sides is compared first with the patient's eyes open and then closed. To detect ataxia and incoordination involving the trunk and neck, one observes the patient's ability to sit up motionless without support. Coordination of the legs in the sitting position may be tested by asking the patient to rapidly tap the toes of one foot against the ground; then the toes of the other foot. Finally, the ability of the patient to stand motionless with feet together and eyes closed, is observed (Romberg's test).

Light touch, pain, and temperature sensations* are usually studied together. Light touch is tested by using a wisp of cotton or tissue, and pain by a straight pin or safety pin. The patient may be sitting or lying on

*Part of the neurologic examination.

his back. He is instructed to close his eyes (or avert his gaze) and to say "yes" whenever he feels the cotton touch his skin and "no" when he does not. The malingerer may say "no" when an allegedly anesthetic area is stimulated. Likewise, the patient should say "sharp" or "dull" when he feels the sharp or blunt end of the pin. In screening, each modality is tested separately. But when an area of sensory deficit is found, all sensory modalities should be checked, including the less important temperature sensation, by using hot and cold water in test tubes. In looking for a sensory deficit, the full length of each limb is tested, crossing all dermatomes. *Symmetrical areas of the right and left limbs must also be compared for minor differences.* If there is an area of impaired sensation, testing should move from decreased to normal sensation and back again. Care should be taken to detect a zone of hyperesthesia at the boundary between normal and decreased sensation. Also, when a sensory abnormality is suspected, the examination should be extended to check sensation of the trunk.

*Vibratory sensation** is tested by holding firmly the end of a 128 cycle-per-second tuning fork against bone in the distal hand and foot. The patient is asked to look away or to close his eyes and to tell what he feels. He should not only report a buzzing or vibratory sensation, but also be able to say when it stops as the examiner damps the tuning fork with his other hand. If the patient is unable to detect vibration distally, the test is repeated over bone at progressively more proximal locations of each extremity.

*Position sense** is tested by grasping the great toe of each foot at its sides. As the patient looks away, the digit is passively flexed and extended varying distances, the examiner being careful not to brush the neighboring toes. The patient is then asked to report the direction of the movement. The same procedure is repeated with the fingers.

*Cortical Function Tests.** A few simple tests may serve to test cortical sensory discrimination. Point localization is determined by touching an area of the body with a dull pointed object as the patient keeps his eyes closed. He is then asked to point to, but not to touch, the area of the body that was stimulated. A similar test is two point discrimination. A paper clip may be opened to provide two points whose distance may be varied like a caliper. Beginning with the two ends close together, they are simultaneously touched to the patient's skin and progressively spread until he can discriminate two points. Certain areas of the skin are more sensitive to small distances, such as the finger pads. Stereognosis is the ability to identify objects by touch. When the patient closes his eyes, different coins may be placed in each hand for him to identify. The extinction phenomenon tests the ability of the patient to detect two

---

*Part of the neurologic examination.

stimuli applied simultaneously to symmetrical areas of the body. In the presence of a parietal lobe lesion, he will not be aware of sensation on the side contralateral to the damaged lobe, even though sensation is present when that side is stimulated alone.

If the orthopedic or neurologic deficit is isolated and minor (for example, a frozen shoulder or diabetic neuropathy), the examination may be readily incorporated into the general physical examination at the time of the study of the extremities. If, on the other hand, there is suspicion that the deficit is widespread, it is usually better first to do the general physical examination and then return to do a complete orthopedic or neurologic examination. In such circumstances more extensive testing is indicated.

THE MALE EXTERNAL GENITAL EXAMINATION

Ambulatory

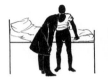

THE EXAMINER.   *Standing before the patient and slightly to his right.*

THE PATIENT.   *Standing, facing the examiner.*

Bed-bound

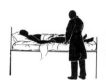

THE EXAMINER.   *Standing at the right side of the bed.*

THE PATIENT.   *Lying on his back.*

The techniques used are inspection and palpation.

The genitalia and surrounding skin are first inspected for any bulges, ulcerations, irregularities, or asymmetry.

The examiner may begin by gently feeling the scrotum. Each hemiscrotum is examined and compared, using one hand to feel the testis, epididymis, and spermatic cord. The presence of fluid around each testis may be looked for at this point; and if present, it should be confirmed by transillumination (this is a diffuse illumination of the underlying fluid-containing tissue when the light of a pocket flashlight is pressed against the organ in a darkened room). Note is next taken of the size, consistency, smoothness of contour, sensitivity, and position of the scrotal structures. Testes are usually smooth, approximately 4 cm. long, and somewhat sensitive to mild pressure, which is felt as a deep "visceral" type of discomfort. The epididymis is found posterolaterally; it is smooth and closely attached to the testis with a palpable sulcus between. The spermatic cord is felt between the thumb and forefinger. It is of variable thickness and contains the vas deferens, which is normally smooth without beading. Any varicosities, spermatic cysts, or other masses are carefully examined.

The penis is next palpated gently but firmly. First, the presence or absence of a foreskin is determined. If present, the foreskin is retracted and the adequacy of the preputial orifice is noted. The entire glans is inspected, especially for the size and position of the urethral meatus and for the character of any urethral discharge. Scars on the glans or in the coronal sulcus are noted, and the foreskin is replaced if it was retracted. The penile shaft is palpated, as is the penile urethra, noting any deviation from the normally smooth contours of each. The perineum is palpated as a continuation of the urethral examination.

When the patient is ambulatory and standing, this is the most convenient time to check for hernias. As the student observes the inguinal and femoral regions, the patient is asked to bear down, which increases intra-abdominal pressure. Any suspicious bulge is palpated as the patient strains. This is the method used in the female examination. In the male, one checks further for inguinal hernias by examining each inguinal canal. Such a procedure is uncomfortable; the examiner should be gentle and the patient forewarned. In order to enter the canal, the index finger is placed on the low scrotum and loose skin is carried up and invaginated into the inguinal canal. One first feels the external inguinal ring, then enters the inguinal canal by following the spermatic cord. Four or 5 cm. in from the external ring, one should feel the internal ring

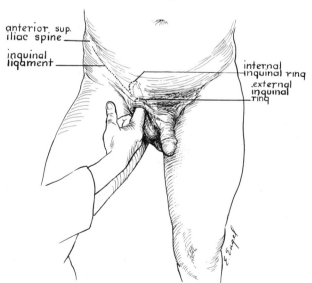

Fig. 4-37 To examine for a right inguinal hernia, the right index finger picks up loose skin low in the scrotum and advances through the external inguinal ring toward the internal inguinal ring.

posteriorly with the pad of the finger tip. The patient is then asked to cough or bear down, the latter being more helpful, as it produces a sustained intraabdominal pressure. A bulge is felt at the finger tip or a soft mass may enter the canal if herniation is present. The same procedure can be carried out with the patient lying in bed, but it is less accurate.

THE PELVIC EXAMINATION

Ambulatory

THE EXAMINER. *Sitting on a stool facing the perineum, and standing for part of the examination.*

THE PATIENT. *Lying on her back on an examining table with both knees flexed and her feet in stirrups.*

Bed-bound

THE EXAMINER. *The same.*

THE PATIENT. *Lying on her back obliquely across the bed, with both legs flexed.*

The techniques used are inspection and palpation.

The pelvic examination done with the patient in bed is much less satisfactory than the one performed on an examining table. If the patient is too ill to be moved to the proper table, she should lie obliquely across the bed; her buttocks are elevated by pillows or an inverted bedpan covered with a blanket.

Because a nurse or attendant must be present during a pelvic examination, the student will be wise to prepare in advance for such assistance. When he approaches the end of the general examination, he may excuse himself to check with the head nurse as to the availability of the examining table and an assistant to prepare the patient. The pelvic examination may have to be scheduled at a different time. If the patient is also to be examined by another physician, arrangements should be made to do the examination together, so that the patient does not have to be prepared twice.

Indications.   The examination of the female reproductive system is an integral part of the general physical examination in the patient who is not a virgin. Where gynecologic abnormality is suspected, the genitalia of virgins are also examined, either by a rectal-abdominal approach or by the introduction of just one finger into the vagina when the hymen permits such penetration without undue pain.

Some women prefer to defer a routine pelvic examination when they are menstruating, and it is reasonable to do so. However, there is no medical reason to contraindicate the examination in the presence of menses. Indeed, if the menstrual flow is abnormal, there may be special reason to examine the patient at this time.

General Considerations. Relaxation of the abdominal muscles is essential for an accurate examination of the female reproductive tract. Not infrequently, unresolved, and perhaps unrecognized, patient apprehension may interfere with the relaxation of the abdominal muscles. The resultant muscle spasm and behavior of the patient during the examination may even mislead the examiner to believe that organic disease is present. Consequently, the ability of the examiner to secure maximum patient cooperation is of first importance. This ability depends on the following specific points:

The introduction of the examination. The student may begin the examination by saying, "I feel it is important to do an internal examination, and the nurse will help you prepare for this." The patient may be asked whether she has had a pelvic examination before, and from her answer one gains some impression of her attitude or concerns about such an examination. If the patient expresses any fears or doubts, the student should carefully explain what he is going to do, that he will not hurt her, and that the internal examination is an important part of the physical evaluation. Rarely will a patient refuse under these circumstances. If she does, her refusal and its underlying reasons may provide important clues to the existence of certain medical or psychological problems.

Preparation of the patient. The student should leave the room while the patient is being prepared. The nurse or female attendant conducts the patient to the lavatory and instructs her to empty her bladder. Ideally she should also have had a recent evacuation of her bowels. She is then asked to disrobe completely and to put on a loose hospital gown. The patient is helped onto the table and her feet are placed in the stirrups. The abdomen and lower extremities are then draped in such a way as to expose only the perineal area, which is covered with a towel until the examiner returns to the room. He removes the towel covering the external genitalia and procedes with the examination. At its conclusion, the student again covers the external genitalia with a towel and leaves the room while the patient is dressing.

The attendant. The presence of a nurse or female attendant is mandatory, and under no circumstances should a pelvic examination be undertaken without such chaperonage. In addition to its obvious legal implications, the nurse's presence further enhances the professional atmosphere that should surround such an examination.

Her attitude should reflect a concern for the comfort and privacy of the patient, and she should be fully capable of assisting the physician. An able attendant is often of great assistance in putting the patient at ease during the examination.

In conducting the examination, the student should proceed in a professional manner, focusing attention at all times upon the patient and the examination. It is not the place for small talk or witticisms that may be acceptable in a social setting. This is so even though the patient's superficial attitude appears to encourage such an approach. It is also unwise to focus the patient's attention upon the examination by repetitive and leading questions as to whether she is, or is not, experiencing pain. If there is pain, it will usually be indicated verbally or by the patient's facial expression.

During the course of the examination, the student should be alert to indications that the patient may be poorly relaxed or apprehensive. Such signs include tensing of the abdominal muscles, contraction of the gluteal muscles, gripping the sides of the examining table, distressed facial expressions, or apparent tenderness in regions not ordinarily painful. For example, gentle pressure just inside the introitus should not cause pain. In instances where the patient is not relaxed, it may help to instruct her to fold her arms across her chest and to breathe deeply and slowly. She may be complimented on how she is trying to relax and encouraged to relax just a little more. A few women for whom the examination is a psychologically disturbing experience may never be able to relax.

The Technique of the Pelvic Examination. This is best learned by demonstration and performance under supervision. Learning will be enhanced by reading a detailed, illustrated description of the technique before and after performing the first pelvic examination. Also, while doing the examination, the student should mentally visualize the anatomic relationships of the pelvis. The general order of such an examination is as follows:

Initial preparation by the examiner. He checks that an adequate spotlight is present and that needed equipment, such as the speculum and cytology slides, is at hand. He puts on a glove and sees that the speculum is warmed under running water. A reassuring word may be given the patient as the examination begins.

The external genitalia are inspected. The patient is asked to spread her knees apart, and the labia are opened with the gloved thumb and fingers. Structures to be noted are the pubic hair, labia, clitoris, introitus, urethral orifice, perineal area, and the anus. One specifically looks for scars, ulceration, inflammation, discoloration, masses, and discharges.

Testing fascial support. The patient is asked to take a deep breath and to bear down. The student notes if there is bulging of the anterior vaginal wall (cystocele), bulging of the posterior vaginal wall (rectocele), or descent of the cervix toward the introitus (prolapse).

Examination of the vagina and cervix using a speculum. The speculum is introduced very gently with the blades closed and with pressure exerted toward the posterior vaginal wall. The instrument is inserted obliquely and then turned when in the vagina so that the short blade faces anteriorly. The speculum should not be opened until it is fully inserted; and when closed, care must be taken not to pinch vaginal tissue. It should be noted that the cervix usually points posteriorly. Water, preferably, is used to lubricate the speculum when specimens are taken from the vagina or cervix for cytology, microscopic study, or culture. After the specimen is obtained, the entire vaginal surface, cervix, and os are inspected for abnormalities: color, erosions, masses, swelling, discharge, and bleeding.

Bimanual examination. This is done by introducing the index and third fingers of the gloved hand into the vagina with the fingers of the opposite hand pressing down the patient's lower abdomen. The abdominal muscles must be sufficiently relaxed so that the abdominal hand may manipulate the organs downward in the pelvis to make them accessible to examination by the fingers in the vagina. The size, shape, consistency, mobility, and tenderness of the following structures are determined: the cervix, fundus, fallopian tubes (palpable only if abnormal), ovaries, general adnexal areas bilaterally, and the cul-de-sac. It should be emphasized that pelvic masses, not originating from the genital organs, may be felt and tenderness elicited. An example would be an inflamed appendix presenting in the pelvis.

The rectovaginal examination. This examination may be done with the index finger in the vagina and the next finger in the rectum. The

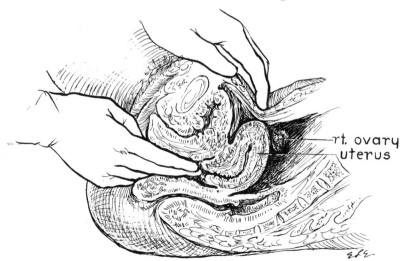

Fig. 4-38 Bimanual palpation of the uterus. The fundus is felt with the fingers of the left hand pressing the lower abdomen inward while the index and third fingers of the right hand press against the cervix to move the uterus toward the left hand. Note that the ovary can also be felt with bimanual palpation as the fingers of the right hand are advanced high in the vagina in each lateral fornix.

fingers palpate the rectovaginal septum and the area of the cul-de-sac, searching for masses. At the same time, the opposite hand presses down on the lower abdomen.

THE RECTAL EXAMINATION

Ambulatory

THE EXAMINER.   *Standing, facing the buttocks.*
THE PATIENT.   *Bending at the hips over the bed or examining table. In the female, done in the position of the pelvic examination.*

Bed-bound

THE EXAMINER.   *Standing at the right side of the bed.*
THE PATIENT.   *Lying on his left side with both legs flexed at the hip.*

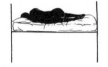

The techniques used are inspection and palpation.

If the patient is very ill and bedridden, he may be turned on one side with his back to the examiner and both legs flexed at the hip. However, a more thorough examination is done by having the male patient bend over the examining table. The more flexion there is, the flatter the buttocks become and the less tissue there is between the examining hand and the anal canal. This position makes the internal study of the pelvis easier for the physician and less uncomfortable for the patient. In the female, the rectal examination usually follows the pelvic examination, with the patient supine on the examining table, her feet in stirrups.

To begin the rectal examination, the student puts on a clean glove and spreads the patient's buttocks. The perineum, anus, the perianal area, and the region of the pilonidal sinus are inspected. Skin color, pigmentation, erosions, edema, fissures, inflammation, or masses are noted. The location of hemorrhoids may be described in terms of the hour hand of a clock, with 12 o'clock toward the pubic symphysis, whether the patient is in the supine or prone position.

The examiner then adequately lubricates his gloved index finger; and after telling the patient what he is about to do, he introduces this finger slowly and gently into the anus with a slight rotary motion. If the patient is asked to bear down when the finger is in the anal canal, the sphincter will relax. While introducing the finger into the rectum, the examiner pays particular attention to the anus and its sphincter tone, to the anal canal, and to the crypts lining the initial 2 or 3 cm. of the anal canal. Note is made of any masses, areas of tenderness, any cord-like structures indicative of thrombosed internal hemorrhoids, or the expression of blood or pus.

In the male, the lobes of the prostate are easily palpated. Their consistency, which is normally firm, should be noted. The size of the prostate is estimated by the number of times it exceeds normal, or its width is determined by the number of fingerbreadths across. The borders of the prostate are palpated to determine whether they are smooth, irregular, well-demarcated, or merged with the perirectal tissue. The median groove is described as being present, shallow, or absent; and the prominence of each lateral lobe is noted. Tenderness of the prostate itself must be differentiated from the general discomfort of the rectal examination. Any increase in the amount of discomfort as the gland is touched or compressed indicates prostatic tenderness. Nodules of the prostate are described as to location and consistency (soft, firm, or hard). The seminal vesicles are not palpable unless they are diseased. Ordinarily, one does not feel resistance or discrete masses above the prostate.

Finally, with the finger introduced as far as possible into the rectum,

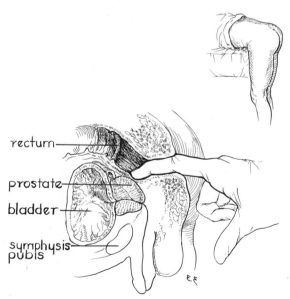

rectum

prostate

bladder

symphysis
pubis

Fig. 4-39 The prostate is palpated during the rectal examination with the pad of the right index finger. The gland lies anteriorly and is felt as a firm slightly compressible structure with two lateral lobes and a median furrow.

the examiner feels for masses as he rotates his forearm and sweeps his finger around the rectal circumference. In the female, the cervix is usually felt anteriorly through the wall as an extrinsic mass. If the patient is able, he should be asked to strain and even squat down so that the examiner may feel for a mass high in the rectum. When there are symptoms suggestive of rectal disease, examination in the squatting position is important in the female as well as the male. A fecal bolus is differentiated from a polyp or a tumor in that it is freely movable and is not attached to the rectal wall. To conclude the rectal examination, the student slowly withdraws his finger. Any stool present on the glove is inspected and then spread on filter paper to be tested for blood.

An anoscope may be introduced if lesions in the anal canal are suspected, such as internal hemorrhoids. It is easiest to insert the anoscope when the patient is in the knee-chest position and no special preparation is required.

Following the completion of the rectal examination, the patient is offered a tissue to wipe himself. The examiner washes his hands, disposes of his glove in the proper receptacle, and steps out of the room, giving the patient the opportunity to wash and dress himself.

THE NEUROLOGIC EXAMINATION

The basic neurologic examination is incorporated into the general examination as has been described in the preceding pages (See General Inspection, the Head, the Back, the Abdomen, and Extremities, where the parts of the neurologic examination have been marked with an asterisk.)

When the patient's problem is primarily a neurologic one, as when he has a stroke, multiple sclerosis, or a spinal cord lesion, a detailed comprehensive neurologic examination should be done after the general physical examination. The order of the examination roughly follows the outline of the neurologic examination in Chapter 5. Because the full neurologic examination is highly detailed, the student should refer to other texts for a complete description of techniques.[11-13]

THE MENTAL STATUS EXAMINATION

A screening mental status examination is indicated when the patient's behavior is abnormal, and it is usually performed during the

---

[11]Bastron, J. A., and other members of the Sections of Neurology and Physiology at the Mayo Clinic: Clinical Examinations in Neurology. W. B. Saunders Co., Philadelphia and London, 1963.

[12]DeJong, R. N.: The Neurologic Examination. The Hoeber Medical Division of Harper & Row Publishers, Inc., New York, 1967.

[13]Denny-Brown, D.: Handbook of Neurologic Examination and Case Recording. Harvard University Press, Cambridge, 1962.

course of the interview. (See Chapter 3.) Occasionally, however, abnormal behavior may not become apparent until the time of the physical examination. Under such circumstances a brief mental status examination should be carried out at the end of the examination. Tact is required lest the patient be offended or embarrassed by too obvious an exposure of his mental incapacities.

If the patient seems *confused* or has difficulty following directions, the student may begin by saying "You seem a little drowsy. Is it difficult for you to understand the directions?" If the patient answers "Yes," he should be reassured that it is often difficult to remember things when one is ill. Questions asked about sleep, drowsiness, and the patient's ability to keep up with his daily activities may lead to more direct questions about memory. "Have you had any trouble with your memory recently?" If carried out with adequate appreciation of the patient's sensitivities and need for reassurance, more formal testing then becomes possible. "I'd like to check how your memory is right now." At this point the student may begin to inquire into the patient's orientation, recent memory, and ability to carry out simple calculations such as the serial subtraction of 3's or 7's from 100.

If the patient appears *depressed* or withdrawn, the student should not hesitate to ask directly "You seem depressed (or 'down in the dumps'). Is that so?" Depressed patients will usually acknowledge their depression and may welcome an opportunity to discuss their problems. Further elaboration should be encouraged.

Bizarre behavior requires systematic study by the student. He should be alert to peculiar gestures, inappropriate smiling, or facetious comments. If the patient appears to be responding to voices or visions, he should be asked what he hears or what he sees. Mental abnormality may be suggested when the patient becomes inexplicably angry or agitated during certain parts of the examination; when he appears suspicious and questions the examiner's motives; or when he appears detached, as if in a trance. Signs of extreme agitation, of a catatonic stupor, or of hysteria may occasionally develop during the physical examination. When syncope or a seizure is due to hysteria (conversion), the patient will demonstrate atypical findings, such as limpness, fluttering of the eyelids, irregular movements, or unconsciousness, without other physiologic changes.

For further details about a more formal mental status examination, the student is referred to a textbook of psychiatry.

THE PHYSICAL EXAMINATION UNDER SPECIAL CIRCUMSTANCES

The method and order of examining and positioning the patient described in this chapter assume that the physical examination is done under ideal circumstances. More often than not, with a seriously ill patient, these ideal conditions will not exist. He may be too ill to communicate or too weak even to sit up. Under such difficult conditions, the student does his best to be as thorough as possible. He can often do a fairly complete examination if he takes his time and particularly if he has assistance in supporting or moving the patient. The student must learn to be flexible, to adjust his examination to the special circumstances, and not to sacrifice good technique because the patient is unable to cooperate. Examples of how to do the physical examination under special conditions are described in the following section.

The Emergency Examination

When the patient has an acute and urgent problem, it is important to approach the abbreviated physical examination with deliberate speed. The interview, physical examination, laboratory work, and therapy are initiated almost simultaneously. For example, if a patient comes in with massive upper gastrointestinal bleeding, a quick general inspection is made, vital signs are noted, and the patient may be put in a head-down position because of shock. Blood is drawn for the hematocrit and crossmatch, while an intravenous drip is started. In the critical situation, only the highlights of the history are taken from the patient or family, usually as the doctor checks the patient at the bedside. It usually takes 5 to 10 minutes to obtain the pertinent highlights of the present illness. (See Chapter 3, "The Approach To The Medical Interview," under "The Brief Interview With Limited Goals.") An abbreviated general physical examination is done in which the examiner searches particularly for clues as to the etiology of such conditions as gastrointestinal bleeding or congestive heart failure and for resulting complications, such as shock. Jaundice, spider angiomas, or an enlarged liver may point to cirrhosis. Pallor, cold clammy skin, tachycardia, and low blood pressure would indicate shock. Evidence of pulmonary congestion, neck vein distention, or a gallop rhythm would be a sign of congestive heart failure that might be precipitated by the hemorrhage.

When the situation has stabilized and the patient has been treated adequately, there will be time to go back and get a fuller history and to do a more detailed physical examination. *Even though there is great urgency and the lesion is obvious, the general format of the interview and physical exam should be conscientiously followed, regardless of how abbreviated.* If the student does not approach the problem in a deliberate and systematic manner, he will miss abnormalities, treat the patient poorly, and eventually waste more time. For example, it is perfectly proper to direct one's attention first to the leg in an older man who fell and fractured a femur, but the general physical examination must also be done; otherwise, the doctor may miss an enlarged, tumor-laden liver which points to the possibility of a pathologic fracture, or the slow pulse of complete heart block which may explain why the patient fell in the first place.

The Uncooperative Patient

There are some patients who are unable and others who are unwilling to cooperate during the physical examination. It is important to differentiate between the two. The former include delirious and demented patients who have difficulty understanding what is expected of them. Ordinarily the patient's defect in attention will have been recognized during the interview; but sometimes it first becomes obvious during the physical examination, as when the patient proves to be incapable of carrying out the examiner's instructions. For example, he may perseverate by continuing to carry out the preceding instructions despite new directions, such as persisting to stick out his tongue when asked to bite down. When such is the case, a rapid check for cognitive defects is indicated. If such defects are present, the examiner must word his directions in the simplest terms possible, with repetition or demonstration utilized as needed.

Refusal to cooperate may have many different origins. An occasional patient refuses the entire examination; others balk at some part. The latter situation most often indicates fear, shame, or embarrassment. Encouraging the patient to express his feelings may often reveal a source of concern that turns out to be quite unrealistic. The examiner should give appropriate reassurance and proceed with the examination in a considerate manner. At times, it may be necessary to delay part of the examination in order to give the patient an opportunity to work through his feelings. One may then return to the troublesome region at the end of the examination or at a later time if delay is permissible.

The patient who absolutely refuses to be examined presents a more complex problem, especially for the student. Sometimes the refusal is based on a misunderstanding of the student's role on the ward. If the patient does not respond to an explanation, the student should seek the assistance of the resident or the attending physician to resolve the difficulty. Often such a patient is emotionally disturbed. Discreet exploration of the issue with him may reveal the irrational anger or fear of the paranoid, the hopeless resignation of the psychotically depressed, the overactive distractibility of the manic, the disordered thinking of the schizophrenic, or the guarding of the malingerer.

Not to be overlooked, however, are cultural determinants, including language difficulties, that influence the occasional patient who is unfamiliar with medical and hospital procedures. If the patient refuses the physical examination because of a language barrier, it may be very helpful to call on a family member to explain the procedure to the patient.

The Patient in Coma

The general examination of a comatose patient does not differ from that of the usual patient, except that it is obviously done in the absence of patient cooperation and must be done with dispatch in order to give the patient prompt care. As soon as the comatose patient reaches the hospital, certain vital functions demand immediate attention even though the cause of coma remains uncertain. Temperature, pulse, respiration, and blood pressure are immediately taken and recorded. Attention is directed especially to the state of the airway, the circulation, and the possibility of a low blood sugar level.

1. The rate, depth, and rhythm of respirations should be noted. Evidence of airway obstruction is sought for carefully. It is manifested by cyanosis, stertorous breathing, and retraction of intercostal spaces.

2. The circulatory status is evaluated immediately by checking the heart rate and particularly the blood pressure for the presence of hypotension or severe hypertension. Signs of peripheral vascular collapse may be seen. These are: pallor, tachycardia, peripheral cyanosis, sweating, and cool skin.

3. Extremely low blood sugar levels, even for short periods of time, can lead to irreversible brain damage. There may be no physical signs pointing to hypoglycemia, and the only clue will be that the patient is a diabetic taking insulin or hypoglycemic agents. If the drop in blood sugar has been abrupt, there may be signs similar to shock that are compatible with catecholamine release: pallor, tachycardia, sweating, and cool, moist skin.

After the above vital problems have been considered and checked, the student is ready to do a more systematic examination. It is rare that no history is available. Information usually can be obtained from the people accompanying the patient, such as relatives, ambulance attendants, the private physician, and the police, or from hospital records, medical alert medallions or cards carried by the patient. It is important to learn what drugs the patient takes, if there has been trauma, a preceding infection, or ingestion of alcohol. The nature of his occupation and place of work may suggest possible exposure to noxious chemicals. The rapidity of onset may be an important clue to etiology. Past illnesses are also important: convulsive disorders, diabetes, hypertension, coronary heart disease, previous gastrointestinal bleeding, renal disease, previous head trauma, alcoholism, narcotic addiction, or psychiatric problems. Among young adults, suicide attempts with drugs are an extremely common reason for coma.

Observation is of particular importance. The student must study the patient thoroughly for any possible clue to disease, and he should be constantly thinking of possible underlying causes. The patient's general appearance is noted, his color, posture, spontaneous movements, and breathing pattern. Very deep breathing, for instance, may suggest diabetic or renal acidosis; and very depressed respiration, drug intoxication. The odor of a patient's breath is a useful clue to diagnosis. One may smell acetone, alcohol, paraldehyde, or fetor hepaticus. Signs of injury anywhere raise the possibility of head trauma. Blood behind an eardrum or spinal fluid leaking from the nose may indicate a skull fracture. Other neurologic signs, such as facial asymmetry, puffing out of one cheek with respiration, saliva drooling from one side of the mouth, or tongue deviation, suggest an organic brain lesion. Evidence that the tongue has been bitten points to a convulsive seizure.

Examination involving all the physical diagnosis techniques proceeds in a logical order, with special emphasis on the likely causes of coma. Such an evaluation need not be time consuming, but is essential before moving on to laboratory or therapeutic considerations. The arms and thighs are examined for needle punctures (diabetes or drug addiction). Lacerations, ecchymoses, and petechiae may be clues to an injury or a bleeding defect. The eyes are carefully studied for pupil inequality, absent reaction to light, dysconjugate movement, nystagmus, or impaired corneal reflex. The fundus should be examined for hemorrhage or papilledema. Asymmetry of facial movement is noted.

The neck is checked for resistance to passive flexion that would be compatible with meningeal irritation, as with meningitis or subarachnoid hemorrhage.

Particular attention is directed to the cardiovascular system, including the heart rate, rhythm, bruits over the carotid vessels, and murmurs.

Spontaneous muscle movements, strength, tone, and resistance to passive stretch are studied. Differences in tone or strength of muscles on either side may be brought out by raising and simultaneously dropping both arms or the flexed legs. The deep tendon reflexes are speedily evaluated. The plantar responses are checked for the abnormal extensor reflex (Babinski sign). Movements can be elicited at times by a noxious stimulus, such as sticking the patient with a pin, by pressing firmly over the upper medial orbital ridges or the sternum, and by squeezing the Achilles tendon. Failure to respond at all to such maneuvers indicates deep coma. In lesser degrees of coma, unequal responses of the face or limbs may suggest a neurologic defect that should be observed. Sometimes the patient will grimace even though there is no other body movement.

Stimuli to evoke pain, for instance, two pins, should also be tested simultaneously on the right and left sides to bring out neurologic differences. Since the patient is unable to protect himself, the student must be careful not to harm him during these maneuvers.

Inaccessible areas should not be forgotten during the examination. For example, the patient should be turned to one side to look for infected bed sores in the sacral area or a possible gluteal abscess caused by prior intramuscular injections.

Finally, the student must make certain that the patient does not harm himself after the examination is completed. Instruments or pins should not be left in the bed; the patient may need an attendant to watch him, and the side rails should be raised so he will not fall out of bed.

For a fuller consideration of the study of patients with coma, the student is referred to the monograph of Plum and Posner.[14]

The Immobilized Patient

There will be many instances when the student must examine a patient who is immobilized; for example, when the patient is in traction, is in the postoperative state, has severe pain on moving, is severely debilitated, or is attached to respirators and suctioning equipment.

If the student plans his order of examination and moves with deliberate speed, he can usually do a thorough exam without undue distress to the patient. It may be wise to examine him following pain medication, if pain is severe, and to seek assistance from an attendant or nurse when moving him. Often, if the patient is told what position is needed, he will prefer to move himself rather than be moved. The house staff or physician-in-charge should be asked whether it is safe to temporarily turn off a respirator or suction equipment.

The usual order of examination may have to be changed for the immobilized patient, but the student should be able to do a thorough study, including that of inaccessible areas. For example, the paralyzed patient can be carefully turned on one side to inspect the sacral area and back of his heels for pressure point skin breakdown and ulceration. Following recent abdominal surgery, the patient may be assisted in sitting up so that the student may properly examine the posterior lung fields. One should not attempt to palpate or listen through the bandages. This

---

[14]Plum, F., and Posner, J. B.: The Diagnosis of Stupor and Coma. F. A. Davis Co., Philadelphia, 1966.

is highly inaccurate; and if an examination is indicated, study should be directed to the area adjacent to the bandages, or the bandages should be temporarily removed after the student receives permission from the resident or surgeon-in-charge.

The Patient in Isolation

If a patient has an infectious disease, he may be put in a single room on "precautions" so as not to spread the infectious organism to the ward personnel or other patients. In special instances, as in the case of agranulocytosis or extensive burns, he will be placed on "reverse precautions," to avoid exposure to infection. Here, the hospital staff will wear masks and gowns so as not to transmit to the patient any organisms they may be carrying.

The isolation procedure is as follows: Before entering the room, the student checks to see what examining instruments are already in the patient's room. If other instruments are needed, such as his stethoscope and flashlight, he selects these. He then washes he hands outside of the room, takes off his white coat and puts on a gown and mask. He makes sure his back is completely covered by securing the ties at the neck and waist. Carrying the necessary instruments, he enters the room and places them on clean paper toweling on the bedside table. If equipment is used for diagnostic tests, it is left in the patient's room after being used and will be picked up later to be sterilized by the ward personnel.

During the patient examination, the student should take special care to avoid contaminated secretions. It is very important to educate the patient in the management of infectious sputum. If he is coughing, he should be told to cough into a tissue or cloth and to turn his head away when breathing deeply. Following the examination, the student uses the sink in the room to wash his hands, the head of his stethoscope, and other instruments that have become contaminated. He should untie the waist band of his gown before going to the sink. After washing, he holds the handles of the taps with paper toweling to turn them off. He may now untie the relatively uncontaminated neck straps of the gown. The gown is then removed by grasping it on the inner uncontaminated side and by rolling it off with the inner clean side kept exposed. It is then dropped in the room hamper. The mask is removed by holding its straps and dropping it in the wastebasket. The student should use a clean paper towel to open the closed door, disposing of the towel as he leaves. Before putting on his coat, he should again wash his hands at a clean outer sink.

References

Bastron, J. A., and other members of the Sections of Neurology and Physiology at the Mayo Clinic: Clinical Examinations in Neurology. W. B. Saunders Co., Philadelphia and London, 1963.

Beetham, W. P., Jr., Polley, H. F., Slocumb, C. H., and Weaver, W. F.: Physical Examination of the Joints. W. B. Saunders Co., Philadelphia, 1965.

DeJong, R. N.: The Neurologic Examination. The Hoeber Medical Division of Harper & Row Publishers, Inc., New York, 1967.

Delman, A. J.: Hemodynamic Correlates of Cardiovascular Sounds. *In* De Graff, A. C., Ed.: Annual Review of Medicine. Annual Reviews, Inc., California, 1967, Vol. 18, p. 139.

Denny-Brown, D.: Handbook of Neurologic Examination and Case Recording. Harvard University Press, Cambridge, 1962.

Haagensen, C. D.: Carcinoma of the Breast. American Cancer Society, Inc., New York, 1958.

Kirkendall, W. M., Burton, A. C., Epstein, F. H., and Freis, E. D.: Recommendations for Human Blood Pressure Determination by Sphygmomanometers. Circulation, *36:* 980, 1967.

Leatham, A.: Auscultation of the Heart. Lancet, *2:*703 and 757, 1958.

Plum, F., and Posner, J. B.: The Diagnosis of Stupor and Coma. F. A. Davis Co., Philadelphia, 1966.

Chapter 5

THE MEDICAL RECORD

In the written medical record, the physician describes the patient's present and past state of health and analyzes his illness in terms of diagnosis and prognosis. In subsequent notes he records the course of the illness, consultant opinions, results of laboratory tests, procedures, and the patient's response to treatment. The primary purpose of the medical record is to document the medical experience of the patient. This information will be used by those concerned with the patient's current and future care. Occasionally, the record may serve in a scientific case study. Legally, it is a public document, available to other physicians, to the court by subpoena, and to insurance companies with the written permission of the patient. *Neither the patient himself nor his visitors have access to the medical record.*

Careful thought should go into every written note. A clear picture of the patient and his illness is given for the benefit of later physicians, including a concise, accurate, and clearly-written history. Sentences are complete and abbreviations are sparingly used, since they are subject to misinterpretation or may become obsolete with time. Proper consideration for confidential material given in the personal and social history is mandatory, because the written history is, legally, public information. The physician's personal emotions should not be written into the record, regardless of how he feels toward the patient. Implied criticism of the patient, or of other physicians, is inappropriate. Opinions should be dispassionate; they should include accurate descriptions, not moral judgments.

All notes are written in ink or typed, with the patient's name and unit number recorded in the upper right hand corner of each page. Every entry is dated and signed by the person who writes the note. A special effort is made to keep the records readily available. On the hospital floor, they are kept in a chart rack in the physicians' or head nurse's office. A record should not be removed from the ward except when it accompanies the patient to a distant area for rounds, consultation, or therapy. It is then signed out by notifying the head nurse or ward secretary. It is inadvisable to permit patients to look at their own records; and when a record accompanies the patient to another hospital area, he should not be given an opportunity to read it. After the patient has been discharged, the record is promptly returned to the Record Room.

THE ORGANIZATION OF THE MEDICAL RECORD

As soon as possible after admission, preferably within 24 hours, the patient's chart should contain the following items which constitute the initial work-up:

1. The History
2. The Physical Examination
3. Admission Laboratory Data
4. Diagnosis
5. Prognosis
6. Plan of Study
7. Plan of Management

See the Outline of the Case Write-up in Table 5-1, which gives the detailed organization of the initial work-up.

TABLE 5-1. AN OUTLINE OF THE CASE WRITE-UP

I. THE HISTORY
   A. Identifying data
   B. Source and reliability of the history
   C. Present illness
       This section of the history is written in narrative form beginning with an orienting statement about the patient's past health; followed by a general description of the present illness; and ending with a concluding paragraph, including pertinent positive and negative information, medications and treatment, weight, and the degree of disability.
   D. Past health
       1. General health
       2. Childhood health
       3. Adult health
           a. Medical Illnesses
           b. Surgical Procedures
           c. Psychiatric Illnesses
           d. Obstetrical History
       4. Accidents and injuries
       5. Allergies and immunizations
   E. Family health
       A family tree is diagrammed and accompanied by a paragraph giving the details of family illnesses, including pertinent negative information.
   F. Personal and Social History
       This section of the history is written in narrative form and includes: (1) Current life situation (home and family; present occupation and economic status; social and community commitments; leisure activities; personal characteristics and pattern of living); (2) Past development (childhood and adolescence; educational and occupational history; marital and family history).

TABLE 5-1. AN OUTLINE OF THE CASE WRITE-UP *(Continued)*

    G. Systems review
        1. Skin
        2. Hematopoietic system
        3. Head and face
        4. Ears
        5. Eyes
        6. Nose and sinuses
        7. Mouth, pharynx, and larynx
        8. Breasts
        9. Respiratory tract
      10. Cardiovascular system
      11. Gastrointestinal system
      12. Urinary tract
      13. Genital tract (male) (female)
      14. Skeletal system
      15. Nervous system
      16. Endocrine system
      17. Psychological status
II. THE PHYSICAL EXAMINATION
    A. Reliability and completeness
    B. General description of the patient
    C. Vital signs
    D. Skin, hair, and nails
    E. Lymphatic system
    F. The head (skull, face, eyes, ears, nose, mouth and pharynx)
    G. Neck
    H. Breasts
    I. Thorax and lungs
    J. Cardiovascular system (heart, peripheral vascular system)
    K. Abdomen
    L. Genitalia (male) (female)
    M. Rectum
    N. The skeletal system
    O. The neurologic examination (general status, cranial nerves, motor system, sensory system, reflexes, spinal nerve irritation)
    P. The mental status examination (behavior, cognitive function, thought content, perception, affect and mood)
III. ADMISSION LABORATORY DATA
IV. DIAGNOSIS
    The section on diagnosis includes the identification of abnormal findings, the interpretation of these findings, and the differential diagnosis of disease, concluding with a list of all diseases affecting the patient.
V. PROGNOSIS
    One writes a paragraph describing the patient's prognosis, including an estimation of the severity of the patient's illness, the expected efficacy of treatment, and the predicted outcome of the illness.
VI. PLAN OF STUDY
    Each major disease requiring study is indicated in a separate paragraph with the relevant tests and procedures that are planned, including chemical determinations, roentgenographic and isotopic studies, microbiologic and immunologic studies, electrographic studies, endoscopic studies, cytologic and pathologic studies, other special tests, and consultation.
VII. PLAN OF MANAGEMENT
    The overall plan of management for each major disease is indicated in separate paragraphs and includes: activity, diet, and fluids; special procedures; special services; drug therapy; surgical treatment; patient education; and preventive medicine.

Usually the patient will reach the hospital floor with a brief note written by the emergency department house officer or by the patient's private physician. Included in this note is a preliminary diagnosis, as well as an account of any treatment or investigation which may already have been initiated. The more complete notes of the ward house officer and of the student will be written shortly after admission. The student's goal should be to complete the seven parts of the write-up within 24 hours of first seeing the patient. When a student is just beginning his clinical experience, he will require a longer time. In all cases, the write-up must be completed before the case is presented to the attending physician.

After this admission work-up, the record will be composed of notes describing the patient's hospital experience:

8. The Patient's Hospital Course
   a. *Progress notes.* These notes describe changes in the patient's symptoms or physical findings during hospitalization and any revision in diagnosis, plan of study, or plan of management.
   b. *Diagnostic or surgical procedure notes.*
   c. *Notes by consultants.*
   d. *End-of-service note.* This is a summary by the house officer or student who leaves the service before the patient is discharged.
   e. *The final note.*

The various sections of the written medical record will now be discussed.

THE HISTORY[1]

The patient's recorded history represents the organization and interpretation of material derived from the interview as well as from other sources, such as previous medical records or outside informants. In order to write down a logical and understandable history, the student must organize his information into the following categories:

1. Identifying Data
2. Source and Reliability of the History
3. Present Illness
4. Past Health
5. Family Health
6. Personal and Social History
7. Systems Review

---

[1]Examples of written histories are found in Appendices A and B.

After the student has completed his interview, he should review his notes and fill out any details that may be forgotten. It is wise for him to write the history and physical examination as soon as possible while the patient's findings are fresh in his mind. The preparation of the written history is more complex than recording the findings of the physical examination. It involves making certain judgments as to what differentiates the current illness from illnesses in the past. It calls for decisions as to the relevance of data and their proper assignment to the major categories. To write a well organized history, it is first wise to review in one's mind the information obtained by interview, noting especially relationships and sequences which seem to have clinical meaning. This mental review must be done with reflection and imagination, and with due attention to the physical and laboratory findings. The data must be examined particularly for completeness; and it may be necessary to go back to the patient for clarification or exploration of issues that were not fully appreciated during the initial examination. The student should also read appropriate references to clarify his thinking. These references may bring up new issues justifying further examination of the patient. Only after the student has completed such a systematic analysis and evaluation of the data is he ready to write the history.

Thought must be given to the clarity and conciseness of language used in the final draft. One must learn to be accurate and complete, yet sufficiently to the point so that the busy physician who next reviews the chart can do so quickly, without being misled by ambiguities, omissions, distortions, or misstatements. The student learns to be economical with words and yet to describe clearly and fully the patient's symptoms. Thought must be given to organizing the material so that it will be readable and understandable. Events are reported in the sequence in which they occurred, and symptoms are delineated in terms of their seven dimensions. (See Chapter 3.) A rigorous effort is made to eliminate unnecessary repetition. Should an item be included in more than one division of the history, cross referencing is used rather than repeating the full description. To make it easier for the reader to check back on a particular fact, key dates, symptoms, or events are underlined for emphasis.

Clinical judgment is required to determine how much of the voluminous data obtained in the interview should be recorded in the written record in order to convey an accurate account of the patient's illnesses. For example, the patient may have described shortness of breath in a variety of experiences. Such detail was necessary in the interview to verify that the symptom was truly dyspnea and not some other disturbance. For the purposes of the written history, however, it is not necessary to record all of the examples provided by the patient. Only a general statement is needed to specify the point of onset and the subsequent course of the dyspnea, perhaps using an example or two to document the symptom (e.g., "Within a week's time the patient became unable to climb one flight of stairs" or "The patient regularly developed wheezing and shortness of breath when he was rushing to class, yet could walk just as rapidly without symptoms when returning to his room.").

Throughout the written history careful distinction must be made between the *description* of data and its *interpretation*. It is improper, for example, to write "The patient is having angina pectoris," rather than to record a complete description of the symptoms in question, allowing the reader to form his own opinion: "The patient felt a mild retrosternal pressure which began abruptly when he was emotionally excited or exerted himself, as for example, when he climbed two flights of stairs at a normal pace. The sensation usually lasted 3 to 5 minutes and was relieved by nitroglycerin. These symptoms have been present for about a year, averaging four to five episodes a month. In the past 2 weeks, during the cold weather, there has been similar chest distress with less activity, averaging once or twice a day. About half the time, he may have an associated dull ache in his left biceps region; and with the retrosternal pressure, he may feel slightly short of breath."

Quotations are used sparingly and only when the patient's exact words contain specific information which cannot be conveyed in any other way. For example, the pain is described "like a red hot poker sticking in my back." Quotes are also used when recording an undocumented medical term used by the patient, such as "nephritis" or "nervous breakdown"; but these should always be followed by a brief description of the condition so named. It is unnecessary when recording data from the patient to write repeatedly "The patient said. . . ." This adds to the length of the history and decreases readability.

Emphasis should be on the description of symptoms and events as these affect the patient, rather than on the patient's report of what the physician said or did. If the patient's statement of what a physician said is recorded, it should be in quotes and clearly distinguished from what the physician may have told the interviewer directly. When information comes from several sources, including the family, the physician, or the old chart, each of these should be identified. For example, "The patient reports that swelling of his ankles appeared for the first time in mid-January 1969, 2 weeks ago, but his wife claims it has been present for at least a month and that he also had ankle swelling briefly in June 1968. No ankle edema was recorded on the clinic visit of November 4, 1968."

The old hospital record, if available, is reviewed before the history is written. The pertinent information is summarized and incorporated into the proper divisions of the new write-up. Especially when the old record is an extensive one, a concisely written summary is not only a valuable experience for the student, but also is of help to others reading the chart. Included might be symptoms and signs, results of laboratory and diagnostic procedures, diagnoses, and treatment. Such a summary gives an overview of what has been happening to the patient over the years and may yield new diagnostic insights.

Finally as he writes the history, the student should constantly keep in mind the future reader, who may not have seen the patient or who may read the chart long after the patient has been discharged. The student should anticipate questions arising in the reader's mind and include pertinent positive or negative information.

Identifying Data

A brief four or five line description serves to introduce the patient to the reader. This description may include the patient's age, sex, occupation, marital status, number of children, race, religion, address, and the number of his hospital admissions. It is also helpful to state the reasons why a patient is admitted. This word picture should be written concisely, in one sentence if possible. For instance, "This is the first Strong Memorial Hospital admission of Mr. Wentworth Davis, a 68-year-old white, retired, widowed electrician with two married daughters, who lives alone in downtown Rochester in a two-room apartment, and who is admitted because of chest pain." Such a concise statement immediately gives valuable orienting information about the patient.

The date that the patient was interviewed should follow this introductory statement. The date the history was written is also noted in the upper right hand corner below the patient's name and unit number.

Source and Reliability of the History

The sources of the history are recorded. They may include the patient, family members, the old chart, and the referring physician. When information is received from another informant, his full name, address, telephone number, and relationship to the patient are obtained. It is particularly important to identify other physicians by name and specialty. The used of the term "L.M.D." (local M.D.) is inappropriate.

Finally, a brief statement is made as to the reliability of the data. A reason is given if information is not reliable. For instance, "The patient had considerable difficulty remembering past events and no other informants were available; hence, the past history in particular is not reliable."

Present Illness

The Present Illness refers to the recent change in health that caused the patient to seek medical attention. The write-up of the Present Illness may be organized in one of several ways, depending on the problem. It is an orderly and usually chronological account that includes all the symptoms, signs, feelings, events, and relationships that are pertinent to the patient's current illness. With experience, the student learns what events in the past are pertinent and should be included in the Present Illness. In general, such information should have a direct bearing on the understanding of the problem that brought the patient to the hospital. It should be appreciated that what is recorded includes not only the data necessary for the diagnosis of the disease, but also an adequate account of the individual patient's illness. (See Chapter 2 for the distinction between disease and illness.) For example, little data may be needed to justify a diagnosis of diabetes, but a great deal of information is necessary to understand the course and characteristics of the diabetes in the patient under consideration.

THE DECISION AS TO WHAT CONSTITUTES THE PRESENT ILLNESS

In many cases this decision is not a simple issue, nor one where there is necessarily agreement among the different physicians examining the patient. Many patients present complex histories, reflecting the presence of a number of concurrent pathological processes. The physician's decision as to what he is going to regard as the Present Illness also reflects an early stage of his diagnostic thinking. The doctor, for example, who is seriously considering hemochromatosis as the explanation of the patient's diabetes, or conversion as the explanation of the patient's headache, is very likely to include within the Present Illness items which another physician, not thinking of these possibilities, might record elsewhere in the history. These are matters of judgment and clinical experience for which no hard and fast rules are possible.

In general, the identification of the Present Illness begins with the symptoms and events that cause the patient to seek medical attention. Usually a reasonably well-defined episode has provoked the patient or the family to seek help. When this episode has developed recently during a period of good health, the decision is simple. When it is a significant event in a series of difficulties, the Present Illness may be more difficult to define. It then becomes necessary to examine how the various symptoms and events relate to each other in order to decide when the current illness began. One must appreciate that the term, Present Illness, does not necessarily refer to a single illness but to *all the disease processes contributing to the patient's clinical condition at the time of the examination.* An example of such a complex present illness might be a 65-year-old man admitted to the hospital with 3 days of chills, fever, cough, and chest pain, which are symptoms indicative of pneumonia. However, this was the culminating event of a month-long bout of unremitting alcohol ingestion and depression, which was the patient's reaction to his wife's death. During a 6-month period, he had also manifested the symptoms and signs of gastritis, malnutrition, polyneuritis, depression, and impending delirium tremens. The account of Present Illness in such a patient would begin with a description of the 3-day respiratory illness. The student would then go back and describe chronologically the related symptoms and events of the preceding 6 months, all of which constitute the Present Illness for this patient. Further, one would make a brief reference to the several previous episodes of alcoholism extending back many years, which would be described in more detail under Past Health.

Judgment as to how the Present Illness is written is also influenced by the reason for the patient's hospital admission. For example, if the same patient were admitted to the hospital 3 months later for treatment of depression and alcoholism, the account of the Present Illness might begin with the death of the wife 9 months earlier. The history of the pneumonia 3 months before, as well as gastritis and polyneuritis might be mentioned briefly in Present Illness, but would be described more fully under Past Health. Previous episodes of depression or alcoholism would be detailed in subsequent paragraphs of the Present Illness.

CHRONOLOGIC ORGANIZATION

Each segment of the Present Illness is organized chronologically so that a logical sequence of events is developed. The time of onset of each symptom or event should be documented and the progressive evolution of these symptoms described, with successive dates up to the time of hospital admission. For example, "In the first week of September, 1968, three weeks before admission, the patient began to have epigastric pain." Calendar dates or clock times as far as possible should be recorded, with the relationship to the date of admission added when relevant. One should avoid the nonspecific, "Saturday before admission," since this time interval will be unclear in the future. Underlining the date or time at the beginning of the sentence serves to highlight it. The student may then go on in the first paragraph to describe in detail the symptoms of epigastric pain as well as associated events. He may start the next paragraph with a new event: "Four days prior to admission on September 25, 1968, the patient first noted pitch black stools." This symptom is then developed in detail.

THE ORGANIZATION OF THE WRITE-UP OF THE PRESENT ILLNESS

The Present Illness can be organized as follows: (1) An initial orienting statement describing the patient's past health. (2) The general description of the present illness. (3) A concluding paragraph that brings in any additional information pertinent to the understanding of the problem.

Initial Orienting Statement. A very brief statement concerning the patient's health prior to the onset of the present illness helps orient the reader to the setting in which the present illness occurred and sometimes indicates the reason for hospital admission. Examples are:

> The patient has been in excellent general health his entire life until January 2, 1969, 2 weeks before admission, when he first noted black stools.

> Except for an episode of hepatitis 4 years ago, the patient has been in good health.

> Diabetes has been known for 5 years, effectively controlled with diet and oral hypoglycemic agents. The patient has felt well until December 26, 1968, 5 days before admission, when after eating heavily over the holidays, he developed nausea, vomiting, and epigastric pain.

> A long-standing chronic alcoholic, the patient has had repeated admissions to this and other hospitals over the past 4 years for delirium tremens, polyneuritis, and cirrhosis. In the last year he has been admitted twice to this hospital (4/2/68 and 8/1/68) with bouts of hematemesis. Two hours before the present admission, he was struck by a car.

> This patient has had poor health for at least 20 years, with multiple hospital admissions, including different diagnoses, and at least six major surgical procedures. (See Past Health.) She is now admitted for investigation of blurring of vision, a new symptom.

> This 69-year-old woman, who had a resection of a carcinoma of the descending colon 4 months ago, now enters for closure of a bypass colostomy.

Some of the items referred to in this initial statement are then written in more detail under Past Health. Those, which in the judgment of the writer have direct bearing on the patient's current situation, are described in more detail in the Present Illness.

The General Description of the Present Illness. As has already been discussed, the description of the Present Illness is organized chronologically by introducing the reader first to the symptoms and events leading to admission, then going back to the apparent beginning of the illness and tracing it up to the present. Each manifestation is fully described in terms of the seven major dimensions: bodily location, quality, quantity, chronology, setting, aggravating and alleviating factors, and associated symptoms. (See Chapter 3.) Successive symptoms and events are developed in sequence, with relevant dates clearly indicated. The entire course of the present illness must be described, beginning with whatever is taken as the point of onset of the current disorder. In addition to symptoms, this description includes what the patient has done about the disorder; other medical investigations or treatments; and indeed, anything which the writer considers contributory to an understanding of the illness. Reactions to specific circumstances in the illness should be incorporated into the body of the Present Illness, including life situations bearing on the course of the illness; as for example, acute anxiety on discovering bright red blood in the stools, depression or hypochondriacal concern upon feeling a lump in the breast, a fight with the boss immediately preceding the onset of a symptom, or grief and mourning following a loss.

When an illness is manifest largely in psychologic or behavioral terms, more extensive description of behavior, feelings, relationships, and life events are necessary. The account of the Present Illness is then likely to include considerable information which might otherwise be recorded in the Family and the Personal and Social Histories.

There is an almost endless variety of patterns to the present illness. Some representative examples follow:

An acute illness in a previously healthy person. When a patient has been in excellent health and develops an acute illness, the organization of the Present Illness is relatively simple. One usually begins with the initial symptoms and events, and systematically describes the progress of the illness up to the time of admission. For example, the Present Illness of a 22-year-old student entering the hospital with symptoms of acute appendicitis of 2 days' duration may begin as follows:

> Two days before admission, beginning around 10:00 A.M. on April 5, 1968, the patient was sitting in a lecture when he began to feel slightly nauseated and noted vague midabdominal cramping. The pain felt like a mild gas cramp lasting 2 or 3 minutes, going away for 5 to 10 minutes; but it gradually increased in frequency and severity over the next 8 to 12 hours so that he was unable to eat dinner and was awakened several times at night.

> The morning before admission (April 6), the patient was more nauseated and vomited once. The vomitus just consisted of his breakfast. Following this, he was less aware of the midabdominal cramps and instead was conscious of a steady, deep moderate ache in his right lower quadrant.

The description of the current illness continues in such a chronologic way up to the time the patient enters the hospital.

A recurring disease with acute episodes. A patient may have a disease characterized by remissions and recurrences, often with symptom-free intervals in between. Examples might be bacterial pneumonia, a peptic ulcer, or depression. The fact that there have been previous episodes is mentioned in the initial orienting statement. Next, a full description is given for the current episode. In subsequent paragraphs, the previous episodes are described briefly, with particular emphasis on resemblances or differences from the current illness. Intervals between acute episodes should not be neglected, since these may clarify what factors were favorable for remission or what contributed to the recurrence. Mild symptoms indicative of possible underlying disease should also be mentioned if they appear relevant; for example, a persistent cough with some sputum may indicate the presence of chronic bronchitis or of bronchiectasis that may in turn be responsible for repeated episodes of pneumonia. Changes in the patient's personal life or environment may play a role in remission or recurrence of ulcer symptoms or of depression and should be noted in the write-up of the Present Illness.

Acute multisystem disease. Occasionally, a patient will have a complicated illness with symptoms involving several systems. One must think carefully how to organize the Present Illness in the best way. Such organization will be influenced by the student's initial diagnostic impression. If the illness is relatively recent and symptoms are few, it may be wise to develop the Present Illness chronologically, beginning with the earliest symptoms or events and to progress to the time of hospital admission. On the other hand, should there be multiple symptoms involving different organ systems all beginning at different times and evolving differently, it may be best to deal with each major organ system in separate paragraphs. Each symptom complex would then be developed chronologically from the time of its onset. For instance, a patient may describe an episode of arthritis experienced 8 weeks before, then a bout of fever and pleuritic chest pain 4 weeks later, and finally convulsions the day before admission. Between each episode, symptoms subsided. The Present Illness should begin with a paragraph describing the neurological syndrome that precipitated hospital admission. A separate paragraph may then be devoted to each of the preceding episodes, beginning with the joint symptoms, detailing the chronology and manifestations of each. Such organization takes experience and judgment, since there may be more than one disease process and the relationship between symptoms may be obscured by such arbitrary divisions.

New events related to a chronic disease. A patient may repeatedly have episodes of illness in the course of a chronic disease. The present problem should be fully described in the write-up, followed by a summary of relevant past events, including data derived from previous admissions. It is wise in the first sentence or two to orient the reader as to the reason for the present hospitalization. Facts of the past history which do not pertain to the current problem are put under Past Health. The summary of past manifestations of chronic disease in the Present Illness should be brief, especially if there are previous admissions recorded in the old chart.

The new events may be a recurrence of a previous manifestation, though not necessarily caused by the same disease. For example, a patient with a past history of duodenal ulcer may enter the hospital with a second episode of massive gastrointestinal bleeding beginning 2 days before admission. The details of the present bleeding episode are given first, with particular attention to features clarifying whether the history is consistent with bleeding from an ulcer or whether some other etiology is suggested. The symptoms preceding bleeding and the setting in which it occurred are described. Then, for comparison, another paragraph summarizes the relevant information regarding the previous hematemesis responsible for the admission 6 months before. Symptoms at that time as well as significant laboratory values and therapy are briefly mentioned. The level of the hematocrit, the finding of a duodenal ulcer by barium swallow, transfusions, and medications are all included as important background information. The Present Illness concludes with any other pertinent information regarding the ulcer; for example, the fact that the patient has been a heavy drinker for ten years, has been unable to stop, and has been recently under stress at work.

There are patients with chronic illness who are uninterruptedly sick for months or years. Some may have a well-defined physical entity like multiple sclerosis or lupus erythematosus; some have chronic psychologic difficulties, such as hysteria, depression, or hypochondriasis; and some a combination of both physical and psychologic symptoms. Such patients also are subject to illness unrelated to the underlying process, including iatrogenic complications due to administered medication. The Present Illness of such patients is very difficult to write. In general, it is best to begin with an account of the most recent episode or symptom complex. One then goes back in time and attempts to identify the beginning of ill health and develops a sequential story of the illness. Sometimes it is necessary to deal individually with symptoms or manifestations and to report the history of each in separate paragraphs, as was described for acute multisystem disease. Thus with blurring of vision and weakness of an arm, as may occur with multiple sclerosis or with hysteria, the history of the visual disturbance might be written in one paragraph and the arm weakness in the next. Due attention should be paid to the interrelationship which may exist between these two symptoms as well as to other symptoms.

On other occasions, it is better to group together the symptoms that occur at a particular point in time and to describe the entire illness chronologically. One may begin, for instance, by discussing a constellation of symptoms occurring 2 years ago, such as vomiting, headache, and blurring of vision of the right eye; then the subsequent period of continuing depression, malaise, and blurred vision; and finally the next incident 6 months ago marked by the recurrence of nausea and vomiting with the addition of arm weakness. When the discussion includes material from the old hospital record, a summary of relevant data should be included in proper chronologic order.

A new and clearly unrelated event in a chronic illness. If a patient with Parkinson's disease develops symptoms of acute cholecystitis, for example, it is not necessary to include a description of Parkinson's disease in the Present Illness. The reader is told of the chronic illness in the initial sentences and is referred to the Past Health for a fuller account. The bulk of the Present Illness should be devoted to a chronologic description of the symptoms of the acute abdomen up to the time of admission.

If, on the other hand, the chronic illness plays a significant role in the management of the unrelated new disease, a brief summary with pertinent information concerning the chronic illness should be included at the end of the Present Illness; and fuller details are included under the Past Health. For example, a patient with chronic rheumatic heart disease and congestive heart failure might enter the hospital with appendicitis. The initial sentence of his Present Illness would mention the previous diagnosis of rheumatic heart disease. The symptoms of appendicitis would come next, followed by a final paragraph describing his current cardiac symptoms and their management. Details of his past heart disease would be recorded under Past Health.

Readmission of a recently discharged patient: the interval history. When a patient is readmitted to the hospital after a brief interval with a continuation of the same problem and the record of the previous admission is available, the history may be abbreviated in the form of an *interval note* to describe what has happened in the intervening time. It is assumed, however, that the student will have first secured his own history of the illness from the patient and also will have later checked this with the recorded history. Any new information antedating the previous admission and not recorded in the previous record should be included in the interval note. Indeed, if one is not satisfied with the completeness or accuracy of the previous record, he will do well to write his own version of the Present Illness.

Data of uncertain relevance. If there is information of uncertain relevance to the Present Illness, it is best included in a separate paragraph rather than under the Past Health or Systems Review. For example, a patient with a one-month history suggesting lupus erythematosus may also have had gross hematuria 3 months before (which may or may not be related to this disease). The hematuria should be mentioned in the final paragraphs of the Present Illness. Any such information which may help in the understanding of the patient's illness is appropriately recorded in the Present Illness, even when one is unsure of its importance. This may include psychological stresses and life events, such as a recent death or job loss where the chronologic relationship with the disease onset justifies consideration.

The Concluding Paragraph. The Present Illness concludes with a paragraph containing additional information important to the full understanding of the patient's problem. It may include the following items:

Pertinent positive and negative information. As one considers the illness, questions will inevitably come to mind regarding a differential diagnosis. These questions should be anticipated by noting positive and negative data pertinent to such diagnostic considerations. Possible exposure to infectious agents or injurious substances would be recorded here, as well as relevant information from the past or family health. For example, in case of upper gastrointestinal bleeding, pertinent positive data might include the following: "The patient has previously bled excessively with tooth extraction; he has an uncle with hemophilia; and he recently has been drinking 8 to 10 cups of coffee a day." Pertinent negative data might include the following: "He had not been taking aspirin or related drugs; he does not drink alcohol; and he did not feel faint or lose consciousness, despite the large volume of blood loss."

Medications and treatment. All of the patient's medications, his diet, restrictions, and other treatments should be detailed here if not already alluded to in the main description. Included are drugs given on a chronic basis for other conditions as well as self-administered medication. Familiarity with the therapeutic program will help in understanding the patient's response to treatment, as well as in deciding whether some of the present symptoms could be caused by drugs. The names of the medications, dosage, frequency, and duration of therapy should all be noted.

Weight. Changes in weight are pertinent to most illnesses and should be recorded at the end of the Present Illness. The current weight, recent changes, as well as prior maximum and minimum weights, should be recorded here.

Degree of disability. Before the Present Illness is concluded, the physician should give the reader some idea of the magnitude of the patient's disability. Has he had to stop some of his regular activities? Does he depend on others for help in carrying out his basic functions? How recent and how progressive have these limitations been? Any pertinent comments or interpretation by the patient about his illness should also be recorded here.

Past Health

The divisions of the history following the Present Illness are organized to give a clear picture of the patient's former health, the health of his family, and his personal development, relationships, and achievements. If this information has been recorded in a recent admission, only an interval history need be written. Included would be data concerning the family or personal history occurring since the last admission or any other information that may not have previously been recorded. When a prior admission was more than a few months past, one should write out in full the Past Health, Family Health, and Personal and Social History.

Newer information may be available. Further, no two histories are the same because of variations in the skill and emphasis of the interviewer and in the memory and clinical condition of the patient. To write simply "See old record" is not adequate. Data could be missing in the old record, or the chart could be misplaced and unavailable.

All major illnesses and injuries, especially those requiring medical attention or hospitalization, are described and listed chronologically under Past Health, which is divided into five major categories:

1. General Health
2. Childhood Health
3. Adult Health
   a. Medical Illnesses
   b. Surgical Procedures
   c. Psychiatric Illnesses
   d. Obstetrical History
4. Accidents and Injuries
5. Allergies and Immunizations

Under each of these major divisions, illnesses are listed chronologically. Confusion may occasionally occur where there is a chronic disease that falls into two categories, such as one treated both medically and surgically. Here, a judgment must be made as to where the illness is best listed. For example, a patient may be under long-term medical management for a recurrent duodenal ulcer with an episode of perforation, which in the past, required surgery. In this example, it is best that the entire illness be listed under Medical Illnesses, including details of the surgery. Under Surgical Procedures a brief notation is then made: "In 1962, surgery was performed for perforation of a duodenal ulcer (see Medical Illnesses)." When there have been an unusual number of illnesses and operations, it may be clearer to list them all in chronologic sequence under Adult Health.

Information under Past Health is recorded in less detail than in the Present Illness but is sufficient to identify clearly past events. Each past illness is listed in a separate paragraph with dates and diagnoses underlined for emphasis. When previous hospital records are available, the essential findings as well as the discharge diagnosis should be recorded. For example, the summary of a previous admission for myocardial infarction should include enough information to indicate the reliability of the diagnosis, the severity of the illness, complications, and treatment. When the problem is simple and uncomplicated, such as a hospital admission for repair of an inguinal hernia, one just records this fact unless there were complications.

The major categories to be considered under Past Health are as follows:

GENERAL HEALTH

A statement is first made about the patient's general health in the past. For example, "The patient has enjoyed excellent health all his life" or "The patient has been sickly all her life with frequent visits to many doctors for varied complaints. These symptoms have included periodic headaches, alternating anorexia and overeating, insomnia, and feelings of depression." Such a general statement is then amplified to give a fuller picture of the patient's long-standing chronic syndrome. Minor, isolated problems, such as occasional headaches, frequent colds, or hemorrhoids, are noted in the Systems Review.

CHILDHOOD HEALTH

Included in this category are first a general description of health in childhood and then a reference to the occurrence of the following: measles, mumps, chicken pox, whooping cough, scarlet fever, rheumatic fever, chorea, diphtheria, poliomyelitis, significant respiratory infections, or diarrhea. Complications of any of these diseases are reported, as is the age at which they were experienced. Birth injuries and congenital or genetic defects are also noted.

ADULT HEALTH

Medical Illnesses.   Those illnesses requiring hospitalization or a physician's care are recorded here; for example, pneumonia, heart disease, hepatitis, diabetes, pleurisy, or infectious mononucleosis. Rarer parasitic or infectious granulomatous diseases are included, such as malaria, amebiasis, hookworm, histoplasmosis, coccidioidomycosis, or cholera. Also noted are descriptions of significant illnesses that are not necessarily diagnosed by name but which need to be described adequately for purposes of identification; for example, a febrile illness that kept the patient in bed 2 weeks, or diarrhea recurring over a 3-month period. The date, the patient's age at the time of each illness, the names of the hospital and physician, symptoms, complications, and treatment are each recorded.

Surgical Procedures.   The patient's age, type of surgery, dates of hospital stay and of the operation, as well as the names of the hospital and the surgeon are recorded. A brief statement is made as to the symptoms, findings, and complications of the surgery. For example: "June 1948, age 35, cholecystectomy done at the Highland Hospital by Dr. Ralph Z. Smith. The patient had right upper quadrant pain for 3 days, was jaundiced, and was told that many small stones were removed." Minor surgical procedures, such as a tonsillectomy or excision of skin lesions, are also noted. *The report of the surgical pathology should always be included.* Operative notes are summarized if there are details pertinent to the patient's present condition. For example, the description from the operative note of a complicated intestinal bypass may be helpful in the interpretation of current x-ray films.

Psychiatric Illnesses. Those illnesses that are primarily psychiatric in nature, such as neuroses, psychoses, or chronic alcoholism, are recorded here. One notes the diagnosis, the major manifestations, the name of the responsible physician, the frequency of office visits, the dates and locations of hospitalizations, special treatments (such as drugs or electroconvulsive therapy), and the general course of the illness.

Obstetrical History. Each pregnancy, whether full term or not, should be listed in order, with the date of each, the mother's age, duration of gestation, type of delivery, complications, and the weight and condition of the baby. Miscarriages, abortions, and their complications are also described. It is particularly important to record the patient's health during each trimester, noting such findings as nausea, vomiting, weight gain, edema, and hypertension.

ACCIDENTS AND INJURIES

Examples of injuries are lacerations, head trauma, sprains, broken bones, or gunshot wounds. When residual changes occur, they should be described. For example, "Head injury: The patient fell from a moving truck at age 15 (1942), was unconscious for several hours, and was hospitalized at Strong Memorial Hospital for 3 weeks with a diagnosis of skull fracture. He had slight weakness of the right arm which cleared in 2 weeks and had recurring headaches for 6 months." When there seem to be an unusual number of accidents or injuries, the circumstances surrounding these should be described.

ALLERGIES AND IMMUNIZATIONS

A final paragraph summarizes the details of the patient's sensitivity to drugs, including the name of the drug, the type of reaction, and the date. If there is a history of drug allergy, this fact should be written in red here, listed under Diagnosis, and noted at the beginning of the physician's orders. The patient should also be advised to tell any doctor or nurse in the future that he has had a prior specific drug reaction. Other allergic disorders, such as eczema, hives, hay fever, asthma, food allergy, or contact dermatitis, are also noted here, although they may already have been described above; if so, only the comment "See above" is necessary.

Dates of smallpox vaccinations, tetanus, diphtheria, polio (type), and other immunizations are noted. If the patient is a child, include

DPT (Diphtheria-Pertussis-Tetanus), mumps, and measles; if the patient has been overseas, include typhoid and yellow fever. Skin tests and serum injections should be described as to type, date, reaction, and reason for their use.

An example of the recorded Past Health of a 48-year-old housewife, admitted with pneumonia, is as follows:

Past Health

1. General Health. Except when limited by her cardiac illness, the patient has been normally active and has had few complaints.
2. Childhood Health. As a preschool child, she had chicken pox and mumps without complications. At age seven, she was kept at home from school for 6 weeks because of painful swollen joints in her arms and legs that limited walking for 2 to 3 weeks. Symptoms subsided in a month, never to recur. There was no scarlet fever or chorea, but she did have frequent sore throats as a child.
3. Adult Health
   A. Medical Illnesses
      1. Infectious mononucleosis 1938, at age 18. The patient was treated by Dr. Frank J. Green at home. She recalls being in bed for 2 to 3 weeks with a severe sore throat and slight jaundice.
      2. First Strong Memorial Hospital Admission (11/2/61 to 11/14/61), age 41, with the diagnosis of rheumatic heart disease, mitral stenosis, and congestive heart failure. She had had exertional dyspnea for 3 months, and entered the hospital with uncontrolled atrial fibrillation and paroxysmal nocturnal dyspnea the night before admission. She rapidly improved with digitalis, diuretics, and salt restriction.
      Second Strong Memorial Hospital Admission, 1½ years later (5/13/63 to 5/16/63), was for cardiac catheterization. She had had slowly progressive exertional dyspnea for 6 months. Pure tight mitral stenosis was confirmed.
      Third Strong Memorial Hospital Admission at age 43 (9/14/63 to 10/10/63), was for a closed mitral valvulotomy. There was no mitral regurgitation at surgery; the valve was flexible, and was opened to 2 fingerbreadths with fracture of the medial and lateral commissures. Her hospital course was uneventful and she has remained well with normal activity, avoiding salt and continuing digitoxin 0.1 mg. daily for atrial fibrillation.
   B. Surgical Procedures
      1. Tonsillectomy, age 12, 1932, Genesee Hospital.
      2. Mitral Commissurotomy, 1963, Strong Memorial Hospital. (See A. Medical Illnesses.)
   C. Psychiatric Illnesses
      None.
   D. Obstetrical History
      The patient had a miscarriage at age 26 (1946) in the third month of pregnancy which did not require hospitalization. Two subsequent pregnancies at ages 28 and 32 were normal full term, and delivery was uncomplicated. She gained 20 and 26 pounds with each pregnancy.
4. Accidents and Injuries
   A. Left wrist fracture, 1930, caused by a fall.
   B. Concussion, April 1955. The patient was admitted to Highland Hospital overnight following an auto accident. X-ray examination

was negative, but she recalls headaches and dizziness that persisted 3 or 4 months.

5. Allergies and Immunizations

    There are no known allergies, including drugs. The only immunization she recalls was polio vaccine in 1957 or 1958.

Family Health

A diagram of the family tree is used to illustrate the family pedigree, which includes grandparents, siblings, and children. The family tree indicates the health history of the family, whether a member is living or dead, and the age of each. For the living, any known major illness is recorded. For the dead, the date and cause of death are recorded. The student should keep in mind that the date of death of a family member may constitute an important psychological stress for the patient; if so, it is discussed in more detail in the Personal and Social History, unless it is clearly part of the current problem, in which case it is included in the Present Illness.

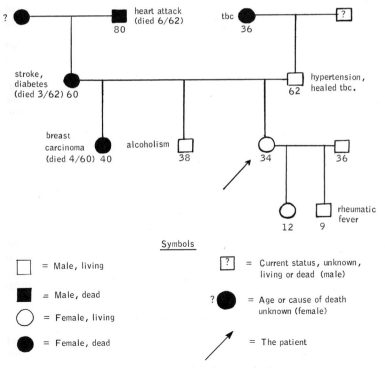

Fig. 5-1   An Example of a Family Tree.

A paragraph follows the family tree, giving fuller details of the illnesses of family members, *including those illnesses not responsible for the death of the deceased members.* Such descriptions are especially important when there is a possiblity that the patient's illness may be related to that of a family member through contagion, a congenital influence, a genetic factor, or the psychological impact of the family member's illness. For example, using the illustrative Family Tree, the respiratory symptoms of the 34-year-old woman patient may be related through contagion to the father's tuberculosis or may represent a conversion based on the patient's knowledge that the grandmother had a heart attack or the father, pulmonary tuberculosis. Accordingly, information about these illnesses, e.g., dates, description of symptoms, the extent of the patient's exposure, may be important for a complete understanding of the patient's illness.

When considering possible familial transmission of disease, brief descriptions of the family illnesses may be more informative than just accepting the name diagnosis provided by the patient. For example, a family history of nose bleeds may suggest the diagnosis of hereditary hemorrhagic telangiectasia in a patient with gastrointestinal bleeding; or a history of anemia and splenectomy in several family members may point to a diagnosis of spherocytosis in the patient; or the recognition of the patient's symptoms as hysterical may be prompted by the description of the mother's life-long hysterical illness. When a genetic factor is a serious consideration, the family tree should be expanded to include siblings of the parents as well as those of the grandparents, and a statement made concerning a history of consanguinity.

At the conclusion of Family Health, negatives pertinent to illnesses that run in families should be recorded. For instance, if the patient is hypertensive, pertinent negatives are: no known hypertension, kidney disease, strokes, or heart attacks in the family.

Personal and Social History

The more personal aspects of the patient's history are best organized under two categories: the *Current Life Situation* and *Past Development.* A narrative account bringing together related matters is more readable and more informative than merely giving a few items in each category. In general, the Current Life Situation is the more important, for this includes factors that may have a bearing on the present illness, knowledge of which will be important for the patient's care. When directly pertinent to the development of the illness, part of the Current Life Situation may have been included under Present Illness, as for example, when a job promotion is associated with recurrence of ulcer symptoms or the development of a depression. When there are major psychologic or social components of the illness, as is particularly the case with psychiatric illness, the Past Development will need to be emphasized. The student may then prefer to write a detailed chronological account beginning with the patient's early childhood.

Current Life Situation

A description of the patient's present situation includes the following:

HOME AND FAMILY. His current living arrangements, marital status, children, and other close family relationships are recorded. The significant persons in his life are identified.

PRESENT OCCUPATION AND ECONOMIC STATUS. The details of the patient's present occupation and related responsibilities are given. With regard to a job, the schedule and the nature of the work, satisfactions, frustrations, and possible chemical exposure are noted. It is important to describe any financial problems or other factors that may influence the current illness and hospitalization. If the patient is unemployed, the reasons are given as well as a description of contacts with social agencies. Also included are financial resources, such as payments from medical insurance, a pension, social security, or welfare.

SOCIAL AND COMMUNITY COMMITMENTS. One describes the patient's social activities that go beyond his daily occupation.

LEISURE ACTIVITIES. These include hobbies, exercise, vacations, and travel.

PERSONAL CHARACTERISTICS AND PATTERN OF LIVING. Information is given concerning the patient's characteristic behavior and patterns of living, including his manner of coping with stress. One also notes socially deviant behavior, eccentricities, or fads. The patient's patterns of diet, sleep, and consumption of tobacco, alcohol, and coffee are recorded here.

In defining the current life situation, most important are unresolved problems and sources of concern reported by the patient, such as marital difficulties and conflicts at work. Also important are recent changes in his life, such as graduation, marriage, births, separations, illness or death of important persons; and changes in his home, job, and economic or social status. The dates of each should be recorded. *Emphasis is always on the patient's reactions and method of dealing with these events, not simply on the event itself.*

Past Development

CHILDHOOD AND ADOLESCENCE. Included are the patient's birthplace, location of childhood homes, parental occupation, religious affiliation, and his relationship with parents and siblings. The parents are characterized and their relationship to each other is noted. When important in understanding the patient's illness, one should describe how the patient dealt with adolescence. One emphasizes particularly the experience of breaking away from the parental environment and the course of sexual development, as indicated by dating patterns, etc.

EDUCATIONAL AND OCCUPATIONAL HISTORY. This includes the following: The full extent of education or training (including dates, the patient's age, and degrees earned); military service (with dates, ranks, nature of service, and discharge status); past work history (including successive jobs, promotions, retirement, successes and failures, and relationships with peers, subordinates, and superiors). The main emphasis is on how the patient adjusted to his work role in terms of personal gratification, interpersonal relationships, economic security, and success.

MARITAL AND FAMILY HISTORY. A description is given of the patient's family life in the adult years up to the current life situation. If married, a history of the marital status is given, stating whether the patient has been separated, divorced, or married more than once, with relevant dates. If the patient has not lived with a husband or wife, it is noted with whom he lived and the conditions of the living arrangements. In the present section, one also records what the important family members' interests and occupations have been, as well as the details of their relationships with the patient. The name, age, and health of the spouse, children, and important family members will already have been described under Family Health. Emphasis is on the patient's feelings and his reaction to changes that may have been brought about by conflict, separation, illness, or death. Especially important is the impact of children leaving home for education, marriage, or military service.

Taking as an example the patient listed in the Family Tree, a 34-year-old woman with respiratory symptoms, the following description illustrates a typical Personal and Social History:

Current Life Situation. Mrs. Carver is living with her husband and two children in an old, but adequate farmhouse in Lima, New York. Her 62-year-old father, who is unemployed, lives with them. There is considerable friction between the family members. The patient's husband, James, runs a small dairy farm; and Mrs. Carver helps with the milking, cooks all meals, and cleans the three story farmhouse. There are two children; Mary age 12, who has been well, and John age nine, who has rheumatic fever. (See Family Health.) John has been in the Children's Convalescent Home for the past 3 months, which has been a source of great concern to the patient. At the present time, the family is heavily burdened with debts related to the son's illness and the husband's limited income. They are receiving help from Aid to Dependent Children and Welfare. (The name of the Social Worker is Mrs. George Black.)

Because of demands of the farm and housekeeping, the patient has had little time for leisure activities, including sewing, which she enjoys. For the most part, she has had a rather resigned, long-suffering attitude toward the hardships of life. She has chronically been a dependent person, being unable to assert herself, and frequently has needed to turn to others for help. She has always seen to it that her family has three good meals a day, usually gets 5 or 6 hours of sleep, and neither drinks nor smokes.

Past Development. The patient was born January 2, 1930, near Albion, New York, the youngest child of a tenant farmer, and spent all her life on a farm. The family suffered considerable hardship during the depression

of the 30's. When she was 9 years old, her father, who drank heavily, was
hospitalized for 3 years with tuberculosis. The family went to live with the
maternal grandparents on another farm, and the mother went to work in
a nearby factory. All three children helped with the farm chores. The patient completed ninth grade at age 17, having lost some time because of
illness (see Past Health) and the necessity of working on the farm. Her
school performance was only average. She then worked in a tile factory.
While continuing to live at home, she met her husband when she was 19
and was married at age 20. He is 2 years older. For the first 3 years of the
marriage, they lived with her parents. The husband then inherited the
dairy farm from his father. The marriage has been a stormy one, the patient having separated twice, first in 1958 and again in 1960 for several
months, because of the husband's aggressive behavior and drinking. Each
time she stayed at her parents' home with her children.

The deaths of the mother and maternal grandmother in 1962 were
severe blows to the patient, who still cries when speaking of them, even
though 2 years have elapsed. Her mother and grandmother were two persons to whom she could go when in trouble with her marriage.

She was never close to her older sister who moved to California when
the patient was 13, and died in 1960 of carcinoma of the breast. The whereabouts of the 38-year-old brother, a chronic alcoholic, is unknown.

The Systems Review

The written history concludes with the Systems Review, which is
organized on the basis of systems. It serves as a final check list on all
other symptoms and minor illnesses the patient may have had. It includes past as well as current symptoms that are not considered part of
the Present Illness. With a little practice, it is relatively easy to commit to
memory the major symptoms associated with each of the bodily systems.
To facilitate this process, it is recommended that with the first few write-
ups the student record all negative as well as positive findings.
Positive symptoms should be briefly described in order to clearly identify
them, especially with respect to their chronology. For example, "The
patient has had difficulty initiating his urinary stream for the past 2
years, and in the past 6 months he has been getting up twice nightly,
compared to nocturia once a night a year ago." The term "pertinent
negatives" means the absence of symptoms that might be expected with
the patient's present or past illnesses, or with other illnesses discovered
in the Systems Review. In the example of prostatism just given, pertinent
negatives are "The patient has had no dysuria, known urinary tract
infection, or hematuria." Symptoms that have already been recorded
in Present Illness or Past Health need not be repeated in the Systems
Review. One simply states "See Present Illness" or "Past Health" but
should go on to record other symptoms in the same system that were
not previously mentioned.

Symptoms to be considered under each system are as follows:
Skin: Color changes, itching, bruising, petechiae, birthmarks,
moles, infections, rashes; hair; nails.

Hematopoietic system: Anemia, transfusions, and reactions (include dates); spontaneous bleeding or excessive bleeding after tooth extraction, tonsillectomy or minor injury; enlarged, tender, or suppurative nodes.

Head and face: Headache, trauma, facial pain.

Ears: Pain, discharge, tinnitus, deafness.

Eyes: Vision, glasses (date last checked), pain, inflammation, infections, diplopia, blurring, scotomata.

Nose and sinuses: Epistaxis, obstruction, discharge, postnasal drip, sinus pain.

Mouth, pharynx, and larynx: Sores, bleeding gums, teeth (abscesses, extractions, dentures, date last checked), sore tongue, sore throat, hoarseness.

Breasts: Lumps, pain, discharge.

Respiratory tract: Cough, change in chronic cough, sputum, wheeze, hemoptysis, pleuritic pain, night sweats, date of last chest film.

Cardiovascular system: Chest pain with exertion, dyspnea on exertion, nocturnal dyspnea, position for sleep, dependent edema, palpitations, high blood pressure, known murmur, calf pain on exertion, varicosities.

Gastrointestinal system: Appetite, thirst, nausea, vomiting, hematemesis, food idiosyncrasies, gas, sour eructations, trouble swallowing, heartburn, abdominal pain, jaundice, bowel movements (frequency, diarrhea, constipation, blood, tarry stools, change in bowel habits, laxatives), hemorrhoids, hernia.

Urinary tract: Dysuria, unusual color, polyuria, frequency, urgency, nocturia, burning, hematuria, stones, trouble with stream, incontinence, enuresis, retention, generalized edema.

Genital tract (male): Penile discharge or lesion; positive serology; testicular pain or swelling.

Genital tract (female):   Menstrual history: Age of onset, characteristics of first periods, frequency, regularity, duration of flow, pads per day, date of last period; associated symptoms; intermenstrual or post menopausal bleeding; discharge or itching. Contraceptive pills or devices. Menopause: Age and symptoms. Venereal disease: Abscess, genital lesion, serology.

Skeletal system: Pain in extremities, back or neck; stiffness; limitation of motion; joint swelling, heat, redness or crepitation; sprains; deformity.

Nervous system: Convulsions, syncope, dizziness, vertigo, tremor, ataxia, speech difficulty, muscle atrophy or tenderness, limp, weakness or paralysis, paresthesias, anesthesia.

Endocrine system: Goiter, tremor, heat or cold intolerance, sweat-

ing, exophthalmos, voice change, polyphagia, polyuria, polydipsia; change in body contour, change in glove or shoe size; hair
distribution; infertility.

Psychological status: "Nervousness," irritability, memory loss, depression, phobias, insomnia, nightmares, impotence, frigidity,
sexual disturbances, criminal or other sociopathic behavior.

THE PHYSICAL EXAMINATION[2]

General Principles

The written description of the physical examination must be accurate and comprehensive so that other physicians reading the record
may clearly visualize important findings. Positive findings deserve elaboration, not just passing mention. Judgment is needed to decide how
much information should be included. Some items in the outline that
follows may be omitted; others must be described in detail.

Just as the written history differs from the interview, so does the
written physical examination differ from the actual examination of the
patient. It is most efficient to examine the patient by regions, whereas
the write-up is more clearly organized by systems. For example, cervical
lymph nodes are palpated during the examination of the neck, and inguinal nodes at the time of the examination of the abdomen or of the
lower extremities. In the write-up, all lymph node abnormalities are included together under the lymphatic system.

In some instances, it may be appropriate merely to write "normal"
when describing findings, such as in the breast examination. In general,
however, even though there is no abnormality, it is best to give a brief
descriptive statement. For example, "Both breasts are small; the tissue is
slightly lobular, and there is moderate retraction of the right nipple."
Not only does this give a clearer picture to the reader, but the necessity
for a description reinforces the care and completeness of the
examination.

Pertinent negatives should be mentioned. If a patient entered the
hospital, for instance, with hemiplegia and mild delirium, under the
examination of the head, one might add: "There was no evidence of
skull injury, no bruits, and no mastoid tenderness."

Abbreviations are avoided since they are subject to misinterpretation. Fresh and varied terminology is sought in order to paint a vivid
picture for the reader. For example, in describing the examination of a
normal thorax and lungs, one might say: "The contour and expansion of

---

[2]Examples of written physical examinations are found in Appendices A and B.

the chest are normal. Diaphragms each move 4 cm.; there is no abnormal dullness, and breath sounds are vesicular." One avoids such a hackneyed phrase as "The chest is clear to P. and A. (percussion and auscultation)." The use of diagrams in describing the physical examination is often very helpful. Wherever possible there should be quantification of findings, with accurate metric measurements.

The Order of the Write-up

The recording of the physical examination may be organized as follows:
1. Reliability and completeness of the physical examination
2. General description of the patient
3. Vital signs
4. Skin, hair, and nails
5. Lymphatic system
6. Head (skull, face, eyes, ears, nose, mouth and pharynx)
7. Neck
8. Breasts
9. Thorax and lungs
10. Cardiovascular system (heart, peripheral vascular system)
11. Abdomen
12. Genital examination
13. Rectal examination
14. Skeletal system
15. Neurologic examination (general status, cranial nerves, motor system, sensory system, reflexes, spinal nerve irritation)
16. Mental status examination (behavior, cognitive function, thought content, perception, affect and mood)

RELIABILITY AND COMPLETENESS OF THE PHYSICAL EXAMINATION

One notes the accuracy and completeness of the physical examination. Any reasons for a deficient examination are given, whether because of the patient's mental or physical state, or because of unfavorable environmental conditions, such as poor lighting or excessive noise.

GENERAL DESCRIPTION OF THE PATIENT

It is very difficult to describe a patient, but one should strive to do it as clearly as possible so that another physician would be able to identify the patient should he see him walking down the hall. When one trains himself to write an accurate and full description, he enhances his own powers of observation. Not only should the patient's characteristics be described, but also how he fits into the ward setting. The questions which should be answered in a brief description are: What does he look like; what is his gait or his position in bed, his behavior, cooperation, voice, apparent age? Is he in discomfort, coughing, cyanotic, wasted, overweight, confused, fearful? Trite phrases, such as "Well-nourished, well-developed, and in no acute distress," are of little value. Examples of general descriptions are:

> The patient is a tall, gaunt, bald, white haired man of 66, who looks 10 years older. He is sitting bolt upright, gasping for breath and holding the side rails for support. He is pale, sweating, slightly cyanotic, and grunting with pain, which he locates retrosternally. He is extremely apprehensive and cooperates poorly in the examination.

> The patient is a bright, attractive, cooperative 25-year-old girl, wearing make-up and her own bed jacket, who does not appear ill, but is obviously blind.

VITAL SIGNS

Included are the *blood pressure* (designate which arm and the patient's position), *pulse rate, respiratory rate, temperature* (designate oral or rectal), *weight*, and *height*. If the blood pressure is measured more than once or in more than one extremity or position, record and specify each measurement and the sequence in which the pressures were measured. Ordinarily, only those vital signs taken personally are recorded; however, if height, weight, or temperature have just been measured, these figures may be used and the source of the information noted.

SKIN, HAIR, AND NAILS

A statement is first made concerning the *general description of the skin*: its color, pigmentation, temperature, moisture, and the presence or absence of lesions. *Skin lesions* are fully described as to their topography, areas affected, tenderness, size, shape, configuration, elevation, color, consistency, fluid content, and characteristics of scales and crusts. A description of the *hair*, including quality and distribution, is also included here, as are any abnormalities of *finger or toe nails*.

LYMPHATIC SYSTEM

The location of palpable nodes is given, including a description of their size, consistency, mobility, and tenderness.

HEAD

The description of the head follows the order of examination:
1. Skull
2. Face
3. Eyes
4. Ears
5. Nose
6. Mouth and pharynx

Any positive finding should be described in full detail. Normal or absent findings need only be noted.

Skull: Size, shape, masses, scars, tenderness, arterial pulsations, bruit.

Face: Color, scars, asymmetry, weakness, tenderness, edema.

Eyes: Visual acuity, glasses, visual fields; prominence, palpable intraocular tension; coordination of extraocular movements, nystagmus; lids, (ptosis, width of palpebral fissures, lid lag, paresis, edema); bulbar and palpebral conjunctivae (color, vascularity, petechiae, lesions, exudate); sclerae (color, pigmentation, lesions); cornea (scars, ulceration, arcus senilis); pupils (size, equality, regularity, reaction to light and accommodation).

Ophthalmoscopic Examination: Iris (color differences, defects), lenticular or vitreous opacities; discs (color, cupping, margins, pigmentation); arteries and veins (ratio, tortuosity, A-V nicking, color, distribution); maculae; retinae (hemorrhages, microaneurysms, exudates, pigmentation, scarring, tumors, detachment).

Ears: Hearing; external ear (pinnae, tophi); canal (wax, discharge, inflammation, tenderness); drums (landmarks, scars, perforations, color, vascularity, hemorrhage, discharge); mastoid (tenderness, scars).

Nose: Mucus membranes (color, discharge, edema, lesions); patency; septum (deviation, perforation); turbinates (color, edema, discharge); frontal and maxillary sinuses (tenderness, transillumination).

Mouth and Pharynx: Breath; lips (color, moisture, lesions, cheilosis); tongue (size, papillation, moisture, coating, movement, lesions); teeth (caries, pyorrhea, number missing, gums, dentures); buccal cavity, palate, tonsillar area, posterior pharynx (noting color, pigmentation, movement, lymphoid tissue, masses, lesions); tonsils (size, exudate, color).

A brief description of findings is given under each category. For instance, descriptions of the examination of the nose would be:

> **Where there is no abnormality,** *"Nose:* Normal mucus membranes, no obstruction and no sinus tenderness." **Where there is abnormality,** *"Nose:* The mucus membranes are pale and granular with a mucopurulent discharge and crusting on the left inferior turbinate. The flow of air is impaired

on that side and the septum is deviated slightly to the left. There is moderate
tenderness over the left maxillary sinus, which fails to transilluminate."

NECK

Neck mobility and strength, tenderness, scars, masses; salivary
glands (size, tenderness); thyroid (size, tenderness, nodules, bruit).

BREASTS

Size, symmetry, tenderness, glandular tissue, masses; nipples (discharge, retraction, ulceration). Diagram and describe any lesion.

THORAX AND LUNGS

Shape, symmetry, masses, scars; tenderness of skin, muscle, ribs,
sternum; tracheal position; expansion, retraction, or abnormal
movement of the chest; the level and measured motion of the
diaphragms. The location of abnormalities by changes in tactile
fremitus, resonance, whispered or spoken sounds, breath sounds. Presence and location of wheezes, rales, or rubs.

In addition to a description, it is helpful to illustrate abnormal pulmonary findings by a diagram. For instance, a patient may have obstructive emphysema and right lower lobe pneumonia:

> The chest shows a moderate increase in the anterior-posterior diameter
> and decreased thoracic expansion, the left hemithorax moving more than the
> right. The accessory muscles of respiration are used, and expiration is pro-
> longed. Except for the right lower chest posteriorly, the lungs are hyperre-
> sonant. The left diaphragmatic dullness is at the level of T10 posteriorly, with
> only 1 cm. of motion. Breath sounds are distant, and there are generalized
> high pitched wheezes in the early part of the prolonged expiratory phase.
> The abnormalities localized to the right posterior chest are as diagrammed
> below:

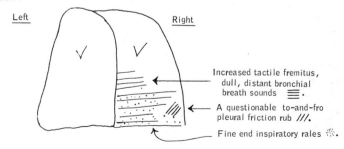

CARDIOVASCULAR SYSTEM

Heart: Character and location of apical impulse (interspace and
number of centimeters to the left of the midsternal line), right ventricu-

lar heave, pulsations, thrills, and area of cardiac dullness. *Heart sounds*: Rate and rhythm; description and comparison of the first and second heart sounds, (intensity of pulmonic and aortic components and splitting); extra sounds; gallops. *Murmurs*: Location, timing, intensity (grade 1 to 6), duration, quality, pitch, and radiation. Any other abnormal sounds, such as a pericardial friction rub.

An example of how one would describe the heart of a patient with pure mitral stenosis is as follows:

> There is a strong heave in the lower left parasternal region. The apical impulse is not palpable, but the cardiac border is percussed 11 cm. to the left of the midsternal line in the fifth intercostal space. The pulmonic component of the second heart sound is palpable in the second left intercostal space, and there is an apical diastolic thrill. The rhythm is regular.
>
> Both the mitral first sound and the second sound in the pulmonic area are considerably accentuated. There is an opening snap close to the second sound. At the apex, one hears a grade 4/6 low pitched, rumbling, full length diastolic murmur with presystolic accentuation, transmitted to the left posterior axillary line. A grade 1/6 early, high pitched decrescendo, blowing diastolic murmur is heard to the left of the midsternum. No systolic murmurs are present.

Peripheral vascular system: Neck: Jugular veins (distention and pulsation, noting distention in centimeters above the clavicle and the patient's position, or the number of centimeters above the sternal angle); carotid arteries (aneurysms, tortuosity, pulsations, bruits, thrills). *Abdomen*: venous pattern, direction of venous blood flow; abdominal aorta (diameter, expansile pulsation, bruits). *Extremities:* Edema, color, moisture, temperature, varicosities, ulceration, calf tenderness. Arterial pulses: The amplitude and contour of the pulse, together with any abnormalities in the vessel wall are noted, such as tortuosity, irregularity, and decreased compressibility. The strength of the pulses may be diagrammed as follows:

	RADIAL	CAROTID	FEMORAL	POPLITEAL	DORSALIS PEDIS	POSTERIOR TIBIAL
Right	+++	++	+++	++	++	+
Left	+++	++	+++	++	+	+++

(Grade 0 = absent; 2+ = normal; 4+ = full and bounding)

An example of how to describe vascular abnormalities in the neck may be illustrated in a patient with aortic stenosis and regurgitation:

> There is a prominent "a" wave in the deep jugular pulse, and both external jugular veins are distended 3 cm. above the clavicles, with the patient's head elevated 45 degrees. The carotid arteries are tortuous, easily seen, and one can feel a forceful pulsation with rapid ascent and collapse of the arterial pulse. There is a bilateral carotid thrill and a grade 4 bruit.

ABDOMEN

Size, contour, symmetry, scars, distention, visible movements, peristalsis, borborygmi, tenderness (location, rebound, cough, costovertebral angle), spasm, edema (subcutaneous, sacral). *Palpable organs*: Liver, gall bladder, spleen, kidneys, bladder, uterus. With respect to an enlarged liver and spleen, dimensions are recorded in centimeters below the costal margin in the midsternal or midclavicular line. The interspace of upper liver dullness must also be noted. Masses (location, size, consistency, contour, tenderness, mobility, pulsations, relation to organs); umbilicus; hernias; peritoneal fluid.

In a patient with a large uterine tumor and with metastases to the liver a diagram may serve to illustrate the major abnormal findings.

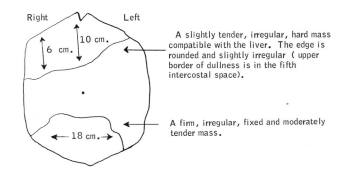

Right / Left

10 cm.

6 cm.

18 cm.

A slightly tender, irregular, hard mass compatible with the liver. The edge is rounded and slightly irregular (upper border of dullness is in the fifth intercostal space).

A firm, irregular, fixed and moderately tender mass.

GENITAL EXAMINATION

Male: Penis: Circumcision, prepuce, urethral meatus, glans, body (scars, discharge, inflammation, masses). Scrotum: Testes, epididymis, spermatic cord, cysts. Perineum.

Female: External genitalia: Labia, clitoris, introitus, urethral orifice, perineum (erosions, scars, inflammation, discharge, masses, perineal support). Pelvic examination: Vagina; cervix; fundus; fallopian tubes; ovaries; adnexal areas; and cul-de-sac (discharge, color of cervix, cysts, scars, erosions, inflammation, masses, tenderness).

When the pelvic examination is deferred or omitted, this fact should be recorded together with the reasons for the omission. For example:

"*Pelvic examination deferred* at patient's request; menstruation"; or "*Pelvic examination omitted* at the request of Dr.＿＿＿＿＿＿＿＿＿ because＿＿＿＿＿＿＿＿＿＿＿＿. Too often the statement "Pelvic deferred," means it was omitted because of inconvenience to the examining physician.

RECTAL EXAMINATION

Perianal area (including pilonidal sinus), hemorrhoids, fissure, fistula, sphincter tone, anal canal. Rectum: Masses, tenderness, blood, appearance of fecal specimen. Prostate: Size, consistency, borders, median groove, masses, tenderness (diagram, if necessary).

SKELETAL SYSTEM

Organize by anatomic regions, i.e., neck, back, hips, upper and lower extremities. Bones: Irregularity, tenderness. Joints: Deformities, swelling (soft tissue or fluid in the joint), redness, heat, tenderness, crepitation, range of motion (limited by pain, contracture or ankylosis), nodules, tophi. Ligaments, bursae, tendons: Swelling, redness, heat, tenderness, tendon contracture.

NEUROLOGIC EXAMINATION

1. *General status*: Appearance, behavior, speech, posture, gait, gross coordination (Romberg's test).
2. *Cranial nerves*: I to XII.
3. *Motor system*:
   Handedness
   Muscle symmetry, bulk, contracture, tenderness
   Tremor, involuntary movements, muscle fasciculation
   Strength
   Tone
   Coordination, ataxia (cerebellar signs)
4. *Sensory system*:
   Light touch, pain, and temperature
   Position and vibration
   Stereognosis, tactile localization, two-point discrimination
   Higher cortical function: aphasia, agnosia, apraxia[3]
5. *Reflexes*:
   Triceps, biceps, radial, knee, and ankle jerks
   Jaw jerk, Hoffmann's sign, grasp reflex and plantar reflexes[3]
   Abdominal, cremasteric, anal reflexes[3]
6. *Spinal nerve irritation*:
   Meningeal signs
   Sciatic pain (straight leg raising)

---

[3]Consult a physical diagnosis book or neurological text for a description of these tests.

If abnormality is present in any of the preceding reflexes, a general description is indicated to include such findings as briskness, slow relaxation, or clonus.

The strength of reflexes may be diagrammed as follows:

	BICEPS	TRICEPS	RADIAL	KNEE	ANKLE	PLANTAR
Right	+++	++	++	+++	+	↓
Left	+++	++	++	0	0	↓

OR

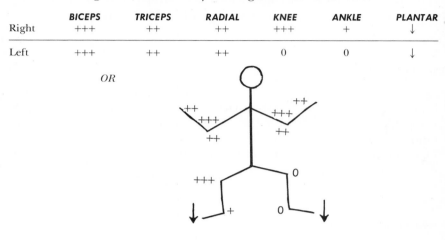

(Grade 0 = absent, 2+ = normal, 4 + = very hyperactive)

MENTAL STATUS EXAMINATION

The patient's general behavior and psychological status ordinarily are included in the general description. When a mental status exam is performed, the findings are recorded as follows:

1. *Behavior*: Unusual or bizarre conduct, mannerisms, tics, gesturing, posturing, catatonic rigidity, waxy flexibility, rhyming, punning.

2. *Cognitive function*: Orientation as to time and place, attention, recent and past memory, serial subtraction of 3's or 7's, interpretation of proverbs, general information, judgment.

3. *Thought content*: Illogical, bizarre, depersonalized; feelings of unreality, persecution, influence or reference; delusions; compulsive, obsessive, or phobic thoughts.

4. *Perception*: Illusions and hallucinations (auditory, visual, gustatory, olfactory, tactile). Describe and specify circumstances.

5. *Affect and mood*: Appropriateness, depressed, hostile, irritable, anxious, panicky, guilty, ashamed, helplessness, suicidal, euphoric, manic.

ADMISSION LABORATORY DATA

Special forms are usually provided for the recording of admission laboratory data, including tests of blood, urine, and stool. When indicated, sputum, spinal fluid, chest fluid, ascitic fluid, and joint fluid may also be examined at the time of the admission work-up. The results of such examinations are recorded, as well as a description of the procedure when needle aspiration is required.

DIAGNOSIS[4]

This section on diagnosis identifies the diseases, and the subsequent section on Prognosis evaluates the patient's illness. Both sections represent the ultimate objectives of the diagnostic process. (See Chapter 2.) They serve as an analysis of previously recorded data and are the foundation for planning diagnostic studies and patient management. Diagnosis concerns mainly the Present Illness but may also involve reevaluation of previous illnesses, particularly if they have some bearing on the current problem. For example, when a patient has abdominal pain similar to an earlier illness diagnosed as appendicitis, it may now be recognized that the past illness was more likely a conversion symptom or regional enteritis, symptoms of which are recurring. Diagnosis may be organized into three parts: The identification of abnormal findings, the interpretation of these findings, and the differential diagnosis of disease, which weighs evidence for and against several specific diseases that might reasonably account for the patient's illness.

The write-up of Diagnosis is based upon the student's interview of the patient and other informants, including the referring physician; the admission physical examination; the admission laboratory data; and a review of available previous hospital records. Conclusions drawn are considered to be provisional and are subject to revision in the form of Progress Notes as additional information becomes available. The length and emphasis of the section on diagnosis will vary with the nature of the problem. Ordinarily, it will require several pages. Considerable thought and preparation are needed before one begins to write about diagnosis, including a review of suspected diseases in the textbooks and a return to the patient to confirm or extend findings.

One begins his discussion of Diagnosis by *identifying* the major abnormal symptoms and signs that pertain to the patient's current illness. A concise summary is written, which includes the abnormal findings in the patient's history, physical examination, and admission laboratory work. This summary should not exceed half a page. Only data needed to identify the present problem are included. Such interpretive terms as "pleuritic pain" or "shock" may be used, since the reader has access to

[4]See Appendices A and B for sample write-ups of Diagnosis and Prognosis.

the previously recorded primary data as well as to the writer's reasoning which follows. Minor abnormal findings are not included unless they have an important relationship to the present illness or cause some problem in diagnosis. When findings of other diseases are present that may influence the patient's primary problem, these are briefly summarized in separate paragraphs.

Once the abnormal findings have been identified, the student must *interpret* them. That is, he must make clear their interrelationship and the sequence in which they have appeared, and relate them, if possible, to an organ system. The purpose of interpreting the abnormal findings is to explain the course of events by reconstructing step-by-step the evolution and nature of the underlying pathologic processes. It is only after this fundamental reasoning has been completed that consideration is given to diseases which are consistent with such a reconstruction. In some patients, the abnormal findings require no interpretation. This may be the case with an admission for an elective hernia repair, unless the symptoms do not correspond to the localized physical findings. Symptoms may also be so generalized or vague as to make discussion unrewarding, such as the patient with an unexplained fever or weight loss. In most patients, however, some interpretation of abnormal findings is required. For example, it may be necessary for the student to clarify the fact that the symptoms of dyspnea and wheezing are due to congestive heart failure, rather than to a primary pulmonary problem; that a loud systolic murmur is organic and orginates from the aortic valve, not from the mitral valve; and that the course of development of the findings is consistent with a valvular lesion of relatively recent origin. If there are abnormal findings in more than one system, it should be made clear whether these represent different pathological processes or the same one affecting multiple systems. When writing this paragraph, the various steps in the student's interpretive thinking should be clearly and succinctly stated. Particular effort must be made to account for the sequence in which abnormalities have evolved.

The *differential diagnosis of disease* is considered next, by naming diseases that could reasonably be responsible for the patient's abnormal findings. Depending upon the nature of the present illness, the differential diagnosis is based chiefly on a major symptom (crushing retrosternal pain), a major sign (abdominal mass), a combination of symptoms and signs (cough, hemoptysis, pleural friction rub), or an identified functional abnormality (congestive heart failure, uremia, anemia). The great variability in the presentation of clinical problems is such that no single format for the differential diagnosis can be recommended. In general, the student should first state which *one disease* best explains the course of development of the patient's findings. He supports his opinion in a few sentences with clinical evidence for and against the diagnosis.

Three or four possible alternative diagnoses are then discussed in order of probability, beginning with the most likely. Clinical evidence is again marshalled for and against each of the alternative diagnoses. The name of each disease mentioned should be underlined to highlight it for the reader. When considering possible alternative diagnoses, it is helpful for the student to consider the various causes of disease (e.g., congential, genetic, mechanical or electrical, immune or allergic, infectious, metabolic, endocrine, neoplastic, psychologic, etc.).

Only those diseases that reasonably pertain to the patient under study should be considered. The differential diagnosis is not an abstract discussion of the literature or a summary of classical disease pictures. Where there are findings in more than one system that may or may not be related, one should consider that more than one disease may play a role. A second differential diagnosis may therefore be required to explain an alternative combination of symptoms and signs. Finally, there are some patients with clearly established diagnoses who do not require a differential diagnosis, such as a patient with gallstones entering for cholecystectomy or a woman with recurrent uterine carcinoma admitted for radiation therapy.

At the conclusion of this section on diagnosis, *all* the diseases affecting the patient are listed. The student begins with what he considers to be the major disease accounting for the present illness and concludes with the least consequential disease. Alternative possibilities are not listed here but belong above in the discussion of differential diagnosis, where they are underlined so that they are easily noted by the reader. "Rule out this disease" "? that disease" or "Diagnosis deferred" are not properly part of the final list of diseases. Even though in some patients there may be little initial evidence to make a clear-cut diagnosis, the student should indicate what he feels is most likely, such as "Unexplained fever, possibly due to bacterial endocarditis." When a physician commits himself to the most probable diagnoses, he helps clarify his own thinking in planning initial studies and management; he clearly indicates to other physicians which diagnosis is considered the most likely; and his learning is enhanced when he later discovers whether or not his diagnoses are correct.

The following example illustrates how a patient's diagnoses should be listed:

1. Pneumonia, right middle lobe, ? pneumococcal
2. Congestive heart failure
3. Chronic rheumatic heart disease with severe mitral stenosis and slight aortic regurgitation
4. Atrial fibrillation
5. Right hemiparesis, secondary to left middle cerebral artery embolus (4 years ago)

6. Chronic depression
7. Bilateral indirect inguinal hernias
8. Internal and external hemorrhoids

PROGNOSIS

In order to determine prognosis, which means to predict the outcome of a patient's illness, one must understand what makes the illness unique for each individual. (See "The Evaluation of the Patient's Illness," Chapter 2.) It is often very difficult to comment on a patient's prognosis because of the many unknown contributing factors, but the student should attempt to do so. Not only will a consideration of the prognosis help him in planning future management, it will also give him an appreciation of the many elements which influence such a judgment. Prognosis may be organized in three parts: The estimation of the severity of the illness, the expected efficacy of treatment, and the predicted outcome of the illness.

Using the information obtained from the interview and admission physical examination, the student first *estimates the severity of the patient's illness.* In a few sentences, he should give the reasons for his opinion. For example, the severity of pneumonia is estimated in terms of the degree of toxicity, the extent of pulmonary involvement, and the virulence of the infecting organism. Heart failure is judged in terms of the duration of symptoms, the extent of physical signs, the degree of functional impairment, and the response to previous treatment. The severity of depression is evaluated by knowing the chronicity of symptoms, the behavior of the patient, the presence or absence of suicidal thoughts, and the reality of the precipitating circumstances. When more than one disease process accounts for the patient's illness, significant interrelationships should be discussed; as for example, the effects of pneumonia on heart failure and vice versa. The student should also be aware of the patient's psychological attitude towards his illness, since the degree of the patient's concern and the severity of the illness may not necessarily correspond; some seriously ill patients may be remarkably casual, while others with more benign disorders may be excessively concerned.

A brief statement is then made regarding the *expected efficacy of treatment.* Prognosis is clearly influenced by the effectiveness of therapy. For example, the natural history of pneumococcal pneumonia has been changed by penicillin, compared to viral pneumonia, for which there is no specific treatment. If there is a choice of therapy, the student should state his preference, give his reasoning, and comment on the expected outcome. An example would be the choice of medical management as compared to cardiac surgery for a patient with mitral stenosis. Not only specific drugs and surgical intervention are evaluated, but all the factors bearing on the current management of the patient. His personality structure must be taken into consideration, especially to estimate how well he will cooperate in following a therapeutic program. Knowledge of his current life circumstances is also important in order to predict how well he will respond to treatment. One must know such information as the patient's financial status, the availability of family and friends, and the adequacy of home facilities.

The section on prognosis is concluded by commenting on the *predicted outcome of the illness.* This judgment is based upon the natural history of the disease, the severity of the patient's illness, and his expected response to treatment. A general statement is made concerning the anticipated duration of the illness and the degree of future disability. It should be recognized that no physician can predict exactly how long a patient will live, and it is unwise to do so. With regard to duration, the student states in general terms whether the illness will be acute and self limited; chronic and remittent; or progressive and unchanging. In estimating disability, he predicts the duration of hospitalization, the time for convalescence, and any expected residual deformity. Since the section on prognosis is written at the time of initial hospitalization and an acute illness may change dramatically in a few days, the student should realize his predictions will need to be revised, and this is properly done in the Progress Notes.

PLAN OF STUDY[5]

Having completed his preliminary analysis of the case, the student must now identify the problems that remain to be resolved and propose a plan of study. He must decide what additional observations and diagnostic procedures are indicated, as well as how and when they are to be carried out. Such studies usually have two main objectives: the further clarification of the diagnosis and the evaluation of the status and course of each diagnosed disease.

The preparation of a Plan of Study derives directly from the considerations that went into the writing of the Diagnosis and Prognosis. In essence, the student examines each of the major items in his list of diagnoses, as well as the conditions seriously considered in his differential diagnosis, and decides what additional tests and procedures would be helpful in verifying or in ruling out pertinent diagnoses. At the same time, he chooses useful indices with which to follow the course of the

---

[5]See Appendix B for a sample write-up of the Plan of Study.

illness. In compiling such a list of tests and procedures, he does not overlook the minor diagnoses or those findings which are not adequately accounted for in the differential diagnosis, the further investigation of which may be overlooked if not made explicit. Further, he weighs the procedures recommended in terms of the urgency of the problem, the clinical condition of the patient, the risk of the procedure itself, and its potential for providing the information sought.

This approach emphasizes the problems to be solved and serves to minimize the use of a "shot-gun" approach to laboratory procedures. At the same time, the student must recognize the usefulness of certain routine tests, such as the hematocrit, white cell count, differential count, study of the blood smear, urinalysis, and stool for blood, which serve a screening function to identify unsuspected disease processes. Careful thought goes into the selection of every test. This involves a clear understanding of the meaning and limitations of the tests. For example, the routine ordering of fasting blood sugars may fail to detect the mild diabetic who is discovered only by a postprandial blood sugar. A bacterial count of a urine culture may fail to detect infection if the patient is having a diuresis and has recently voided. When a procedure carries possible risk, such as an angiogram or a renal biopsy, one should carefully weigh what the expectation is of making the diagnosis against the risk of the procedure to the individual patient.

The student begins with the least complex and most comprehensive studies, then proceeds to the more detailed. In studying anemia, for example, he should initially determine the hematocrit, study the blood smear, look for blood in the stool, and determine the reticulocyte count before examining the bone marrow or estimating the glucose-6-phosphate dehydrogenase activity. Finally the laboratory work must be kept in proper perspective. Interpretation of laboratory data must always be carefully balanced in terms of the physician's own clinical findings and reasoning. Laboratory error is not uncommon, and tests may need to be repeated. The review of biopsy material, roentgen films, or electrocardiograms in person with the specialist is also excellent practice.

When the patient has several illnesses, the student should organize his plan of study so that the tests and procedures for each major disease are listed in separate paragraphs. In each of these paragraphs, the name of the disease should be underlined, and the planned studies should be listed in the order in which they will be performed. Such a problem solving approach has been advocated by L. L. Weed.[6]

The general categories of tests and procedures to be considered are:
   1. *Chemical determinations.* e.g., blood sugar, serum urea nitrogen,

---

[6]Weed, L. L.: Medical Records That Guide and Teach. New Eng. J. Med., *278*:593 and 652, 1968.

serum electrolytes, arterial oxygen content, urine catecholamines, urine 5-hydroxyindole acetic acid.

2. *Roentgenographic and isotopic studies.* e.g., chest film, intravenous pyelogram, gastrointestinal series, radioactive iodine uptake, isotopic scanning of the brain.

3. *Microbiologic and immunologic studies.* e.g., Gram stain of a sputum smear; tuberculin skin test; serologic test for syphilis; cultures of sputum, blood, urine, or other body fluids; serum electrophoresis; tests for the L.E. cell or rheumatoid factor.

4. *Electrographic studies.* e.g., electrocardiogram, cardiac monitoring, electroencephalogram, echoencephalogram.

5. *Endoscopic studies.* e.g., gastroscopy, bronchoscopy, cystoscopy, sigmoidoscopy.

6. *Cytologic and pathologic studies.* e.g., cytologic study of a cervical smear, bronchial washings, or gastric aspirate; biopsy of kidney, liver, or lymph node tissues.

7. *Other special tests.* Included are tests of organ function such as cerebral spinal fluid analysis, gastric analysis, pulmonary function tests, cardiac catheterization, blood reticulocyte count, platelet count, or hemoglobin electrophoresis.

Should there be controversy as to the indications for a given test or procedure, the student should briefly give the reasons for his choice. Finally, one should also list in the plan of study the need for *consultant opinion* should it be indicated.

PLAN OF MANAGEMENT[7]

Before concluding the initial patient write-up, it is helpful to list in general terms an overall Plan of Management. Not only will it help to clarify one's own thinking, but the Plan of Management also serves to summarize the proposed course of therapy for those sharing in the care of the patient. The specific day-to-day details of treatment are written elsewhere in the Physician's Order Book. (See Chapter 6.)

As with the Plan of Study, it is wise in planning management to first identify all the problems that need to be considered. Where there is more than one disease, each major diagnosis should be underlined and its plan of management described in a separate paragraph. Such organization will help one avoid overlooking important issues, as for example, the care of diabetes in a patient who enters with a stroke, or the consideration of suicide precautions in a depressed patient with cirrhosis.

---

[7]See Appendix B for a sample write-up of the Plan of Management.

The plan of management may be organized under the following headings:

1. *Activity, diet, and fluids.* The overall plan for the patient is described. For example, in the patient with hematemesis and an ulcer: "Bed rest. Transfusions and intravenous fluids, to be followed by hourly milk and antacid when the patient stops vomiting."

2. *Special procedures.* Suction, the type of traction, inhalation therapy, urinary catheterization, gastrointestinal intubation, or electro-convulsive therapy would be mentioned here.

3. *Special services.* Social service, speech therapy, physiotherapy, or occupational therapy are examples to be considered.

4. *Drug therapy.* The names of the important medicines to be used are mentioned. If the patient has congestive heart failure: "To be digitalized over 3 days with digitoxin, continue long term warfarin and add chlorothiazide."

5. *Surgical treatment.* The timing and type of operation planned are briefly described if a patient has a surgical problem. For example, in a patient with cirrhosis who is bleeding from esophageal varices: "When the patient has stabilized after transfusion, provided there is no deterioration in liver function, a side-to-side portacaval shunt will be done."

6. *Patient education.* When a patient has a chronic disease, it is most important that he be educated about his illness and its management. With diabetes mellitus, for example, the patient should be informed about the nature of the disease, its inheritance, and possible complications. How much should be told the patient requires clinical judgment, and it is the responsibility of the physician-in-charge. He should also talk with the patient about diet, medications, urine testing, foot care, see that the patient carries identification stating that he is a diabetic, and answer any questions he may have. Further instruction should be arranged with the Dietary Department and Nursing Service.

7. *Preventive medicine.* One should consider what can be done to prevent future disease in the patient and others. This would include such procedures as immunizations, the reporting of infectious disease to the responsible community health agency, or the examination and treatment of family members who may also be afflicted with the patient's disease.

Where management presents special or controversial problems, these should be discussed briefly. Such problems might be the reasons for the choice of an antibiotic, the benefits and risks of elective surgery in an elderly patient, or the patient's ability and motivation to undertake therapy at home.

When the Plan of Management has been completed, the initial patient write-up is concluded. The student signs his name at the end of the record followed by the title, Clinical Clerk. The medical orders are then written in the Physician's Order Book. However, some of the orders may need to be written before the student completes his work-up in order to provide continuing care. These orders include the patient's activity, diet, fluids, and needed medications.

THE PATIENT'S HOSPITAL COURSE

Progress Notes

Progress notes record the changes in the patient's symptoms and findings during his hospitalization as well as the physician's revised impression and plans. Pertinent historical or physical examination data not obtained on admission should be included in the progress notes. The patient may have been too ill for a complete interview or a physical examination when admitted, or new information may have come from the family, the referring doctor, or other hospitals. In general, progress notes highlight only one or two important points, and they should be written frequently in order to summarize briefly the patient's status. These notes should not be merely a description of planned laboratory procedures or their results; they should also emphasize the patient's current findings and include the student's most recent diagnoses. Each note should be dated and identified with the student's name.

Progress Notes may be organized as follows:

1. *The Patient's present symptoms*: Only a few lines may be needed to say how the patient feels, how the presenting symptoms have changed, or what new symptoms have appeared.

2. *Pertinent physical findings*: A brief description is made of the positive findings or changes in findings. Often, only the region containing the abnormalities need be described. One may also wish to record the patient's vital signs.

3. *Impression*: It is most important that the student indicate his current diagnostic thinking, which may have changed since the admission diagnosis. There is a need for continuing reformulation, and this must be communicated to others reading the chart. Interpretation of the results of important laboratory and diagnostic tests should also be included.

4. *Plan*: It is appropriate to indicate the current diagnostic and therapeutic plan, which may have changed since admission.

When a patient has multiple diagnoses, progress notes may be organized by using the problem solving method of Weed, in which each diagnosis is listed in a separate paragraph.

Well-written progress notes are not only helpful to others in under-

standing the patient, but they are also most valuable in promoting critical examination and thinking by the student. When he knows he must
enter historical and physical findings in the chart, his accuracy of examination at the bedside is reinforced. When he trains himself to write a
diagnostic impression, he will be more apt to consider a differential diagnosis to explain new findings. Also, when he writes a plan of study and
management, he will give careful thought before ordering new laboratory work or medications. Further, the writing of progress notes serves
to keep attention focused on the problems that remain to be solved.

The following is an example of a progress note written about a
patient with infectious hepatitis:

October 20, 1968   The patient continues to have a
J. G. Smith, Clinical Clerk   severe loss of appetite but no further
                                          vomiting since admission. He com-
                                          plains of weakness, is only able to
                                          take soft solids, and has continuing
sharp, right upper quadrant pain when he moves suddenly. A daily rectal
temperature up to 39.4° C. persists.

Physical examination: BP (Right arm) = 112/64. P = 104, regular. The
patient is listless. Since admission he has become more icteric and his urine is
the color of Coca Cola. A right upper quadrant mass, consistent with an
enlarged liver, has a sharp edge which is moderately tender; and on inspiration descends 5 cm. below the costal margin in the midclavicular line. A
tender mass compatible with a spleen, can easily be felt on deep inspiration 2
cm. below the left costal margin in the anterior axillary line.

Impression: The acute phase of viral hepatitis with increased jaundice.
Liver function tests confirm parenchymal disease.

Plan: Continue bed rest, high calorie soft foods and liquids, as tolerated.
Gamma globulin prophylaxis for the patient's children.

Diagnostic or Surgical Procedure Notes

All procedures performed should immediately be entered in the
chart in red ink and identified with the date and the responsible physician's or student's name. These procedures may include lumbar
punctures, bone marrow aspirations, "cut-downs," thoracenteses,
paracenteses, cardiac catheterizations, biopsies, and other operative
interventions. A careful description is given of the premedication, the
local preparation, the instrument used, the site of needle puncture or
incision, the amount and description of material obtained, and what
studies were ordered. Any associated symptoms and the patient's status
after the procedure are also reported. Where a surgical procedure is
performed, the written permission of the patient is required. An
example of a diagnostic procedure note for a lumbar puncture is:

November 1, 1968   The patient lay on his right side;
S. S. Jones, Clinical Clerk   his back was initially cleaned with
                              .   alcohol and iodine, and the skin
                                          and subcutaneous tissues were in-
                                          filtrated with 1% procaine. A #21

L. P. needle was easily introduced between L3 and L4 on the third attempt. Ten cc. of fluid, crystal clear in all three tubes, were slowly removed, and the patient had no complaints. The opening pressure was 130 mm. of water and closing pressure 100 mm. The Pandy's test was negative, and the cell count showed five lymphocytes per cm. without red cells. The fluid was sent for serology, total protein, and sugar content together with a simultaneous blood sugar.

Notes by Consultants

Consultants are asked to see the patient by the physician-in-charge. Their notes focus primarily on the special problem in which they are expert, with specific recommendations as to diagnosis, proposed studies, or details of management.

End-of-Service Note

When a student or house officer rotates off a ward, it is good practice for him to write a note summarizing the patient's problem and hospital course. The highlights of the patient's illness will then be underscored for the oncoming intern or resident, and a smoother transfer of care will ensue.

The "End-of-Service" note should be brief. In general, the following four areas should be covered: A summary of the admission findings, the patient's hospital course, his present status, and a statement regarding future plans for study and management. Attention is particularly directed to any therapy that is potentially hazardous and to any anticipated future emergencies.

The Final Note

At discharge, a definitive note should appear in the chart to sum up the hospitalization. The act of writing this summary gives the physician an opportunity to review the record and to see if any important data may be missing or if there are additional points in the patient's management that he may have missed. Such a note summarizing the patient's problem and his discharge management will be of value to other doctors when the patient returns for a follow-up visit or if he should reenter the hospital unexpectedly. The discharge note follows the plan of a well-written progress note.

1. A summary of the history and physical findings on admission.
2. A summary of the hospital course, including treatment.
3. The patient's status at discharge.
4. Final diagnoses.
5. Discharge plan, which includes the following:

a. *Place*: home, nursing home, with relatives, transfer to another hospital.
b. *Activity*: bed and chair, house-confined, fully ambulatory, date when patient may return to work, restrictions.
c. *Diet*: regular, low sodium (state mgs.), diabetic (state calories), ulcer, low residue.
d. *Special instructions*: visiting nurse, physiotherapy, exercises at home, soaks, dressing change.
e. *Medications*: a list of drugs, including dose, route, frequency, duration (if limited), and number of pills given.
f. *Follow-up plan*: the date and time of return to the Out-Patient Department, or the name of the referring physician and the date of the patient's follow-up visit.

It is most important that the physician-in-charge discuss the discharge plans with the patient and his family, that he solicit any questions and make sure the instructions are clearly understood. It is helpful for him to write down specific instructions, including the time and date of the return visit and the name and dose of each medicine. Should a patient not survive hospitalization, one describes the terminal circumstances, findings, and final diagnosis. This final note should also state whether or not an autopsy was done.

Reference

Weed, L. L.: Medical Records That Guide and Teach. New Eng. J. Med., *278*:593 and 652, 1968.

Chapter 6
MEDICAL ORDERS

The beginning clinical student does not have the primary responsibility for writing medical orders for his patients. Nevertheless, he must begin to familiarize himself with the proper method of writing orders. Institutions differ in details of procedure. What follows in this chapter is meant to provide an outline of generally accepted principles. By observing where and how the house officer writes his orders and how the nurse-in-charge communicates them to her staff, the student will learn many of the practical aspects of order writing.

As he gains clinical experience, the student may write the definitive orders for his patients, but these orders are not official unless they are reviewed and countersigned by the house officer or the physician-in-charge, who is then legally responsible. The student himself is not legally entitled to leave written orders.

The continuing care of the hospitalized patient is in the hands of the nurses and assistants. The written medical orders constitute the physician's explicit directive to the nursing staff as to the care and treatment of the patient. It is the physician's responsibility to see that his orders are clear, accurate, and complete; it is the nurse's responsibility to be certain that the orders are correctly interpreted and properly executed. For clarity, as well as for reasons of legal responsibility, orders are written in a designated place and are dated and signed by the physician. In turn, the nurse reviews the written orders, clarifies details or ambiguities with the physician, and indicates by her signature or initials that the orders have been noted and properly implemented.

GENERAL PRINCIPLES CONCERNING MEDICAL ORDERS

Communicating with the Nurses

It is important for optimal patient care that the physician discuss his orders with the nurse-in-charge at the time they are written, especially when they involve matters which are urgent or unusual. This will give him an opportunity not only to clarify and highlight specific orders, but also to discuss the patient's illness and any problems which may be antici-pated during hospitalization. In turn, the Head Nurse may have ques-tions or suggestions concerning the practical management of the patient. The student must also remember that nurses other than the nurse-in-charge will be involved in his patient's care. Usually, all orders left during the 8 hour nursing shift are reviewed by the charge nurse with the incoming group of nurses as they report for duty. This ongoing discussion of the objectives of therapy and the patient's problem with each group of nurses is as important as communication at the time orders are first written.

The needs of the patient are of primary concern in determining what orders should be written. At the same time, practical considerations require that the routine and availability of the nursing staff be kept in mind. For example, the timing of the administration of medications should fit the schedule according to which nurses routinely give drugs. It may be more helpful to write "Give every 6 hours," leaving the choice to the nurses, rather than to write an order for 3 P.M., 9 P.M., 3 A.M., and 9 A.M. When the drug is needed four times a day and is not required exactly every 6 hours, writing "q.i.d." will fit easiest into the nurses' schedule and will not interrupt the patient's sleep. Orders for frequent determinations of blood pressure, the recording of fluid intake and output, or for daily weights should be reviewed periodically to avoid placing an unnecessary burden on the nursing service.

Communicating with the Patient

Patients differ as to how much they should be told about the plan of management, and these differences will influence how orders are written. Many factors are involved, not the least of which is the patient's capacity to comprehend what he is being told. Certainly the critically ill patient is not in a position to deal with any detailed explanation, espe-cially if he is delirious or demented. For such a person it is important to convey by word and behavior one's intent to act promptly and effectively to relieve discomfort and resolve the problem. Because of limited attention span, explanation and reassurance should be confined to what is being done at the moment, such as the insertion of an intragastric tube, the administration of O_2 by nasal catheter, or the giving of an intramuscular injection.

With patients who are not as ill, the interview serves as a guide to indicate what each individual should be told about the treatment program. For instance, a patient may reveal in one way or another that he does not want to know the details but prefers to place himself entirely in the hands of the doctor and will do whatever he is told. Such a patient expects the doctor or nurse to know when he needs medication, and he does not want to have to ask for it. Hence the order is written in such a way that the nurse knows to administer the drug without waiting for the patient to ask. Another patient may be clearly apprehensive about what is going to happen and needs to know in advance the rationale for each procedure and medication. His cooperation is enlisted when the physician takes the time to outline plans, answer questions, and convey his intent to mitigate the patient's concerns. Still other patients are very uncomfortable unless they feel that they have some control over what is being done. Such people need to understand the rationale of each procedure; and they cooperate best when they can exercise an option, such as the privilege of asking for a sleeping pill, analgesic, or cathartic. By granting these minor requests, the physician makes it easier for the patient to accept other more necessary orders.

Questions that may arise in a patient's mind concerning restrictions, equipment, or drugs should be anticipated by the physician. For example, the patient should be given some idea as to his activity in the hospital and any dietary restrictions. When special equipment, such as a positive pressure breathing apparatus, is to be used, its purpose and function must be explained to the patient. If he is placed on sedation, he should be told that he may feel sleepy for a few days because the medication is intended to help him rest. Likewise, the patient in pain is told that medication is available, that he may have it at certain intervals, and that he should call the nurse if he needs the drug for relief.

When patients are given important information or instruction, the student should make sure that it is clearly understood. Instructions should be kept simple, and patients should not be given too many at one time. Repetition is helpful. It is a common error on the part of physicians to underestimate how preoccupied or inattentive the sick person may be.

Although the beginning student may help communicate with the nursing staff and may answer some of the patient's questions about his daily care, it is the function of the house staff or physician-in-charge to discuss the plan of management and specific medications with the patient.

Writing Orders Clearly

The student should strive to write his orders as clearly as possible. When his handwriting is not legible, he should make an effort to print or even use a typewriter. Abbreviations are kept to a minimum. If there is potential confusion in the names of two drugs, such as digoxin and digitoxin, it is helpful to write the name in capital letters and underline it: DIGOXIN. When the daily dose of a medication varies or is complex, it is helpful to make a chart with the date and dose of the drug. Such charts apply particularly to anticoagulant dosage or to insulin and fluid administration and may be put in the record on a separate sheet or written as a progress note.

Individualizing Orders

Every order must be written with the individual patient in mind. One is not treating the disease but the patient afflicted with illness. Close attention to the details of management will often determine whether success or failure is the outcome in a critically ill patient. In addition, the attention paid to small details of the patient's comfort is important not only in making his hospital stay more tolerable, but also in putting the patient in a frame of mind more conducive to recovery. For example, orders for medications should be written so that the patient will not be awakened in the middle of the night to take a pill; a bedside commode may be far more tolerable than a bed pan for the patient restricted to bed; or a board placed under his mattress may make the difference between sleeping or spending an uncomfortable night. Indeed, all "routine orders" should be critically evaluated, including sleeping medications or preoperative orders. Preoperative sedation, for instance, may sometimes need to be progressively increased because of mounting patient apprehension. On the other hand, sitting down with the patient and discussing his concerns may reduce his apprehension and eliminate the need for more sedation. Consultation with the anesthesiologist may be helpful in choosing the best drug to complement the planned choice of anesthesia. Preoperative orders for bladder catheterization or nasogastric intubation should also be timed properly in order to prevent undue patient discomfort.

When feasible, the patient should be consulted and his preferences followed if there are no serious or practical contraindications. Thus, some patients have dietary likes or dislikes, and arranging for them to talk with the dietitian can be very helpful. Others prefer to use medications with which they are familiar and have had good results in the past, especially hypnotics, analgesics, cathartics, and antacids. If the patient has been under the care of another physician before entering the hospital and is accustomed to some medication or therapeutic regimen, the reason for any change should be discussed.

Reviewing Orders

A repeated review of orders is mandatory. By doing this, the physician will avoid errors and will be able to modify treatment as the course of the illness varies and he learns more about his patient's individual needs. The review actually begins immediately after the first orders are written, for the physician must reread the orders before signing them. He should check the nurses' medication sheets daily; this is of special importance if more than one doctor writes orders for the patient. Orders covering several pages should be completely rewritten even as frequently as once a week when there is a complex and changing illness. Only by rewriting the orders can the physician easily review all aspects of the patient's management, eliminate unnecessary procedures, remove possible competing drugs, and fully comprehend what treatment is being given.

Orders are always completely rewritten postoperatively or when a patient is transferred to another service. When postoperative orders are written, the preoperative ongoing medicines, such as digitalis or insulin, must be reestablished; and in the early period of rapid change following surgery, the orders of each preceding postoperative day should be carefully reviewed.

Selecting Drugs

Before a student writes an order for medication, he must be sure of the dose, route, and frequency of administration. He should consult the hospital formulary to learn what drugs are available. If there are questions as to the action of the medication or its side effects, the student is obligated to review the drug in a standard pharmacology text. The manufacturer's circular packaged with the drug also contains important up-to-date information. If there are specific questions about a drug, particularly a new one, a call to the pharmacist may be helpful.

The possibility of an allergic reaction must be kept in mind for every drug ordered. One should consult the old hospital record for previous reactions and check with the patient when a medication is given that has allergic potential. The student should be familiar with the variety of drugs capable of provoking reactions, such as penicillin or chloramphenicol, and not overlook such substances as iodine compounds, which may be administered as radiopaque dyes. He should realize that not all "reactions" to drugs reported by patients are allergic. Also, the student should individualize the type or dose of medication in a patient whose constitution or illness makes him susceptible to an adverse drug reaction; for example, the use of sulfa in a patient with glucose-6-phosphate dehydrogenase deficiency, morphine in a patient with respiratory insufficiency, or digitalis where the serum potassium is low.

The number of drugs used should be kept to a minimum. The student should strive to order only those medications which are necessary and to preferentially select only the well established ones, which will help prevent confusing side effects and deleterious interactions. When a patient is admitted to the hospital, all his current medications should be carefully reviewed to eliminate those that are unnecessary. New drugs prescribed in the hospital should be discontinued as soon as their effect has been achieved or their ineffectiveness demonstrated.

THE CONTENT OF THE WRITTEN MEDICAL ORDERS

The nursing staff has three main responsibilities in the care of the patient: the enhancement of his comfort, the treatment of the disease, and the preparation of the patient for special procedures and diagnostic tests. Later in the hospital stay, the nurse will also be involved in convalescent and rehabilitative measures. In writing his orders, the physician keeps these main objectives in mind. The orders should be written as soon as the admission work-up has been completed and the physician has arrived at his diagnosis, plan of study, and plan of care. Even before the work-up is completed, it is often necessary to write a few initial orders, such as those for urgent medications, diet, or fluids. Orders are reviewed daily and are changed as indicated by the course of the illness. The following are the categories that the physician keeps in mind when he writes his orders. Learning these major headings will help the student in his organization so that he will not omit an important order:

1. Special information concerning the patient
2. The patient's activities
3. Diet
4. Fluids
5. Vital signs and weight
6. Special instructions to the nurses
    a. Notification of the house officer
    b. Patient care
    c. Special equipment
    d. Diagnostic or therapeutic procedures
    e. Collection of specimens
7. Medications

Special Information Concerning the Patient

The first few lines of the orders highlight any special problems that should be brought to the attention of the nursing staff.

It is helpful to indicate a diagnosis, particularly when this will alert the experienced nurse to urgent problems that may arise, e.g., "Acute pulmonary edema," "Diabetic acidosis," "Suicide attempt with barbiturates," or "The patient is delirious." The general condition of the patient at admission may also be indicated, such as "Acutely ill," "Stable," or "Satisfactory."

Other information that should be included are a known drug or food sensitivity with the name of the substance being indicated in red (e.g., Allergic to penicillin); the need to keep the airway clear by suction; the requirement for some type of infectious precaution; or a special status, such as "On the danger list."

The Patient's Activities

The physician should indicate whether the patient may be up and about, have bathroom privileges, be at complete bedrest, use a bedside commode, or have bed and chair privileges. If his activities are limited, it is important to state how long the patient may be up and whether he needs assistance getting in and out of bed. Also, if there are restrictions when the patient is at complete bedrest, they should be stated, e.g., "The patient may not bathe himself, may not shave, but may brush his teeth." Occasionally, one must specify whether visitors are allowed, and if so, who they should be.

Diet

The specific diet order is written, such as "House diet," "Clear liquids," "Low residue diet," or "Nothing by mouth." When diets are restricted, the orders should describe the exact content of the food substance allowed; e.g., a 40 Gm. protein diet, 500 mg. sodium diet, or 1800 calorie diabetic diet (150 Gm. carbohydrate, 75 Gm. protein, 100 Gm. fat). The hospital diet manual is usually available on the ward, and it is instructive for the student to refer to it. When a patient's problem is complex, a dietitian should be consulted before the order is written.

Other instructions under diet orders include in-between meal snacks, restriction of special food items, calculation of caloric intake, and the use of salt or sugar substitutes. When a discharge diet is anticipated and the patient will need instruction by a dietitian, specific orders, including the date of discharge, should be left at least 24 hours in advance.

Fluids

Orders to restrict or encourage fluid intake will be needed for some patients; e.g., "Restrict fluids to 1500 cc. per 24 hours." If a record of fluid balance is needed, one may write: "Record intake and output." In many patients, orders for parenteral fluids will be required. The following should be included: the volume of the solution; its composition (e.g., 5 per cent dextrose and water); the rate of administration, as cc. per hour; and if medications are added, the dose, in what volume of fluid, and the rate of administration. The bottle should also be labeled with the name and dose of the drug. When a patient will require several different parenteral solutions for more than one day, it is helpful to number these bottles sequentially. For example:

#1. 1000 cc. 5% dextrose and water I.V. at 100 cc. per hour.

#2. 1000 cc. 5% dextrose and ¼ normal saline I.V. with 40 ml. KC1 at 100 cc. per hour.

#3. 500 cc. 5% dextrose and saline I.V. with 2 cc. multiple vitamin solution at 75 cc. per hour.

Vital Signs and Weight

A statement is made as to the frequency of measuring blood pressure, pulse, respirations, temperature (route), and weight, if there is special need beyond the ward routine. Special modifications should also be indicated: apical pulses in atrial fibrillation, bed scales to weigh a bedridden patient, or recumbent and standing blood pressures when a patient is on sympathetic blocking agents.

Special Instructions to the Nurses

Orders for the care and study of the individual patient may be organized into five categories:

Notification of the house officer

Patient care

Special equipment

Diagnostic or therapeutic procedures

Collection of specimens

NOTIFICATION OF THE HOUSE OFFICER

Special instructions are often indicated when a change in the patient's condition is anticipated. For example, "Notify staff if feces become bloody" "Call house officer if systolic blood pressure drops below 100 mm. Hg" or "Call house officer if temperature exceeds 40° C."

PATIENT CARE

Orders for nursing procedures beyond the ward routine, such as bathing, mouth care, or feeding the incapacitated patient, should be made explicit. For example: "Change dry sterile dressing on right leg ulcer once daily," "Irrigate bladder twice daily with 300 cc. sterile saline," "Put lamb's wool boots on patient's feet," or "Keep head of patient's bed raised to 45 degrees and use bedside rails."

SPECIAL EQUIPMENT

Included are specific instructions as to the use of equipment, such as an orthopedic frame, positive pressure machine, cardiac monitor, oscillating mattress, or suction apparatus.

DIAGNOSTIC OR THERAPEUTIC PROCEDURES

Orders are needed to prepare the patient for procedures, such as a barium enema, angiography, liver biopsy, cardiac catheterization, fulguration of a bladder tumor, or the changing of an orthopedic cast. Most hospitals will have specific instructions for roentgen procedures, such as an upper gastrointestinal series, intravenous pyelogram, or oral cholecystogram. The student should consult the hospital manual or head nurse for guidance in such orders. One should write not only the order for the roentgen procedure, but also orders for the preparation of the patient, which occasionally may need to be modified because of his condition. A member of the Radiology Department can give helpful advice in this regard. For example, when ordering an intravenous pyelogram for a patient with renal insufficiency, the recommended fluid restriction and cathartic may adversely affect an already dehydrated patient. For such studies as biopsies, cardiac catheterization or cystoscopy, it is important that each step in preparation also be carefully considered; in particular, sedative or narcotic drug dosage may need to be altered because of the clinical status of the patient.

COLLECTION OF SPECIMENS

Specific instructions are written stating what specimen should be obtained and where it should be sent. Any special information is also included: whether, for example, the specimen should be collected over a given time period, whether under sterile conditions, or whether any special determinations should be performed.

Medications

Those drugs that are most urgent are usually written first, such as narcotics, antibiotics, mercurial diuretics, or digitalis. The *generic name of the drug should be used*, the dose (in the metric system), the route and frequency of the drug; and, if indicated, the limitation as to the number of days it should be given. For example: "Morphine sulphate 10 mg. s.c. every 4 hours, if needed for severe pain. Limit the order to 3 days." Hospital regulations may automatically cancel orders for drugs such as narcotics or barbiturates after 48 or 72 hours and require new orders. Some medication orders need to be written each day, as in the case of anticoagulant dosage.

Warning to the nursing staff about possible toxic or side effects of drugs, including the action that should be taken, may sometimes be necessary. For example, if the patient has previously bled on anticoagulants "Watch for gross blood in the urine"; in a cardiac patient "Omit the daily digitoxin dose if the patient's pulse is 50 or below"; or in the hypertensive patient "If the patient's systolic blood pressure when standing is 100 mm. Hg or below, please withhold the guanethidine dose and call the house officer."

Medications which are less urgent, including those given only if needed (p.r.n.), should be listed last; for example, oral contraceptive pills, chronic thyroid replacement, or aspirin for pain. Orders for sleeping medication or laxatives, which are usually written on a p.r.n. basis, may be included here.

EXAMPLES OF WRITTEN MEDICAL ORDERS

Four examples of written orders are given below. Common abbreviations that are used are as follows:

b.i.d.	twice a day	ml.	milliliter
cc.	cubic centimeter	p.o.	by mouth
da.	day	p.r.n.	when needed
Gm.	gram	q.	every
h.s.	at bedtime	q.i.d.	four times a day
hr.	hour	s.c.	subcutaneous
I.M.	intramuscular	stat	at once
I.V.	intravenous	t.i.d.	three times day
mg.	milligram	u.	units
min.	minute	x	times

Case 1.   A 24-year-old girl with a known duodenal ulcer and 4+ guaiac stools:

11/7/68
R. V. Smith, M.D.

A. *Special information.* Diagnosis: upper gastrointestinal bleeding. Condition: stable.

B. *Activities.* May use bedside commode with assistance.

C. *Diet.* 90 cc. of whole milk on the hour and 30 cc. of magnesium and aluminum hydroxides antacid suspension on the half hour. (Bland A. diet)

D. *Fluids.* 1000 cc. 5% dextrose and saline I.V. at 50 cc. per hour. Please keep I.V. open.

E. *Vital signs.* Take q. 4 hr. Take blood pressure and pulse with patient lying and sitting.

F. *Special instructions.* (1) Notify house officer if the systolic blood pressure falls below 100 mm. Hg, or if the pulse is above 120 beats/min., or if the blood pressure falls and the pulse rises more than 20 beats/min. on sitting up.

   (2) Schedule an upper gastrointestinal series on 11/8. Nothing by mouth after midnight, and call house officer to insert a nasogastric tube at midnight.

   (3) Save one stool a day for the house officer to examine.

G. *Medications.* (1) Phenobarbital 32 mg. p.o. q. 6 hr.
   (2) Pentobarbital 100 mg. q. h.s. p.r.n.

Case 2. A 76-year-old man with a fractured hip and chronic bronchitis:

12/6/68
H. M. Brown, M.D.

A. *Special information.* Diagnosis: Intertrochanteric fracture right hip. Condition: satisfactory.

B. *Activities.* Bed rest.

C. *Diet.* Nothing by mouth.

D. *Fluids.* 1000 cc. 5% dextrose and water I.V. at 85 cc./hr.

E. *Vital signs.* q. 4 hr.

F. *Special instructions.* (1) Surgical prep of right hip stat. Use hexachlorophene solution.

   (2) Send a clean catch urine for quantitative culture and antibiotic sensitivities.

G. *Medications.* (1) Atropine 0.4 mg. I.M. ⎫
   (2) Pentobarbital 100 mg. I.M. ⎭ on call to O.R.

POSTOPERATIVE ORDERS

12/7/68
H. M. Brown, M.D.

A. *Special information.* Discontinue all previous orders.

B. *Activities.* Bed rest. Assist patient to sit in chair 1 hr. t.i.d. beginning 12/8.

C. *Diet.* Nothing by mouth.

D. *Fluids.* (#1) 1000 cc. 5% dextrose and water I.V. at 100 cc./hr.

   (#2) 1000 cc. 5% dextrose and ¼ normal saline I.V. at 100 cc./hr.

E. *Vital signs.* Take q. 15 min. until stable, then q. 1 hr. × 4, then q. 2 hr. × 2, then q. 4 hr.

F. *Special instructions.* (1) Turn patient from side to side q. 2 hr. and encourage coughing and deep breathing.

    (2) Warm saline mist by mask q. 2 hr. for 15 min. while awake.

    (3) Endotracheal suctioning q.i.d. and p.r.n. for loud respiratory noises.

    (4) Foley catheter to closed drainage.

    (5) Tap water enema on 12/8 if no bowel movement.

    (6) Send sputum sample for culture and antibiotic sensitivities.

G. *Medications.* Meperidine 50 mg. I.M. q. 3 hr. p.r.n. for pain.

Case 3. A 65-year-old man with lobar pneumonia and benign prostatic hypertrophy:

1/9/69
3 P.M.
W. L. White, M.D.

A. *Special information.* Diagnosis: Lobar pneumonia. On danger list. Allergic to sulfa.

B. *Activities.* Bed rest. Bedside commode.

C. *Diet.* House diet or full liquids as tolerated.

D. *Fluids.* 1000 cc. 5% dextrose and water followed by 1000 cc. 5% dextrose and saline I.V. at 100 cc. per hr. Keep open with 100 cc. 5% dextrose and water. Record intake and output.

E. *Vital signs.* Take q. 1 hr., except rectal temperatures q. 4 hr. Weigh stat. and q. da.

F. *Special instructions.* (1) Call house officer if temperature is greater than 40° C. or if there is respiratory distress.

    (2) Special duty nurses around the clock.

    (3) Elevate the head of the bed to 30 degrees. Footboard.

    (4) Assist patient to stand and void q. 4 hr. while awake.

    (5) O_2 by nasal catheter at 8 liters/min. with saline humidification. Change catheter to opposite nostril q. 12 hr.

    (6) 10% propylene glycol by mask 20 min. q. 4 hr. while awake.

    (7) One sputum for culture and antibiotic sensitivities, and send three deep cough early a.m. specimens to the Cytology Lab.

    (8) Send a urine and stool specimen to the House Officer's Lab.

G. *Medications.* (1) *After* sputum is collected for culture, aqueous penicillin G 600,000 u. I.M. q. 6 hr. for 24 hr., then procaine penicillin G 600,000 u. I.M. q. 12 hr.

    (2) Elixir of terpin hydrate 4 cc. p.o. q.i.d.

(3) Codeine 60 mg. p.o. q. 4hr. p.r.n. for chest
    pain.
(4) Chloral hydrate 500 mg. p.o. q.h.s. p.r.n.
(5) Milk of magnesia 30 cc. p.o. q. da. p.r.n.

Case 4. A 72-year-old woman with diabetes mellitus, depression, coronary
heart disease, and an infected left ankle ulcer:

2/11/69
G.F. Black, M.D.
A. *Special information.* Diagnosis: Diabetes mellitus
   and infected leg ulcer. The patient is depressed.
B. *Activities.* Bed rest. The patient may use bedside
   commode.
C. *Diet.* 1500 calorie diabetic diet (150 Gm. carbohydrate, 75 Gm. protein, 70 Gm. fat), 500 mg.
   sodium diet, and include a bedtime snack.
D. *Fluids.* As desired.
E. *Vital signs.* Rectal temperatures q. 4 hr. Weigh
   every other day.
F. *Special instructions.* (1) Foot cradle. Elevate left leg
   with pillow placed under the calf. Allow patient
   to dangle legs only 15 min. four times a da. Soak
   left foot and ankle in tepid hexochlorophene bath
   15 min. t.i.d. Then remove as much exudate as
   possible with sterile cotton swabs. Lightly cover
   ulcers with sterile dressings. Place cotton between
   toes of both feet. Both heels should rest on a
   lamb's wool pad.
      (2) Collect urines t.i.d. before meals and h.s.
          to test for sugar and acetone.
      (3) Send a clean voided urine specimen to the
          Bacteriology Lab. for quantitative culture
          and antibiotic sensitivities.
G. *Medications.* (1) Mercaptomerin 2 cc. I.M. stat.
      (2) Ampicillin 250 mg. p.o. q. 6 hr.
      (3) Lente insulin 30 u. s.c. q. A.M.
      (4) Regular insulin s.c. by sliding scale q.i.d.

Urine Sugar	Insulin
0+	0 u.
1+	2 u.
2+	4 u.
3+	6 u.
4+	8 u.

      If acetone is present, please notify house
      officer.
      (5) <u>DIGOXIN</u> 0.25 mg. p.o. q.da.
      (6) Nitroglycerin 0.3 mg. sublingually p.r.n.
          for chest pain. The patient may have five
          tablets at bedside.
      (7) Amitriptyline 25 mg. p.o. t.i.d.
      (8) Aspirin 600 mg. p.o. q. 4 hr. p.r.n. for pain.
      (9) Secobarbital 100 mg. q.h.s. p.r.n. Report
          if patient becomes confused.
     (10) Milk of magnesia 30 cc. p.o. q.da. p.r.n.
          for constipation. If no bowel movement
          with milk of magnesia after one da., 4 cc.
          cascara sagrada p.o. p.r.n.

Chapter 7

THE PRESENTATION
OF THE PATIENT

Central to teaching rounds is the case presentation or verbal report of the patient's history, his physical examination, and the analysis of his illness. Such rounds are of value to all concerned. The student who presents the patient benefits from the criticism of his interview and physical examination techniques, has the accuracy of his data checked, and learns how to analyze clinical information in the presence of others. Fellow students learn not only from the instruction given during the presentation, but also from the patient's illness, which is a specific example of disease. The staff physician or preceptor has the opportunity to evaluate his own teaching techniques and methods of case analysis. The patient profits as well through the interest and concern expressed on his behalf and the knowledge that any new findings will be shared with the physicians-in-charge.

GENERAL PRINCIPLES OF PRESENTATION

It is important to acquire skill in the oral case presentation. Every physician is called upon to present patients, whether he is a house officer, a faculty member at a specialty conference, or a practitioner at a medical meeting. The keys to success are preparation and mental visualization of the details which others, who have never seen the patient, will need in order to have a clear picture of the clinical problem. The emphasis and content of the presentation will vary with the patient's illness, the goals of the conference, and the personal desires of the preceptor. The student must train himself to give an appropriate presentation under a variety of circumstances. There are certain general principles which underlie any case presentation:

There Is a Logical Order to the Presentation

In reporting his findings, the student should follow the classical divisions of the history and physical examination. (See Chapter 5.)

The Focus Is on the Patient's Present Problem

The student must clearly explain the chronology of the present illness and the interrelationship of current symptoms so as to be able to reconstruct step-by-step the pathophysiologic sequence of symptom development. Those physical findings relevant to the current problem should be described in detail. Enough information should be given in the interview and the physical examination to allow the listeners to form their own opinion.

Information Other Than the Present Illness Should Be Reported Selectively

Only the highlights of the remainder of the history and the physical examination should be given. If the audience wishes to know more about certain aspects of the work-up, they may ask questions after the presentation. Large areas of the patient's past history or physical examination should not be omitted, however, since these frequently have relevance when considering a differential diagnosis or the circumstances influencing the patient's illness.

Information Presented Must Be Objective and Accurate

The presentation should be based on what the patient said and what was actually found by the student at examination. The emphasis is on the data, not on its interpretation. If the student's findings differ from what others have reported, he should make this known. There should be neither distortion to what the student expects to find, nor mere conformation to a textbook description or the written record of the house staff. Dates and ages should be reported numerically, as should quantitative information, such as the duration of a symptom, the amount of sputum, and the number of flights of stairs climbed before shortness of breath is experienced.

Language Used by the Student Should Be Concise, Clear, and Vivid

When a presentation extends beyond 10 or 15 minutes, it becomes increasingly difficult for the listener to concentrate. Careful organization is particularly important if the history is long and complex. There should be clear identification of the major issues with a strict adherence to proper sequence and chronology. The student should strive for a concise presentation. However, accuracy must not be sacrificed for brevity; otherwise, a misleading picture of the patient's illness may be given, and the student is deprived of the opportunity to learn the relevance of the material being presented. If he organizes his presentation well and conveys a vivid picture of his patient's illness, he will have little difficulty holding the attention of the group, regardless of how long the presentation takes. It is the disorganized, rambling account, or the rapid-fire report of a series of symptoms that quickly loses the audience's attention.

The style of delivery and the choice of language are also important. The student who conveys a sense of interest about his patient's problems will more readily generate a similar interest in his audience. Hackneyed, repetitive statements, such as "Examination of the abdomen revealed" or "The chest was essentially normal," are not only dull but also add unnecessarily to the length of the presentation.

There Should Be an Accurate Choice of Terms

Some medical terms are used commonly yet are inaccurate. The student should strive for precise terminology. For example, "liver function tests" should be used instead of "liver chemistries," "agglutination tests" instead of "febrile agglutinins," "symptoms" instead of "symptomatology," or "abnormality" instead of "pathology." Abbreviations such as "protime" for prothrombin time or "lytes" for electrolytes should also be avoided.

Preparation

An effective presentation requires practice, experience, and careful preparation. It will help to jot down an outline of the highlights of the history and the physical examination and to orally rehearse the presentation before repeating it to the preceptor and fellow students. Even for brief follow-up presentations, the student should review the chart before giving interval findings. It is particularly helpful in identifying one's shortcomings to record the presentation on tape and to listen to the recording before reporting to the group. When one hears his own presentation, he becomes aware of repetitious and imprecise language and can better analyze the organization and clarity of what is said.

The Use of Notes and Visual Aids in the Presentation

The student should use as few notes as possible in his presentation and refer to them sparingly. Not only is it impressive when a physician can stand up and deliver a clear, well-organized case history without notes, but also the audience is not distracted by his frequent reference to them. When notes are used, they should contain only the highlights of the presentation, including important dates or laboratory data that might be forgotten. This information can be outlined on a small sheet of paper or index card. In most instances, careful preparation eliminates the need for notes.

Should the problem be especially complex or should there be many pertinent laboratory tests, such as frequent changes in serum electrolytes or liver function tests, it may be helpful to list these results on a blackboard. The purpose of such a list is to clarify the presentation for the audience, not to serve as a crutch for the student. He should be prepared to discuss the case history with only minimal reference to the blackboard. The presentation of a case is an active learning process. It should not be a slick, abbreviated, or preconceived summary. The student must always strive to highlight the significant relationships in the history and point out the minor as well as the major deviations from normal in the physical examination. With experience and time, he will learn to be concise, to give relevant data, and to deliver a brief presentation.

THE ORGANIZATION AND CONTENT OF THE PRESENTATION

1. The Orienting Statement
2. The History
   a. Present Illness
   b. Past Health
   c. Family Health
   d. Personal and Social History
   e. Systems Review
3. The Physical Examination
4. Admission Laboratory Data
5. Diagnosis

The Orienting Statement

In order to orient the group, the student should give an initial summary statement that identifies the patient, indicates the nature of the current problem, and highlights any significant past illnesses. When describing a patient who is not present one might say, for example, "This is the third admission of a 53-year-old white, married, unemployed janitor who is separated from his wife and who lives downtown alone in a furnished room. He has a long history of chronic alcoholism and now enters with acute upper gastrointestinal bleeding." Such a statement immediately focuses on the important medical issues and identifies some of the patient's personal and social attributes which may have bearing on understanding and managing his illness.

The History

By using the patient's descriptive terminology and avoiding interpretive terms, the student relates the present illness in detail with strict attention to chronology and sequence. For example, the patient may have a long-standing duodenal ulcer with an acute exacerbation of pain. Rather than saying that he has a known duodenal ulcer and comes in with a flare-up of pain, it is better to describe in detail the recent symptoms in terms of the seven dimensions. (See Chapter 3.) Then, one may say that the past episodes consisted of similar pain, and some idea is given of the severity, chronology, and complications in the past. As is done in the write-up, it is helpful to conclude the presentation of the present illness by mentioning pertinent positive and negative findings, medications, changes in weight, and the degree of disability.

The remainder of the history is given in outline form, highlighting only the important findings under each major subsection (Past Health, Family Health, Personal and Social History, and Systems Review). In describing illnesses in the past that are not related to the present illness, interpretive or diagnostic terms may be used, for example, "The patient had a cholecystectomy at Genesee Hospital 25 years ago for cholecystitis and multiple gallstones." If the audience wishes more detail about a past illness, they may ask questions at the end of the presentation. It is assumed that the student knows the details of past illnesses, which justifies his use of interpretive rather than descriptive terms. If an illness of a relative has any bearing on the patient's present problem, it should be mentioned under Family Health, including the nature of the family member's illness, and, if deceased, his age and date of death. The current life situation under Personal and Social History should be described briefly. Knowledge of the patient's current circumstances is important not only in understanding his present illness, but also in planning for his care after discharge. Only those findings that bear an important relationship to the patient's present problems should be mentioned in the Systems Review.

Judgment and experience will help the student strike the proper balance when reporting parts of the history other than the Present Illness. He must learn to avoid excessive detail yet not dismiss findings and events as "noncontributory" when they may have relevance to understanding the patient's problem. Considerable thought should be given to what information is not significant and need not be told and what findings should be mentioned. For example, if the patient is a newly discovered diabetic, the fact that he fractured his wrist as a child may be omitted; however, it is of considerable importance to state that there is no family history of diabetes or that a diabetic uncle had gangrene and lost a leg.

The Physical Examination

By following the general outline of the written physical examination, the student will present his data in a clear and organized manner. He should begin with a general description of the patient, including any gross abnormalities in order to give the audience a vivid and accurate picture. Vital signs are described next. Each major system is then touched upon, starting with the skin and ending with the nervous system. If an abnormality related to the current illness is present or is expected to be present, the physical findings in that given system should be fully described. Those systems without abnormalities, or those that do not bear on the present illness, are mentioned only briefly. For example, the abdominal findings of a patient who has had a chest injury in an auto accident may be briefly presented as follows: "No abnormalities were found in the abdomen." On the other hand, if a steering wheel injury could have affected the abdomen, the pertinent negatives of possible abdominal as well as of chest trauma should be mentioned: "There was no abrasion of the abdominal wall; no tenderness or muscle spasm. The liver and spleen were not felt, and peristalsis was normal."

Admission Laboratory Data

The student should give the values for the admission hematocrit, white blood count, differential count, a description of the blood smear, and the results of the urinalysis and the stool examination for blood. Other known laboratory data significant to the patient's problem may or may not be mentioned at this time depending on the desires of the preceptor.

Diagnosis

The presentation concludes with the student giving the diagnoses that were listed in his write-up. The diagnoses should not be mentioned in the presence of the patient. Following the presentation, the other students in the group are encouraged to ask questions, should they not have had an opportunity to do so previously. Further discussion of the case will be guided by the preceptor. The student who is presenting the patient should also be prepared to give his reasoning for the diagnoses, discuss the differential diagnosis, evaluate prognosis, and describe his plan of study and management.

THE TYPES OF PATIENT PRESENTATIONS

The form, content, and location of presentations will vary. The preceptor will usually indicate what he wants done. If a student is inexperienced and only one patient is to be seen, the presentation may take place in a classroom. Other presentations may be given at the bedside. In order to be most effective, teaching rounds must focus on the patient and his problem.

Examples of different types of presentations are as follows:

The Classroom Presentation Before a Small Group

There are several types of classroom presentations. One is with the patient present and differs little from the bedside presentation, except that there is less occasion for distraction by other patients in the room or interruption by ward personnel. Another type of classroom presentation is given in the absence of the patient, who is seen afterwards either at the bedside or in the classroom. When the student first begins to present patients, it may be helpful to do so without the patient, in a classroom where the student has adequate time to organize his thoughts and to express himself. Interruption by the patient or others will be avoided; the highlights of the case work-up may be put on a blackboard; and the preceptor is able to intervene with comments about the student's presentation.

The disadvantages of classroom presentations without the patient are that there is no opportunity for interaction with the patient and there is a tendency for the discussion to focus more on the disease process than on understanding the individual and his illness. Hence it is most important that the patient be seen later by the group so that such interaction can take place, the accuracy of the student's information can be checked, and his skills in data gathering observed.

Another approach is for the student to introduce the preceptor and the other students to the patient at the bedside. The instructor or another student may spend 2 or 3 minutes inquiring about the patient's problem, following which the presentation is given in the classroom and the patient is informed that the group will return in 20 or 30 minutes. Because of the initial contact, all are better able to visualize the patient as his story is related in the classroom. When the presentation is completed, the group returns to the bedside for further interview or demonstration of physical findings.

Occasionally a student may be asked to tape record his interview of the patient and give the tape to the preceptor who listens to it before the presentation. This enables him not only to check on the skill of the interviewer, but also to evaluate the student's presentation in terms of data selection, accuracy, and organization.

In the event that the patient is brought into the classroom, every effort should be made to indicate a personal interest in him and to avoid the implication that he is a curious example of disease. Any blackboard notes which may disturb him should be kept from his view.

The Bedside Presentation

The student should judge beforehand whether a given patient is suitable for presentation at the bedside. In general, most presentations are appropriate at the bedside and are particularly valuable when an intelligent patient may amplify and clarify his symptoms or where there are physical findings to be observed. However, there are several circumstances where the presentation must be abbreviated or some of the information must be withheld to be given later in the patient's absence. Such instances include: the patient who is critically ill and may be fatigued by a lengthy presentation; the delirious or demented patient who may be further disturbed by hearing his history; the manifestly anxious or hostile patient; the patient whose presence would interfere with the presentation of pertinent personal information or disturbing medical details. Since the student knows the patient best, it is his responsibility to inform his preceptor of the need to alter the presentation at the bedside. The instructor will then decide whether he wishes to have the patient presented at the bedside or in the classroom. Learning how to present in the presence of the patient is valuable preparation for the bedside rounds traditionally carried out by the house staff. The student learns to be brief and to the point, to make observations while reporting, and to maintain a tactful and supporting relationship with the patient. Few serious problems are likely to arise as long as the well-being of the patient remains the central concern of all involved. One must observe the patient closely and respond at once to any indication of distress. The risk of offending the patient comes when the group forgets his presence and engages in a technical or pedagogical discussion that is of more interest to them than the patient's welfare. Even though comments made in such a discussion may not be directly applicable to the patient, he quite naturally assumes that whatever is said at the bedside refers to him. Hence, discussion of the patient, and especially of the disease process, should always take place away from the bedside.

The Follow-up Presentation

During their hospital stay, patients are usually seen on repeated follow-up visits after the original presentation. The student will need to bring the instructor and fellow-students up to date on his patient's hospital course. This may be done briefly, before the group enters the patient's room. In order to refresh everyone's memory, the student gives the patient's name, age, and date of admission, followed by a few sentences reviewing the present illness, physical examination, and admitting diagnosis. Then, any new findings are briefly given in the form of a progress report, beginning with a few words about the patient's current symptoms and physical findings. Pertinent new information about the present or past history should be reported, along with the results of laboratory tests and diagnostic procedures. Any revision in the diagnosis or in the plan of study or the plan of treatment should also be mentioned.

One reintroduces the preceptor to the patient by saying "You remember Dr. so-and-so, Mr. Adams, and the other doctors who saw you yesterday." Then an inquiry indicating personal concern is made "We are all interested to see how you are doing. How are you today?" After the patient has had an opportunity to express himself, further questions may be asked by the group, or physical findings may be demonstrated.

The Formal Presentation Before a Large Group

On occasion, a student will have the opportunity to present his patient before a large group of students and senior physicians. Advance preparation is of particular importance, since there will usually be a time limit for the case presentation. Consequently the data must be carefully selected and the presentation rehearsed. It may be helpful to write the highlights of the work-up on the blackboard, and sometimes the case history is outlined on slides. If a projector will be needed, one should check to be sure it is in proper working order, that a projectionist is available, and that the slides are labeled properly. Any data projected or written on the blackboard must be concise and of adequate size for all to see. Only the essentials should be recorded. A large mass of data may overwhelm and confuse the audience. As in the smaller classroom, the patient's chart should be handed to the physician-in-charge, and notes should be used sparingly. One should speak loudly and clearly, using a microphone if necessary. Before the conference begins, the student should check to be sure the patient has arrived from the ward.

STUDENT RESPONSIBILITIES AND CONDUCT

Advance Notification of the Patient and Ward Staff

Whenever a patient is to be presented, he should be told of this in advance. Usually a simple explanatory statement is all that is needed. For example, "Tomorrow, I am going to bring in several other doctors who are interested in your problem" or "The senior doctor-in-charge will be seeing you, and I will tell him your story." The patient should be given the expected time of the visit so that he may prepare himself. He should also be informed of the presence of others: "There will be several other student-doctors" or "The doctors on the ward will also be there." When the patient is to be formally presented before a large group, it is especially important that adequate time be spent in advance telling him about the conference, its purpose, and the approximate size of the audience.

The head nurse and ward secretary should be informed of the time of the presentation. The nursing staff will then be able to complete the care of the patient, and he will be washed and his bed made before the visit. If feasible, the secretary should schedule procedures, such as radiological studies, to avoid conflict with the presentation; and the patient should be seen at a time that does not interfere with his meals. When the case presentation is to be given in a conference room away from the ward, arrangements must be made with the ward secretary to have the patient sent there at a specific time. Consideration is given to the means of transport, whether it be a wheelchair, stretcher, or bed. A very ill patient should have an attendant with him constantly and should be away from the ward for only a minimal time.

Preparing for the Teaching Rounds

The student who presents his patient at the bedside has the responsibility of seeing that the teaching exercise goes smoothly. The group of students should assemble promptly to meet the instructor. The student presenting should hand his work-up and the ward chart to the preceptor and should remain standing for the entire presentation. Any necessary examining instruments should be available for the instructor's use. The student-in-charge should lead the group to the patient's bed. It is his responsibility to see that the patient's room is quiet, that there is adequate lighting, and that privacy is assured by shutting the door or closing the curtains about the bed.

In the classroom, any materials that will enhance the teaching rounds should be available, such as the patient's x-ray films, blood smears, sputum slides, pathology slides, or a fresh urine sediment. Pertinent source material from journals or textbooks may be at hand for the benefit of the other students. If a blackboard is present, the student may wish to outline information of significance, in particular, complicated laboratory data.

Introducing the Patient

When a patient is presented to a large group in a formal conference, it is especially important that a personal interest be demonstrated towards him and that he not be quickly wheeled in after the presentation, asked one or two questions, and then wheeled out when his abnormal findings have been shown. He should be made to feel as comfortable as possible, with an introductory word of welcome: "Mr. Smith, we appreciate your coming. These are the doctors I was telling you about who are interested in your story." It may help to sit down next to the patient to put him at his ease. He should also be given the opportunity to tell briefly about some aspect of his illness. If the patient is there during the presentation, the student should stand next to him as he relates the history, and he should be constantly attentive to the patient's comfort and feelings.

When at the bedside, the student should introduce his preceptor and fellow students to the patient: "Mr. Smith, this is Dr. Jones who is in charge." The other students are also introduced by name: "This is Dr. White, Dr. Green, and Dr. Black." A brief explanation is then given for the visit: "As I mentioned to you yesterday, we are all interested in your problem. I am going to tell the doctors your story, so you just sit back and relax" or "Dr. Jones has just heard about your illness, and will want to ask you a few questions and check some of your physical findings."

The preceptor goes to the patient's right so that he will be in the best position to interview and examine. It is usually most convenient for the presenting student to be at the patient's left. Here, the group can see the student easily as he gives the story, and he is in a position to make the patient comfortable. The student should help the patient undress, see that he is properly draped and that the bed is elevated to the proper height for the examination.

The other students should stand quietly at the foot of the bed, wholly attentive to the patient and the presentation. Conversation, reading notes and charts, or leaning on the patient's bed are discourteous and distracting. When television sets or radios in the room are too loud, they should be turned down. It may also be necessary to ask patients in adjacent beds to speak more softly.

The Presentation in the Presence of the Patient

After the introduction and attention to the patient's comfort, the student may give the history. He should begin on a personal note: "Mrs. Smith is 29 years of age and has three children. She was admitted 2 days ago with vaginal bleeding." Impersonal phrases stating the obvious, such as "White female" should be avoided. Plain English is preferred to Latin medical terms that may upset the patient. For example, one avoids such terms as "This case is 29-years-old, gravida 4, para 3, with menorrhagia." The use of notes at the bedside should be kept to a minimum. If the student refers sparingly to notes, the patient will feel that the student is more interested in him than in his own performance before his instructor and peers.

Care must also be taken at the bedside to avoid terms that may be misinterpreted by the patient. Although innocent to the physician, words may have a far different connotation to the patient. To say "She aborted in her third week of pregnancy" may imply criminal abortion to the patient; "Heart failure," though mild, may be misinterpreted as a terminal condition; or "I felt a thrill on examining her chest" could have disturbing connotations to the young hysteric. In general, when the student uses the patient's own phraseology and avoids diagnostic medical terms, there should be little problem in causing patient apprehension. Confidential information that might embarrass the patient before the group of students or the other patients in the room should be omitted and can be mentioned later away from the bedside. Any physical findings that might be disturbing to the patient, such as the level of blood pressure or the finding of an unsuspected mass, may also be held back, but most findings can be given. After the student has presented the patient's history and physical findings, the instructor will usually take the lead in indicating the direction of the teaching exercise. He may question and examine the patient further, ask the student to demonstrate his techniques, or invite questions from the other students. Discussion about diagnosis or laboratory data should take place away from the patient.

Patients respond to a presentation in various ways. Some listen quietly; others may interrupt frequently to correct the student or add comments. With the latter type of patient, the student should give him a brief opportunity to express himself and should not argue. He should gently intervene to resume the presentation: "Thank you for reminding me of that. Why don't I go on and give the highlights of your story, and you can add anything else after I have finished." It is important to ask the patient at some time during the visit if he has any questions or if there is anything else he would like to add. The student should always be alert to any concern on the patient's part during the presentation. If the patient shows apprehension, the student should interrupt at that time to reassure him lest there be misinterpretation. For example, if the patient has reacted to an innocent medical term, the student should clarify the meaning and attempt to resolve the patient's concern.

Concluding the Visit to the Patient

Following the examination, the student should help the patient get dressed and see that the bed is returned to the proper level, the side rails replaced, the lights turned off, and the curtains opened. Used equipment, such as tongue blades or tissues, should be disposed of, instruments picked up, and the chart removed from the bedside. A chart should never be left alone with a patient.

It is not necessary to thank the patient at the conclusion of the bedside presentation, especially since such a discussion is in his interest. However, a brief encouraging word by the student or preceptor should be given the patient before leaving: "We all hope you will be feeling better" "We are glad the pain is gone" or "We are now going to go over the studies you have had and see what we can do to help." When the patient has been seen at a formal conference, it is appropriate to thank him for coming. He should be accompanied outside the conference room, and it is the student's obligation to see that he is promptly sent back to the ward.

After the teaching exercise has been concluded, it is considerate to return later to tell the patient that it has been helpful to go over his story with the other doctors and that any conclusions reached will be passed on to the physician-in-charge. At this time, the patient may have questions or he may voice misapprehensions which can be answered or referred to the appropriate physician.

APPENDIX

Two patients were interviewed and examined by the authors whose case write-ups appear below as illustrative examples. Both patients were selected because of their complex medical histories that included neurological illnesses. In addition, both presented problems in interviewing. The first tended to minimize and deny her symptoms; the second patient was mildly demented and had a poor memory for details of past events.

By choosing such examples, the authors are better able to illustrate problems in interviewing and difficulties in organizing the case write-up. Not all cases seen by a student will be as complex. Many patients will give straightforward histories of clear-cut illnesses. The length and content of the write-up will vary with the complexity of the patient's problem and with the student's selection and interpretation of data. Write-ups will also vary according to one's individual style of writing. It is most important in any case write-up that the student make an effort to express himself clearly so that persons reading the medical record will have an accurate understanding of the patient's problem.

In Appendix A, the first patient's interview is recorded verbatim and is followed by a case write-up that includes the History, Physical Examination, Diagnosis, and Prognosis. The clinical problem is reasonably clear-cut and does not involve consideration of several alternative diagnoses, so that the section on diagnosis deals more with the interpretation of findings than with a differential diagnosis.

In Appendix B, a complete patient work-up is recorded, including the History, Physical Examination, Admission Laboratory Data, Diagnosis, Prognosis, Plan of Study, and Plan of Management. Here, the

243

diagnosis of the current illness is more uncertain, and a differential diagnosis is described in detail.

Both case write-ups are organized so as to conform to the outline of Table 5-1, which is at the beginning of Chapter 5.

Appendix A

A VERBATIM INTERVIEW AND CASE WRITE-UP

This section illustrates the course and sequence of an interview and demonstrates how the data so obtained are organized into the case write-up. The physical examination, the diagnosis, and the prognosis are included for completeness and indicate what the examiner considers to be the most important issues of the patient's illness.

The patient is a 52-year-old, married woman, who was admitted to the hospital from another city for an evaluation of symptoms of dyspnea, orthopnea, edema, and rapid heart action. She had recently suffered right-sided weakness. This much was known to the interviewer before he met the patient. The interview was tape recorded and is transcribed verbatim here, except for minor editing to make it more readable and to protect the anonymity of the patient and of her physicians. The interview took approximately one hour. Not all of the necessary information was obtained in the one session, and it would be necessary to see the patient again to completely cover the details.

For the guidance of the reader, a running commentary is printed to the left of the transcript. The commentary highlights the steps of the interview that are outlined in Chapter 3, describes the thought processes of the interviewer, and identifies the principal findings of the patient's history.

Step 1: Introduction
Defining the interviewer's role.

Dr. How do you do, Mrs. Curtis. I'm Dr. Engel. Dr. Morgan has asked me to see you. (extends hand)
Pt. You'll have to take this hand (smiles and offers left hand)
Dr. Uh-huh. Would you sit down here, please? I'm recording this so I don't have to take notes. Do you mind?
Pt. Oh no.
Dr. Good.
Pt. If it all comes out good. (laugh)

Step 2: Defining current status

Interviewer questions "fine."

Dr. How are you feeling?
Pt. Fine! (with emphasis)
Dr. Fine?
Pt. Well, good. (pause) The heart beat is fast, but I'm the same. As long as I don't suffer from it, I don't pay much attention to it. (pause)

245

Dr. When you say fine, what do you mean?
Pt. Well, I don't have anything to complain about. I have
no pain. Nothing like that.
Dr. And during the week that you've been here, how
have things been?
Pt. Oh, fine. I'm getting stronger with the hand every
day.
Dr. Your hand is getting stronger?
Pt. Yes.
Dr. Mm-hmmm.
Pt. So yesterday I went to physical therapy. And they
showed me some exercises to do, you know, that
would make it stronger, so that I can do that myself.
Dr. What was the reason for your coming *here* a week
ago?
Pt. Well, I was supposed to come here for an operation. I
originally was supposed to come sometime in January.
The 1st of January my husband took the month off
and in December I had the stroke, so I couldn't come.
So my physician got in touch with Dr. Y. and told him
that he felt perhaps I was over it sufficiently to have
the operation. And so Dr. Y. made the appointment
and I came.
Dr. When was it originally suggested that you should
come here to have an operation?
Pt. In November.
Dr. Before you had the stroke.
Pt. Oh yes. Dr. W. at the clinic at home gave me a thor-
ough going over and he wasn't satisfied.
Dr. This was in . . .?
Pt. November.
Dr. When in November?
Pt. I think it was the 7th?
Dr. The 7th?
Pt. It was on Election Day.
Dr. Mm-hmmm.
Pt. And so he consulted Dr. Y, who agreed that I should
come back in January to consider having an operation.
Dr. Well, when did this all start then?
Pt. Well, during the hot weather, it always bothered me.
Dr. What bothered you?
Pt. The heat. I can't stand heat, and it's just gotten worse
with the years. I was working, you know, as a teller
with the First National Bank. And so this first time was
in August, on a Friday. I worked under air condi-
tioning. It was, you know, very comfortable. That
noon when I went out the door, oh, it was so stifling,
and I got a pain in my arm and such pains in my chest!
And I couldn't breathe very well. I walked about a
block, and I felt so terrible that I turned around and
came back to the bank and came in. But then I felt
better, so I worked the rest of the day and that night
when I went home I said to my little girl that I thought
that I'd go see the doctor.

So far the patient emphasizes improvement and tends to minimize symptoms.

Step 3: The problems leading to hospitalization

The patient gives a literal response with little clinical information. She continues to avoid speaking of symptoms.

Chronology.

Chronology—Election Day as reference.

Interviewer brings patient back to general question about symptoms. Her response is vague, so again the interviewer has to press.

First mention of specific symptoms, pain in arm and chest and dyspnea.

Interviewer indicates interest in child.

Dr. Your little girl is how old?

Pt. Ten years old.

Dr. Ten years old. What is her name?

The patient resumes her account herself.

Irregular heart beat.

Pt. Lois. I went to the doctor and he gave me some quinidine. He said that I apparently had some irregular heart beat, influenced by hot weather. So I took it and I was to go back on Monday. And when I went back Monday, he said that it was fine. So I went back to work that week. The following week the girls weren't feeling too well in the bank. They were having some kind of a virus, like the 24-hour virus or something. And I guess I got it. Three days I had it.

"24-hour virus."

The patient seems reluctant to dwell on symptoms. She hurries through her story. The interviewer tries to encourage her to give more details by bringing her back to the beginning again.

Dr. Let me get this clear in my mind. The preceding period was in August?

Pt. August.

Dr. Did you give me a date, when in August?

Pt. No, I think it was the first part. Say it was the 3rd of August, or something like that.

The interviewer is trying to impress on the patient the importance of dates.

Dr. The first part of August of this past summer, 1967. And you had been working regularly?

Pt. Yes.

Dr. And on that particular day was there some reason why you went out at that point?

Pt. Well, yes, it was my lunch hour.

Dr. And how were you feeling that morning?

Patient continues to minimize symptoms. By this time the interviewer knows he will have to press for details if he is to discover the range of the patient's symptoms. Hence he moves into Step 4.

Pt. I didn't notice anything different. I didn't have any pain or anything.

Step 4: The delineation of present illness

Dr. No pain. You were getting around?

Pt. Yes. In the hot weather I'm used to it. This thing always beats so fast.

Dr. It beats fast in the hot weather?

Pt. Yes.

Dr. So this was something you had noticed prior to that.

Pt. Yes. But I had been to doctors before in the summertime. It seems as though I go to the doctor in the summertime. I tell him that something's wrong with my heart, and the doctor'll say, "No, I can find no defects in the heart." So I go along with it. I think that there's nothing wrong with it.

The doctors are reported as supporting her use of denial.

Dr. Up to that point no one had said there was anything wrong with your heart?

Pt. No.

Dr. How old are you?

Pt. Fifty-two. I'll be 53 on April 11.

Recapitulation to get patient to resume account.

Chronology.

Dr. April 11, uh-huh. So you walked out of the bank and went from the cold to the hot. And what was the first thing wrong you noticed?

Again she is vague and has to be asked.

Pain; location.

Pt. It hit my arm. (the patient indicates her left arm)
Dr. What hit your arm?
Pt. It just pained, my left arm. And, oh, it felt such pains in it, and it felt just like it was beating *so fast.* (puts hand to left upper chest)
Dr. That is where you felt it?
Pt. Yes.
Dr. How did that pain come on?
Pt. It came just like that, it happened.
Dr. All of a sudden.
Pt. Yes, just as I stepped out of the bank, I thought, "Whew, it's so hot, oh boy." It went like that and I didn't know what to do with it, you know. (The patient indicates pain going from chest down arm)

Pain; quality (open-ended question).
Patient has difficulty describing pain.

Dr. And what kind of pain was it?

Pt. Oh, I don't know. It's the kind of pain you have with—sharp pain like, you know . . . well . . . it's something you just can't stand hardly, you know. It's just like that, you know.

Interviewer was going to give her a choice of adjectives, but she selected the first with conviction.

Dr. Was it aching or . . .
Pt. *Yes, yes,* like that. But then it stopped.

Interviewer is echoing her responses as a means of indicating his interest.

Dr. But then it stopped.
Pt. But this didn't stop. (indicates chest)
Dr. The pain in your chest did not stop?
Pt. No.

"This" is vague—must be defined.

Dr. Well, when you say "this," do you mean the rapid heart, too?
Pt. The rapid heart, too. This pain didn't stop immediately. (indicates chest) But then when I was back in the bank, when it got cooler, then it stopped. But the fast heart beat didn't stop.

Pain; duration.

Dr. How long did the pain in your arm last?
Pt. Oh, I went from the bank down into the next block before it stopped.
Dr. Walking slowly?

Pain: aggravating factor
Pain; location (open-ended question).

Pt. Yes, I had to walk very slow because it was so painful.
Dr. Now where in the arm did you feel it?
Pt. It seems as if it was everywhere. (laugh)
Dr. As if it was the whole arm?
Pt. Yes.
Dr. Did it seem to be inside or on the outside of the arm?
Pt. Well, I don't remember that. It just hurt so bad that I don't remember . . .

Pain; location (specific question).

Dr. Did it go into your hand?
Pt. No, I don't think so. . . I don't know.

Interviewer invites patient to speak of the other symptoms: palpitation and dyspnea.

Dr. You don't remember that. And then you came back in, and you noticed that your heart was beating fast. You also mentioned that you were short of breath.
Pt. Yes.

Dyspnea; quantity.

Dr. How short of breath were you?

Pt. Well, I sort of had to take a deep breath in order to draw it, you know.

Pain; duration.

Dr. Uh-huh. So then you came back into the bank and you say your arm pain disappeared. How soon did the chest pain disappear?

Pt. Oh, it was . . . about 20 minutes.

Dr. About 20 minutes.

Pt. Mm-hmmm.

Palpitation; duration.

Dr. And what about the pounding of the heart?

Pt. No, that didn't let up. I went home, and then I went to the doctor's.

Noting the tendency to minimize, the interviewer wants to explore the fact that the patient stayed at work after her attack.

Dr. Uh-huh. But you continued to work.

Pt. Yeah, yes . . . for a few days.

Dr. No, I mean that day.

Pt. Oh yeah. I worked until 5 o'clock.

Dr. You were going out for your lunch, but you didn't have lunch?

Pt. I didn't eat.

Dr. You just came back to the bank and went back to your window?

Pt. Mm-hmmm.

Dr. How come?

The patient is revealing a personality style, to ignore or minimize disability. The interviewer knows this will have to be taken into account if he is to obtain a full history

Pt. I don't know. The doctor had told me there was nothing wrong with my heart. So I thought, well, there's nothing wrong with it, so I continued to work. I didn't know what else it could be.

Dr. Is that like you, just to go on about your business if you can?

Pt. Yes.

Interviewer recapitulates to encourage the patient to resume her account. In so doing he also emphasizes his interest in details.

Dr. Mm-hmmm. So you went back to your job without your lunch. The arm pain subsided, then the chest pain; but your heart continued to beat fast. You went home at five and told your little girl that you were going to the doctor's.

Pt. Mm-hmmm.

Dr. And he gave you the quinidine.

Pt. Mm-hmmm.

Dr. Can you pick up the story from there?

Pt. Then Monday I went back to him, as he asked me to.

The patient skips the weekend.
The interviewer brings her back.

Dr. Well, how were you over the weekend?

Pt. Fine! (said with vigor) The quinidine made it calm down.

Chronology.

Dr. The quinidine calmed it down how soon?

Pt. Oh . . . I don't remember how long. It was fine when I went to the doctor's on Monday.

The interviewer doubts the patient's "fine!"

Dr. Well, how did you spend the weekend, do you recall?

Pt. It was an ordinary weekend. Of course, I couldn't go out. On Saturdays I always do, but that day I just couldn't. Sunday was quiet.

Setting.

Dr. Who was at home that weekend?

Pt. My husband and my son and my daughter.

Brief exploration of family.

Dr. You have two children?
Pt. I have three.
Dr. Three.
Pt. One is married. One's 16 and one is 22 and one is 10.
Dr. The 22-year-old is a boy or a girl?
Pt. Boy.
Dr. What is his name?
Pt. Bob.
Dr. He's married?
Pt. Mm-hmmm.
Dr. And lives where?
Pt. In the same town.
Dr. What is the 16-year-old's name?
Pt. Mark.
Dr. So there were the four of you at home, you, the two younger children and your husband.
Pt. Mm-hmmm.

Resume account of illness.

Dr. And it was an ordinary weekend.
Pt. Mm-hmmm.
Dr. And Monday you went back to work?
Pt. Mm-hmmm. But I didn't feel so good.
Dr. What was the trouble?

Patient again bypasses details of symptoms.

Pt. Well, I was apparently coming down with the virus. And so I worked all that Monday. Tuesday morning I went to work, but I only worked an hour and I felt sort of sick.

Interviewer insists.

Dr. Well, how did you feel, coming down with the virus?

Patient again skips details.

Pt. I had cold chills and such fever. First you have a chill and you'd be so cold. So I went upstairs and I told the personnel manager that I wanted to go home, and he said all right. So I was sick Tuesday . . . all of the rest of the week. And so the next Monday I went back to work.

Interviewer presses for more details.

Dr. You had cold feelings . . .
Pt. Mm-hmmm. And, oh, I sweated so, I dripped sweat, ooooh!

Open-ended question.

Dr. And what else did you notice that week?
Pt. That's the type of thing that I had.

Finally asks specific questions when patient does not elaborate.

Dr. Aching?
Pt. No.
Dr. Sick to your stomach?
Pt. No.
Dr. Diarrhea? (patient shakes head "No"). Were you short of breath?
Pt. Yes.

Open-ended question.

Dr. Tell me about being short of breath.
Pt. Well, I was just awfully short of breath and . . . (pause)

Dyspnea; quantity.

Dr. How short? What could you do?
Pt. I didn't do anything. I stayed in bed and finally got over it, at least I thought I was over it and then Monday . . .

Patient evades discussion of dyspnea; interviewer insists.

Dr. I want to know a little bit more about the shortness of breath in that week. How much could you do without getting short of breath?

Pt. Well, very little. (hesitantly)

Dr. Very little?

Pt. Very little.

Dr. Did you do the kitchen work, for example?

Pt. Very little. (laugh)

Dr. In what position did you rest in bed? Could you lie flat?

Pt. No, I had two pillows.

Orthopnea.

Dr. Two pillows. How long have you had two pillows?

Pt. Oh. . .quite a while. Especially in the hot weather.

Dr. Was this a matter of years or . . .

For the first time she indicates a longer duration. The interviewer notes this in his mind to come back to later. He continues with the current episode.

Pt. Oh yes, well, I would say a couple of years.

Dr. A couple of years?

Pt. Yes.

Dr. Was there any change in that week in terms of the number of pillows?

Pt. Well, I don't know if there was any change or not, but it felt more comfortable to sleep with the two pillows.

Dr. Did you wake up at night feeling short of breath?

Pt. Yes, in hot weather.

Dr. Did the shortness of breath wake you up?

Nocturnal dyspnea.

Pt. Yes.

Dr. And what would you do when you woke up?

Pt. Nothing. I'd just wake up and be there. There's a small window behind my bed, and my husband put a screen in and it would open and I used to have it hooked back.

Interviewer checks associated symptoms.

Dr. Did you have any wheezing in your chest?

Pt. No.

Dr. Or coughing at night?

Pt. No.

Dr. I gather this shortness of breath is something that goes back some time.

Since the patient has mentioned dyspnea, orthopnea, palpitation, and chest pain, the interviewer now inquires directly about other cardiac symptoms. Edema.

Pt. Yes, a couple of years.

Dr. A couple of years. Did you notice any swelling of your ankles?

Pt. Yes. By 6 o'clock at night my ankles would look like, yeoww. (laugh) They'd get so big!

Dr. How far back does that go?

Pt. Well . . . in the hot weather it was worse. Well, it's been increasing, you know.

Dr. Since?

Now acknowledges 3 or 4 years of symptoms.

Pt. Oh . . . I would say about 3 or 4 years.

Dr. Three or 4 years.

Pt. It would come off and on. But then this past year by the time summer came, every night.

Edema, aggravating and alleviating factors.

Dr. Every night. So there was a change this past summer in that you noticed that by evening your feet would be swollen every night.

Pt. Yes.

Dr. And by morning, how would they be?

Pt. By morning it would be gone.

Dr. Be gone. Now let's come back to after this flu episode.

Pt. Well, after the flu episode I went back to the bank to work on Monday, and on Tuesday I was to go down to the . . . doctor and see if this was taking effect. I didn't think it was taking effect because I could feel it beating so fast.

Dr. When did you first begin to feel this beating again?

Pt. Well, I felt it all weekend.

Dr. But it had gone the first week?

Pt. Yes, before then. So I went down to him and said, "I don't think the medicine has taken effect." Well, he didn't know, of course, that I had the virus, so he asked me a little bit about it and he took my blood pressure and my pulse and he said, "Where is your husband?" And I said, "He's home." And he said, "Well, go to the hospital." So I went up to the hospital and he put me in Intensive Care. He thought I had a heart attack.

Dr. On what date was that?

Pt. I think it was the 15th or 16th . . .

Dr. Of August. Who is your doctor?

Pt. Dr. Jones. And then he called in Dr. Watson, who is a heart specialist, and he gave me a cardiogram. And then they decided I didn't have a heart attack. They didn't know what it was. And so after Dr. Watson had given me two or three goings over, he decided that I had leakage or something like that.

Dr. And is this the first time that anyone had ever mentioned leakage or a murmur or anything of that sort?

Pt. Yes.

Dr. So you were in the hospital how long?

Pt. I was in 2 weeks, until September 3.

Dr. And during the time you were in the hospital, how were you?

Pt. Oh, it was the same, the rapid heart beat and so forth, that I had at home.

Dr. You continued to have the rapid heart beat.

Pt. And then I went home and I had a rapid heart beat and I had one digitalis pill — a digoxin?

Dr. When did you begin the digoxin?

Pt. In the hospital. I was also on blood thinners when I was in the hospital, but then they took me off it. And I didn't take any more. I just had the one digoxin. And when I went home Dr. Jones found out that my heart was beating too fast, so he went to Dr. Watson, who said I should take two digoxins.

Dr. At the time that you left the hosptial, what recommendation was made?

Pt. Well, it was that I should go home and just do light housework and see how I got along.

Dr. Was there any discussion of surgery at that time?

Pt. Yes, he said I would possibly have closed heart surgery but he said, "We'll let this go for the time being." But by November, when I didn't get any better, he called Dr. Y. and arranged for me to come up here in January.

Interviewer explores reaction to prospect of surgery.

Dr. Uh-huh. What was your feeling about that proposal at that time?

Patient minimizes.

Pt. I didn't care.

Interviewer presses.

Dr. You didn't care. What do you mean, you didn't care?

Pt. Well, if I'm gonna get better, I would have to have an operation.

Open-ended question.

Dr. And what was your life like during those weeks at home?

Pt. Well, I didn't go out, except once a week. I used to go to the grocery store with my husband, but that's all. And I got along all right. I knitted, oh, I don't know, about that high pile of sweaters and that sort of thing. I knitted right along and did light housework. And December 11, boom, I had the stroke!

Stroke, December 11, 1967.

Open-ended question.

Dr. Tell me about that.

Pt. Well, it was 11 o'clock at night, which was a little late for me to be up, but I was making a carton to put on the door to fit the newspaper in. 'Cause I didn't want the boys to throw it in the snow and get it damp. And so I thought I would put a little fancy paper on it so it would look better, because I was using a milk carton. And I put the staples on the outside. Sometimes the staple gun sticks, so I was trying to fix that stapler so it would not stick. And I went to put in a second staple and my fingers felt all tingly, you know. (massages right hand) I thought, "Gee, that's funny." I didn't know why they should go to sleep when I was using it. So I just put it on my lap like that, and, gee, it felt, you know, it felt terrible! And then I felt as though I was drooling. So my son had gone to bed and for some reason he got up to get a drink of water and he said, "Mother, what are you doing?" and he looked at me. He said I looked so funny. So he ran to the telephone and called my father — my husband. "You better come home. Mother's sick."

Slip of the tongue.

Interviewer notes husband was not home at 11 p.m. and wonders why.

Dr. Where was your husband?

Pt. He was at the New York Central Railroad. He's a car inspector.

Dr. He works at night?

Pt. Well, he works different hours. And so my husband came right home. And in the meantime my son said, "You'd better get on the bed." And I didn't know the leg had gone. So I got up and I fell on the floor. It was just too much, you know. So he picked me up. I don't remember him picking me up but they did, and took me into the bedroom and then I . . .

Establishing duration of unconsciousness.

Dr. You don't remember them picking you up?

Pt. No, but I became conscious of the fact that I was on the bed and I kept going in and out, you know. And they said both sides of my neck swelled way out.

Dr. Uh-huh. So you were unconscious just between the time that you got up and fell down and the time they picked you . . .

Pt. Well, I kept going unconscious. I remember going to the hospital. . .

Dr. You remember falling?

Pt. Yes.

Dr. Now who carried you in?

Pt. My husband, I guess.

Dr. Your son had called your husband. And had he already come before you had fallen?

Pt. I don't know. He came home within 10 minutes.

Dr. Within 10 minutes.

Pt. Uh-huh.

Dr. So you were unconscious for not more than 10 minutes.

Pt. That's right.

Dr. Then when you were on the bed you were sort of in and out of consciousness.

Pt. Yes. It was the same thing in the hospital. I remember going to the hospital, but I don't remember taking my clothes off.

Dr. Did you have trouble speaking?

Aphasia.

Pt. Yes.

Dr. What was the trouble?

Pt. Well, I couldn't make anybody understand. (laugh) Nobody could understand me for about 3 days.

Dr. Would the words form in your own mind?

Pt. Yes.

Dr. Did you know what you wanted to say?

Pt. Yes.

Open-ended question.

Dr. Well, how were these 3 days for you?

Pt. Well, time went by so fast that I couldn't believe that 3 days had gone by. And then time kept going and things kept coming better and I moved my leg in the bed. So after 6 days I left Intensive Care.

Details of the course.

Dr. When did you first begin to speak understandably?

Pt. The third day.

Dr. By the third day.

Pt. Yeah.

Dr. Uh-huh. And your leg was the first to come back?

Pt. Yeah.

Dr. First your leg improved, then your speech?

Pt. Uh-huh. They didn't all improve, you know, but I could make my husband understand what I wanted.

Dr. How were you feeling during those days in Intensive Care?

Pt. All right.

Interviewer checks cardiac status.

Dr. You felt all right? What about your heart circulation? Were you aware of anything?

Pt. Well, I didn't suffer any pain or anything.

Dr. Were you short of breath?

Pt. No.

Dr. Were you having a rapid heart?

Pt. Well, as I say, I'm so used to having a rapid heart that I don't pay any attention to it.

Dr. So then you were in the hospital for how long?

Pt. Let's see, 4½ weeks.

Interviewer inquires about experience of being away from home during holidays, since this is often upsetting to patients.

Dr. That brings us up to January — you must have been there over Christmas and New Years.

Pt. Oh yeah, all the holidays.

Dr. All the holidays?

Pt. Oh yes! I nearly had a fit to have to stay in the hospital over New Years and Christmas.

Dr. Why?

Pt. Oh, I wanted to be home, you know, with my children, but then I got sick.

Dr. You nearly had a fit?

Pt. Well, I felt terrible, you know. I — well, I cried. (laugh)

Dr. You cried. That's understandable.

Pt. But I got over it.

Patient acknowledges upset but minimizes it.

Recapitulation.

Dr. You felt sad and unhappy at that point?

Pt. Sad for myself, probably.

Dr. Uh-huh. Let me go back now. The stroke was December 11, and you had been discharged from the hospital in September?

Pt. September 3, I think it was.

Dr. So it was about a 3-month period that you were home.

Pt. Yeah.

Open-ended question to elicit more information about illness since September.

Dr. And you told us that you took it easy and you knitted that pile of sweaters and things. What *were* these 3 months like for you?

Pt. Well, at first I thought it was kind of boring, but then I put up with it because I thought, "Well, it has to be done. And after I have the heart surgery, well, I'll be all right."

Dr. You felt you'll be all right.

Pt. So I just took it.

Dr. What restricted your activity? Was it what the doctor said you could do or was it . . .?

Pt. The doctor said what I could do.

Dr. You did what the doctor said.

Pt. Yes.

With indication that patient has been an active person, interviewer wonders how she adjusts to enforced inactivity.

Dr. And I have the impression that ordinarily you're a fairly active person.

Pt. Yes, very much so! (with emphasis)

Dr. Very much so. Can you say a little bit more about that?

Pt. Well, I'm a person who walks a great deal. I'd walk from here to Timbuktu. (laugh) I like to walk.

Dr. You like to walk.

Patient emphasizes activity.

Pt. I mean I go to church every Sunday, and I always walk. I do *all* my grocery shopping, I do *all* my other shopping downtown and everything. And last September I never went downtown or went any place, but I thought, "Well, I want to go but I'll do something else."

Evaluation of disability by exploring daily activity.

Dr. And the two children were at home?

Pt. Yeah.

Dr. And how much of the housework did you do?

Pt. Well, I just did—running dustmops and that sort of thing. When it came to mopping or something, then my husband would do that.

Dr. Your husband would do that.

Pt. Mm-hmmm.

Dr. Did you try to?

Pt. No.

Dr. Why not?

Pt. My doctor said not to. (laugh)

Dr. The doctor said not to. Do you have stairs in your house?

Pt. Yeah.

Dr. Did you climb stairs?

Pt. The doctor said not to go up and down stairs any more than I could help and so I didn't.

Dr. And when you did go upstairs . . .

Dyspnea, one flight of stairs.

Pt. It would make me short of breath, even if I went up slowly.

Resume chronologic account.

Dr. It would make you short of breath. Okay, then let's come back now to the date of your discharge from the hospital, which would have been January . . .

Pt. Oh, I don't know, about the 17th.

Second hospitalization:12/11/67-1/17/68.

Dr. In other words you were in the hospital from the 11th of December to the 17th of January?

Pt. Yeah.

Dr. And what did you do after the 17th?

Pt. Nothing, I can't use that right hand, you see. Although, I couldn't even do this much when I was home. (demonstrates that she can raise right hand almost to chin) So my husband got all the meals and gardening.

Dr. You're right-handed.

Pt. Yes.

Interviewer returns to earlier piece of information.

Dr. You mentioned earlier that your husband was going to take off the month of January.

Pt. Yep! He did!

Dr. He did. He had already planned that.

Pt. Yeah.

Dr. Uh-huh. When had the admission to this hospital been scheduled for?

Pt. In January.

Dr. No definite date, but sometime in January.

Pt. Yeah.

Course after discharge from hospital.

Dr. Uh-huh. Then you were home from the 17th until this past Friday, the 26th. Were you in bed or in a chair or walking around?

Fatigue.

Pt. I got up every morning and during the day I would lay down twice, because if I didn't, I'd be so shook up, you know, so tired.

Clarify term, "shook up."

Dr. Shook up—what does shook up mean?

Pt. Well, you just can't go on. (laugh)

Dr. Uh-huh. Fatigue.

Pt. Yeah.

Fatigue; location, quality.

Dr. How do you feel the fatigue?

Pt. Well, it wouldn't be so much in my chest. I was just all in, you know.

Dr. All in.

Pt. Yeah.

As a point of reference interviewer comments on how patient walked in.

Dr. Uh-huh. Well, you walked fairly well when you came in the room here this morning.

Pt. Yes, that has improved, too.

Dr. That has improved since you are here?

Pt. Yeah.

Interviewer explores patient's reaction to stroke.

Dr. Mm-hmmm. What is your understanding of the stroke?

Pt. An artery or something burst back there on this side, I guess, and it affected this side. (indicates left side of head)

Dr. Have you had any knowledge or experience with stroke?

Pt. Yeah, well, I have had from other people, you know.

Dr. Who?

Pt. My aunt.

Family history of strokes: aunt, father

Dr. Your aunt?

Pt. Mm-hmmm. But she's still living; she's 82.

Dr. Uh-huh. When did she have her stroke?

Pt. A couple of years ago. And I took care of my father, and my father had a stroke.

Dr. Your father had a stroke, too?

Pt. Yes.

Dr. When was that?

Pt. Oh . . . let's see, he was 74. It was about 16, 17 years ago. And I took care of him. So I knew about it then too.

Dr. Mm-hmmm. How long did you take care of him?

Pt. Oh, from March until the last of August.

Dr. Till August.

Pt. Mm-hmmm.

Interviewer takes opportunity to explore early relationships and Family Health while getting details of father's stroke.

Dr. He lived with you?

Pt. No, I lived with him.

Dr. You were married at that time.

Pt. Yeah, oh yeah.

Dr. So you and your family lived. . .

Pt. With my father, uh-huh.

Dr. With your father. Uh-huh. And on which side was he paralyzed?

Pt. This side. (indicates left)

Dr. The left side.

Pt. His stroke was in his leg mostly.

Dr. More in his leg.

Pt. It was just terrible.

Dr. Terrible, how do you mean?

Pt. And in his voice.

Dr. Voice.

Pt. He couldn't get up. He used to try to get up to go to the bathroom, and he couldn't stand up at all.

Dr. This was quite a problem in nursing him.

Pt. Yeah.

The closeness of the relationship to the father prompts the interviewer to explore this further.

Dr. How did you happen to be the one who took care of him?

Pt. Well (laugh), I'm next to the oldest one of five children, and for some reason my father, my people have always depended on me. My brothers and sisters always depended on me and so I've always taken care of them, help 'em get whatever they want.

Patient second of five children.

Family always depended on her.

Dr. Are you the oldest girl?

Pt. No. There's another older girl, but she is . . . well . . . let's say immature. She's married, but she just isn't mature.

Dr. Uh-huh. How do you mean she's not mature?

Pt. Well, the doctors have said that as she grows older, she will grow more immature. At times she has the maturity of a 15-year-old girl.

Older sister mentally defective.

Dr. Mm-hmmm. How much older than you is she?

Pt. Two years.

Dr. Two years. So did you have to help her out when you were young?

Pt. Yeah. (laugh)

Dr. But she did marry.

Pt. Yeah.

Dr. Had children?

Nephew has Down's Disease, institutionalized.

Pt. She had two. And one boy was Mongolian. He's still living, but he's in a home.

Dr. Uh-huh. And the other boy?

Pt. The other boy's all right.

Interviewer now returns to explore the period prior to August, 1967.

Dr. Well now, let me go back to before this past August. You say for a couple of summers you had noticed this intolerance of the hot weather, that your heart beat fast, and that you had been getting short of breath. Can you tell me now how far back this goes, that you were having any trouble at all?

Pt. Well . . . (sigh) I don't know. It's . . .well, it could be 4 or 5 years.

Dr. It might be 4 or 5 years.

Pt. It came gradually . . .

Chronology.

Dr. And what was the first thing you noticed, do you think?

Pt. You mean this past summer?

Dr. No, going back 4 or 5 years.

Tachycardia.

Pt. Well . . . It was just the heart beat got rapid.

Dr. A rapid heart beat.

Dependent edema.

Pt. And the swelling of the legs.

Dr. Under what circumstances?

Sudden increase in edema 2 years ago.

Pt. A couple of years ago I had . . . an accumulation of water. I put on 13 pounds in a couple of days.

Dr. Two years ago?

Pt. Yeah.

Dr. When?

Pt. In the summer.

Checking dates.

Dr. In the summer. Which summer?

Pt. 1966, I think. In June or July; I don't remember. And I went to the doctor's. I got up one morning and I

Swelling of abdomen.

couldn't even put a belt on. So I thought, "My God!" I didn't know what had happened to me. So I went down to the doctor and he said, "Well, I'll give you some water pills and I'll give you a couple of days to take that off and if you don't, we'll send you to the hospital," And gee, I went right at it and I took it right off. It never happened again.

Response to diuretic.

Dr. You urinated it.

Pt. I had to stay right near the bathroom. (laugh)

Dr. Were your legs swollen at that time, too?

Pt. Everything.

Dr. Were you short of breath?

Pt. Well, I don't remember. I suppose I was. It was in the summertime.

Dr. You emphasize the summertime. In the wintertime . . .

Relation of symptoms to hot weather.

Pt. The wintertime I don't pay any attention to it, because in the wintertime I like the cold weather. You can breathe so much easier, and you don't have the hard time to do anything. But the doctors have always said there's no trouble, so I forget about it.

Interviewer challenges patient's minimizing.

Dr. You say you forgot about it. I'm not sure what that means.

Pt. Well, I just didn't pay any attention to it.

Dr. You mean you had the symptoms, but you didn't pay any attention to them?

Pt. Yeah.

Dr. So you might have a fast heart rate in the winter as well as the summer . . .

Pt. Yeah.

Dr. . . . and your feet might get swollen in the winter.

Pt. They don't get swollen *so bad*, up until the last winter. They didn't swell near as much.

Dr. But they *did* swell some?

Pt. Some, yes.

Interviewer tries to establish onset.

Dr. When was the first time that you ever noted any swelling of your feet?

Pt. Oh . . . gee, I don't know. It's . . . a long time. I just can't tell you how long it's been. It's been a long time, because it comes gradually, you know.

Dr. Uh-huh. And would the swelling always go down at night again?

Pt. Yes.

Dr. So you're simply not sure when, but it's a number of years, maybe 4, 5 years that you've had the swelling, more in the summer than in the winter, but you *do* have it in the winter but it just doesn't trouble you as much.

Pt. Yeah.

Dr. And so, too, with the fast heart rate. You have that in the winter, but it doesn't bother you so much.

Pt. Mm-hmmm.

Interviewer tries to clarify whether true orthopnea or paroxysmal nocturnal dyspnea has occurred.

Dr. And for how long is it that you've been sleeping on two pillows?

Pt. A couple of years.

Dr. What does a couple mean?

Pt. Oh, two, I guess.

Dr. What started that? Why did you start moving to two pillows?

Pt. Well, because I thought I could breathe easier.

Dr. You thought you could breathe easier. And did you?

Pt. I thought I could.

Dr. Uh-huh. Did it ever occur at any time that you awakened at night extremely short of breath and had to sit up or stand up?

Pt. No, I didn't ever do that.

Dr. You mentioned your husband fixing the little window.

Pt. Mm-hmmm.

Dr. I don't have clear what that was for.

Pt. Well, it's a dormer window, a small window. So he opened that and I slept right beside that, you see.

Dr. So that you would have more air?

Pt. Yeah.

Dr. I see.

Patient emphasizes association between summer and dyspnea.

Pt. It's the summertime that it seems that something cuts off the air. (laugh)

Step 5: Past Health
Because of the patient's reluctance to speak of illness, the interviewer focuses on her work and life activities, anticipating that these may have been interrupted by illness.

Dr. Mm-hmm. During this 4- or 5-year period, up to this summer, aside from what you've told me, what was your health like?

Pt. All right.

Dr. All right? No other illnesses?

Pt. Nothing has been wrong.

Dr. No other illnesses, no hospitalizations . . .

Pt. No.

Dr. And during that time, have you been working?

Pt. Yes.

Dr. How long have you been working at the bank?

Pt. A year.

Dr. Hmmm. Had you worked before that?

Pt. No. I worked before I had the children, for 7 years or so. I worked at a paper company.

Dr. I see.

First pregnancy — baby died of heart disease.

Pt. And then I had a baby, but it lived only 6 hours because he had a . . . well they said a bad heart.

Dr. This was the first child?

Patient avoids mentioning symptoms.

Pt. Yeah. And then I went back to work after that and I worked for about . . . 2 months. And then I thought I had heart trouble. So I went to the doctor . . .

Interviewer asks.

Dr. What trouble did you have?

She still avoids.

Pt. The doctor said he thought I had thyroid trouble. So I went into the hospital and had a basal metabolism test, and it turned out negative.

Chronology.

Dr. When was this?

1943, 25 years ago.

Pt. Oh . . . let's see . . . 25 years ago.

Dr. Twenty-five years ago. And this was a few months after the birth . . .

First mention of possible valvular defect.

Pt. Yeah. And then after they said that was negative, the doctor said, "Well, go to Dr. E., he's a heart specialist." So I went and he said, "Well, the only thing I can say is that you've got a little scar tissue in there because of having rheumatic fever when you were 8 years old." So I didn't go back to him. It didn't seem necessary. I only came back to him for a corrective, you know, to see if it was all right. So I went back to him for a few times and he says, "Well, it's all right." And the last time I went he said, "Well, gee, I can't find anything wrong; you're all right."

Still no mention of symptoms.

Interviewer repeats question.

Dr. What symptoms were you having that led you to see the doctor?

Pt. I was having rapid heart beat, and I was short of breath.

Setting.

Dr. Rapid heart and you were short of breath. You noticed the shortness of breath under what circumstances?

Pt. Oh . . .well, I don't know. It was so short, you know, all the time. When I was young like that and I thought, well, maybe that I had heart trouble. But the doctor . . .

Dr. I didn't follow that.

Pt. He—I thought that I had heart trouble because I had such short breath.

Duration.

Dr. How long had you been having short breath?

Pt. Well, since I had that baby.

Establishing time of onset.

Dr. Were you short of breath during the pregnancy?

Pt. No.

Dr. Not during the pregnancy.

Pt. I didn't think so.

Dr. Uh-huh.

Pt. And I told the doctor that I thought I had heart trouble and he said, no, that he thought that I had a little scar tissue.

Dr. Were you short of breath in bed?

Dyspnea; quality,
"frequent sighing."

Pt. No . . . well, I don't remember all that.
Dr. You don't remember.
Pt. You know, it's been so long and all, but I remember that at the time I had frequent sighing.
Dr. Frequent sighing?
Pt. Yes. I felt I could hardly get a long breath. You just want to get a long breath like that and that's what really made me wonder if I did have heart trouble.
Dr. Was that what you mean by shortness of breath at that time?
Pt. Yeah.
Dr. The sighing?
Pt. Yeah.

Dyspnea; setting.

Dr. And did this come on at any particular times?
Pt. No . . .
Dr. It could be while you were sitting as well as standing or walking?
Pt. Mm-hmm. Yeah.

Dyspnea; quality.

Dr. You just feel you have to get in a deep breath.
Pt. Mm-hmmm.

Dyspnea; chronologic association with death of baby with heart defect.

Interviewer explores patient's reaction to the loss of baby.

Second pregnancy, 1946.

Dr. And you say the baby, they said, had heart trouble.
Pt. Yeah.

Dr. How did it affect you, to have lost that first child?
Pt. Well, it was something that I had planned on and I, you know, I felt bad that I had lost it. So then 3 days — 3 years later I had a son. And my children are all right.
Dr. Did you cry?
Pt. Yeah.
Dr. You felt sad? (patient nods head) How long did it take before you got over it?
Pt. Well . . . probably a year.
Dr. Probably a year. Were you trying to get pregnant in the interim?
Pt. No.
Dr. You were not.
Pt. No, I was told not to.
Dr. You were told not to? Why?
Pt. Well, I don't know. The doctor that delivered the baby said I should wait a year and a half, at least, before I'd even attempt to.
Dr. Did he say why?
Pt. No.
Dr. And to this day you don't know why.
Pt. No.
Dr. And then after a year and a half did you try?
Pt. No, my husband wasn't too much in favor of my having another one so soon.
Dr. Why not?
Pt. Because he didn't want me to go through it again.
Dr. He didn't want you to go through what again?

First acknowledgment of symptoms during pregnancy. Nausea, vomiting.	*Pt.* Well, every time I get pregnant I get very sick. For 9 months I'm throwing up and everything. After a while I convinced him that I probably wouldn't have it again. So I had another one. But I was just as sick!
Open-ended question.	*Dr.* Uh-huh. Throwing up and what else?
Epistaxes.	*Pt.* And I had terrible nosebleeds. At the time I threw up, I'd lean over the toilet like this and I—once something happened to my eye and it all turned black. I don't know what it was.
Check chronology.	*Dr.* This was the first pregnancy?
	Pt. No, the second.
Since the patient has opened the subject, interviewer will pursue obstetrical history.	*Dr.* The second one. *Pt.* And I had to go to the doctor frequently every week or so and then the baby was all right when it was born.
Interviewer explores specific symptoms during pregnancies.	*Dr.* What happened to your weight during these pregnancies? Did you gain or lose or . . .? *Pt.* That first one, I didn't gain too much.
	Dr. Didn't gain too much.
Edema.	*Pt.* No. The second one, I gained. Oh, I had an awful lot of water.
	Dr. The second one you gained a great deal.
	Pt. Oh yes.
Edema; quantity.	*Dr.* How much? Do you remember?
	Pt. Oh, about 20 pounds. My legs swelled so—and my feet—that I couldn't get anything but bedroom
Third pregnancy, 1951.	slippers on. The next, that was 5½ years later, I was so sick in the third month that the doctor put me in the hospital and I had glucose, I guess. And then when I came out, the same thing happened all over again. So he said, "Well, the only thing that I can do is take the baby." But I didn't want him to do that so I said I would get through it somehow. So I went along and I got through it all right but I didn't lose the swelling of the legs there, oh, it was a long time. It was
Edema; duration.	all of—he was born in July. It was October or something like that.
	Dr. This would be 16 years ago.
	Pt. Yes.
Specific symptoms: dyspnea.	*Dr.* Were you short of breath during that pregnancy? *Pt.* Yeah.
	Dr. How about the first two pregnancies? Were you short of breath?
	Pt. I don't remember whether I was short of breath or not.
	Dr. But you remember well that you were short of breath with the third one.
	Pt. Yeah, uh-huh.
	Dr. Did you have high blood pressure with any of these?
	Pt. No, he said it was low blood pressure.
Low blood pressure.	*Dr.* Low blood pressure.

Headache, vomiting.	*Pt.* It would hurt the top of my head, you know, when I would throw up and I thought I had high blood pressure. And so I spoke to him about it; he said, "No," he said, "it's low blood pressure."
	Dr. Did he ever say you had anything in your urine?
	Pt. He never took any.
Asks about fourth pregnancy.	*Dr.* Now what about the last pregnancy, 10 years ago?
	Pt. I thought I had lost it. At 2 months I think it was, I had a hemorrhage and I had big, big blood clots, *big* blood clots. The doctor came and said, "Well, I think you've passed it." So after about 3 or 4 days in bed he said, "No, you're still pregnant." So I went home and I was home another month, then I had another hemorrhage. And he said, "Well, we'll go to the hospital again." So he thought I'd lost it again. So he examined me and I was still pregnant. I went home after a week and I stayed home until the baby was born.
Bleeding.	
	Dr. Did you gain as much weight this fourth time?
Edema.	*Pt.* No, I didn't, but my legs swelled.
	Dr. Your legs did swell.
	Pt. Yeah.
	Dr. Were you short of breath this time?
Dyspnea.	*Pt.* A little.
	Dr. A little bit.
Edema, duration.	*Pt.* But then afterwards I stayed swollen around my middle and I still had swelling in my legs until quite a while afterwards.
	Dr. Both legs.
	Pt. Mm-hmmm.
Interviewer wonders about thrombophlebitis to account for edema of legs.	*Dr.* In any of the four pregnancies, was there any difference in the size of the legs?
	Pt. The third one, it was worse.
	Dr. No, I mean was there any difference in swelling between the left leg and the right leg.
	Pt. No, I don't think so.
	Dr. Were your calves ever tender?
	Pt. They always have been.
	Dr. They always have been.
	Pt. If you pinch 'em like that.
	Dr. Was the fourth pregnancy planned?
	Pt. No. (laugh) We were kind of surprised.
	Dr. Uh-huh. You were already 41, 42.
	Pt. Yes, 42.
Fourth pregnancy unplanned. Interviewer inquires about patient's reaction.	*Dr.* Uh-huh. How did you feel about it at the time?
	Pt. Well, I wasn't planning on it and I was a little bit . . . skeptical whether I'd carry it through. And my husband felt terrible about it. He thought it . . . was gonna be kind of hard on me. But I said, "We'll let what's to be, so don't get upset about it."
Resume survey of Past Health.	*Dr.* Any other illnesses during these years?
	Pt. No.
	Dr. Have you been in the hospital other than the pregnancies and the times that you told me?

Tonsillectomy, age 9.	*Pt.* I had my tonsils out when I was about nine.
	Dr. Uh-huh. Any injuries?
	Pt. No.
	Dr. Or accidents?
	Pt. No.
Interviewer brings patient back to "rheumatic fever" at age eight.	*Dr.* Tell me about the rheumatic fever when you were eight.
	Pt. Yeah, since I've grown up they call it rheumatic fever, but of course they didn't call it that then. They just said rheumatism because they didn't have the know-how then. I didn't go to school all one winter, my legs
Swelling of legs.	swelled so. And I couldn't get my shoes on. And I don't remember what went on there, but I know that I went to get the tonsils out because I don't remember whether I had sore throats or not, but they said that as a result of this I should have my tonsils out.
Edema, location.	*Dr.* And your legs swelled where?
	Pt. From the ankles up to the knees.
	Dr. The whole leg was swollen.
	Pt. Yeah.
	Dr. Both legs.
	Pt. Mm-hmmm.
Inquires about symptoms of acute rheumatic fever.	*Dr.* Was it sensitive? Were your joints sore or painful?
	Pt. I don't remember.
	Dr. You don't remember that. Did you have swelling of any other parts of your body?
	Pt. No, no.
Checks other features of edema.	*Dr.* Was your face puffy when you woke up in the morning?
	Pt. I don't remember.
	Dr. Did you have rheumatism anywhere else?
	Pt. No.
	Dr. Do you remember whether you had fever?
	Pt. No, I don't remember.
Childhood illnesses.	*Dr.* Any other illnesses in childhood?
	Pt. No.
	Dr. Did you have St. Vitus Dance . . .
	Pt. No.
	Dr. Did you have sore throats when you were young?
	Pt. If I did have, I don't remember.
	Dr. You don't remember. Scarlet fever?
	Pt. No.
	Dr. Diphtheria?
	Pt. No.
	Dr. Do you remember any other childhood illnesses?
	Pt. No. I remember I had mumps and measles, that sort of thing, but they were light, you know.
Not satisfied with story of "rheumatic fever," interviewer returns to it.	*Dr.* You say you had to stay home from school that whole winter.
	Pt. Yes.
	Dr. Why?
	Pt. Because I couldn't get my shoes on, just bedroom slippers. So I had to stay home.

Dr. And did you stay in bed or around the house?

Pt. Well, no, I stayed around the house, you know.

Step 6: Family
Health

Dr. Uh-huh. Where were you living at that time?

Pt. In Geneva.

Dr. You lived in Geneva all your life?

Pt. Yeah.

Dr. And your family comes from Geneva?

Pt. Mm-hmmm, mm-hmmm.

Interviewer begins with
known information —
father's death.

Dr. Your father, you say, was 74 when he died, 17 years
ago?

Pt. Yeah.

Father's work.

Dr. What did your father do?

Pt. He was truckdriver for Roberts Hardware.

Dr. And he worked until when?

Pt. He worked right up until March, until he had his
stroke.

Father's health.

Dr. What was his health like?

Pt. He was wonderful.

Dr. Always in good health?

Pt. Yes.

Dr. And do you know what was the cause of his death?

Pt. The stroke . . . only.

Dr. The stroke, that's all?

Pt. Mm-hmmm.

Dr. And when he was young, what did he do?

Pt. He was an auto mechanic.

Mother.

Died at 49.

Dr. And your mother?

Pt. My mother was very sickly. My mother died at 49.

Dr. Forty-nine. You were how old?

Pt. Oh, let's see, I was 23, 24. Oh no, let me see, 27.

Dr. Twenty-seven.

Pt. Yes.

Interviewer recognizes
mother died same year as
did first baby.

Dr. Twenty-five years ago.

Pt. Yes.

Dr. When was your mother's death in relationship to
your first pregnancy?

Pt. Oh, it was about . . . I became pregnant just a few
months before she died.

Dr. She died before you delivered?

Pt. Yeah.

Two losses, mother and
baby.

Dr. So you had two losses that year, didn't you, the baby
and your mother.

Pt. Yeah.

Dr. What was the cause of her death?

Mother's health: leukemia,
hysterectomy,
cholecystectomy,
appendectomy, chronically
sick.

Pt. She had *so many* sicknesses! She finally died of cancer
of the bloodstream. But before that she had had a hysterectomy and she had had her appendix out and then
she had gallbladder trouble. Just sickness all the time.

Dr. One thing after another.

Pt. Yeah.

Interviewer links mother's
chronic ill health and
patient's role as the helper.

Dr. So was this the reason why you were the one who was
taking care of everybody?

Pt. Yeah.

Mother's symptoms.	*Dr.* Did she have shortness of breath?
	Pt. I don't remember. I don't believe so.
	Dr. Or weakness?
	Pt. She took some kind of digitalis or something; I don't know what it was now.
	Dr. Did you help take care of your mother?
	Pt. Yeah.
Inquires how mother's death affected her.	*Dr.* How did her death affect you?
	Pt. Well, we felt very sad when she died, because, well, she's my mother.
	Dr. Do you think about her still?
	Pt. Not . . . I don't think . . . it don't bother me.
Siblings.	*Dr.* Now the five of you, the oldest one is a girl.
Begins with sister already mentioned: Bessie.	*Pt.* Bessie.
	Dr. And you told me about her. Bessie is married and she lives where?
	Pt. In Geneva.
	Dr. And the one after you is . . . ?
Brother: John.	*Pt.* That's John.
	Dr. John.
Heart attack, March, 1961 or 1962.	*Pt.* And he has a heart attack — a heart condition. He had pneumonia 6 — 7 years ago, the 16th of March.
	Dr. The 16th of March.
	Pt. Mm-hmmm, and as a result of the pneumonia, he got a heart attack. I don't know why, but he has blood clots, so many of them that he has to take blood thinner. And he has to go every week for a blood test. He doesn't work.
Work.	*Dr.* Has he worked since then?
	Pt. No.
	Dr. What did he do?
	Pt. He worked in a machine shop. He was a grinder, I guess you'd call it.
Age.	*Dr.* How old is he now?
	Pt. He's 51.
	Dr. He's a year younger than you.
	Pt. Yeah.
Marital status.	*Dr.* And he's married?
	Pt. Mm-hmmm. He has a little girl.
	Dr. Little girl.
	Pt. Eleven years old.
	Dr. Uh-huh.
Sister: Geraldine.	*Pt.* And then I have a sister, Geraldine, that's in good health. She had a hysterectomy, but she's fine.
	Dr. She's how old?
	Pt. She's 47.
Marital Status.	*Dr.* She's married?
	Pt. Mm-hmmm. She has five children.
	Dr. Five children.
Brother committed suicide, March, 1967. Patient breaks down.	*Pt.* Mm-hmmm. I have another — I did have another brother, and he committed suicide last March. He had a lot of trouble. He had a lung out and . . . well, that was just all. (crying)

Interviewer allows patient to cry; expresses understanding. She then spontaneously gives more details.

Dr. It's hard. (pause) Still affects you deeply, doesn't it? (patient crying for about 2 minutes) It must have been quite a shock at the time.

Pt. A terrible shock.

Dr. Mm-hmmm.

Patient uses present tense, "lives."

Pt. He lives in Westford, Virginia. And he had come to see us the last of March because he said he hadn't seen John, who was my brother who had the heart attack, 'cause he hadn't seen him in such a long time and he wasn't too well at the time. And he says, "Well, I think I'll come over and see him while he's alive." But he never did.

Dr. Did you have warning of this, or . . . ?

Pt. No.

Dr. Was he married?

Pt. Yeah, he has three children.

Dr. Three children. How old was he?

Pt. He would be 45 in April.

Dr. Uh-huh, he was the baby. What was his name?

Pt. Merlin. He was full of spirit, lots of good laughs, you know, and everything.

Dr. Any understanding of what happened?

Pt. No. You see, I live here and he lived down there. He used to call me about once a month. And that month he didn't make that call to me and then I got a telephone call. (pause, sniff) I didn't go down for the funeral because I said that I couldn't go down and meet his wife. You know, we never got a chance to go down there. He used to come home every summer and so I said to myself, "Well, I can't do him good anyway. Because if I got down there I would be *sick* and . . .

Interviewer responds to patient's comment that she would get "sick" if she went to funeral.

Dr. You would be *sick*?

Pt. Yeah. I was afraid I would be sick, so I would rather stay home.

Dr. When you say "be sick," what did you have in mind?

Pt. I don't know. I don't know.

Dr. You just had the feeling that you would be sick.

Pt. Yeah.

Dr. So you did not go to the funeral.

Pt. I did not go.

Dr. Mm-hmmm. How do you feel about that now?

Pt. I still wouldn't go.

Dr. You still feel that was the right thing to do.

Pt. Mm-hmmm.

Inquiry into grief reaction.

Dr. You cried at the time?

Pt. Yeah.

Dr. And you still cry.

Pt. Well, occasionally. (smiles weakly)

Interviewer comments on evidence of close relation with brother.

Dr. So it's almost a year now, isn't it? The first year is always the most difficult. I have the feeling that you and your brother were quite close.

Pt. Oh yes! I always — he's my little brother and whenever he'd get in trouble and would want to talk to somebody, he always called me.

Inquires as to patient's health at time of brother's death.

Dr. Always came to you, uh-huh. How was your health at that time?

Pt. I was good. I was working for an insurance company at the time.

Dr. This was March of '67?

Pt. Yeah, I told you that I was working for a year for the bank. I should have told you I worked for an insurance company before that and then I began work for the bank last April. And the insurance company had about as good as folded.

Further query about brother's death.

Dr. How did your brother commit suicide? Do you know?

Pt. He shot himself.

Dr. Shot himself. (pause) What was his work?

Pt. He was in marketing with the GE company.

Dr. I see. Had he been depressed?

Pt. I don't know.

Dr. Had he ever been depressed?

Pt. Not that I know of.

Dr. But you say he had had problems.

Pt. Yes, he had had with his lung.

Dr. With his lung.

Brother's chronic lung disease.

Pt. I would say about 12 years ago he had a lung removed because — it wasn't a lung cancer. They said it was something that had made it porous. So they took off everything up to about here (indicates midchest), and they sewed it up and left it like that. And so he came home and only about 2 weeks later it started a whistling sound. It was terrible! So then they said, "You'll have to go back to the hospital." The thing had leaked into the cavity, and they put this big tube in his back and he lay for 8 weeks and then they pulled that out of him. And gosh, it was terrible. And I went to see him almost every day.

Dr. He lived in Geneva at the time?

Pt. Uh-huh. But he got over it. He was fine.

Dr. What symptoms did he have?

Pt. Mostly he coughed up a lot, sometimes he had blood in it. And he'd get pneumonia.

Dr. He was married at that time?

Pt. Yeah.

Dr. But he had other troubles more recently?

Pt. No. Well, just that. I don't know now. I heard the doctor had told him that his other lung was starting to get that *same* disease. The doctor told me at the time that if that ever happened again he would suffocate. And so if the doctor had told *him* that, perhaps that's why he committed suicide.

Dr. He didn't leave a note?

Pt. No. Not that I know of.

Dr. Not that you know of. Are you in contact with your sister-in-law?

Pt. Yeah.

Dr. How has she been?

Pt. She's been fine.

Dr. She's been all right.

Pt. They've got a beautiful home down there, three teen-age daughters.

Resume Family History — marriage.

Dr. Now, you've been married how long?

Pt. It'll be 30 years in November.

Dr. Thirty years, and your husband is how old?

Husband.

Pt. He's 50.

Dr. Fifty.

Pt. He'll be 51 . . .

Dr. Uh-huh, he's just a little younger than you are.

Pt. Yeah, two years.

Husband's health.

Dr. Two years younger. And how has he been?

Pt. Fine.

Dr. He works for the railroad?

Pt. Uh-huh.

Work.

Dr. And has for how long?

Pt. All the time.

Dr. And what is his job?

Pt. He's a car inspector.

Dr. That's a big New York Central yard there, isn't it?

Pt. Yeah. Well, It isn't so big any more since they're merging, you know, so what they're going to do now, we don't know.

Dr. Is his job in any jeopardy?

Pt. No.

Dr. Being a car inspector means what?

Pt. Checking the air brakes and all that sort of thing.

Dr. Uh-huh. So he's had long years with New York Central.

Pt. Uh-huh. It takes another year, February I think it is, a year from this February, he will have 30 years in under the present pension system.

Dr. And you say he's been well?

Pt. Yes.

Husband's reaction to patient's illness.

Dr. How is he taking your sickness?

Pt. He's doing very well. (laugh)

Dr. He's doing well.

Pt. He's a good housekeeper. (laugh) And he's taking care of the children.

Children.

Dr. And the children, how have they been?

Pt. Fine.

Lois.

Dr. Lois?

Pt. She's just fine.

Dr. And she is in school?

Pt. Mm-hmmm.

Dr. And has she had any illnesses?

Pt. No.

Mark.	*Dr.* Any problems? (shakes her head, no) And how has Mark been?
	Pt. Oh, he's a big guy. He's about 6 foot now and he's never had any problems.
	Dr. He's in high school?
	Pt. Yeah, He's a junior; he'll be a senior.
	Dr. And how is he doing?
	Pt. Fine.
	Dr. Fine. His grades are good?
	Pt. Oh, good.
	Dr. Any problems?
	Pt. No.
	Dr. His health has been good?
	Pt. Fine.
	Dr. Uh-huh. And what's he heading for?
	Pt. Well, he doesn't know. First he's going to be a teacher and then he's going to be something else, but the most he's talked about is being a teacher.
	Dr. Then he'll probably go on to college, you think?
	Pt. I think so.
Robert.	*Dr.* And your oldest boy, Robert, is 22.
	Pt. Yeah.
	Dr. Is he married?
Navy 4 years ago.	*Pt.* He's married. He's very well. He joined the Navy Reserve when he was 17, and he's been away in the service after he graduated high school for 2 years and then came home and he got married before he finished the service.
	Dr. When did he marry?
Married 2 years ago; baby, 7 months old.	*Pt.* He's been married 2 years. He was 20 when he got married. And now they have a little—7 months old now.
	Dr. Seven months old, uh-huh. And his wife?
	Pt. She's well.
	Dr. Uh-huh.
	Pt. And the baby's cute.
	Dr. Your first grandchild!
	Pt. Yes. (smile)
	Dr. And his wife's name is what?
	Pt. Judy, she was a little Italian girl.
Patient indicates poor relationship with daughter-in-law.	*Dr.* Uh-huh. And do you see much of them?
	Pt. Not too much. (smiles)
Interviewer inquires.	*Dr.* Uh-huh. How come?
Patient opposed marriage.	*Pt.* Well, (laugh) when he wanted to get married, I didn't want him to get married until he was 21. But he insisted no matter what I said to him. And so finally I said, "Well, as long as you want to get married, get married. I'll sign for you."
	Dr. Uh-huh.
	Pt. So his father and I signed for him. But his wife was a little bit—she's very, well . . . Italian people are like

that. They're very much for their own family, for the sisters and brothers and father and mother, you know. And, well . . . she's always nice enough to us when Bobby would bring her over. We're always nice to her and she's nice to him—to John (sigh). But, I don't know, there's something strange about it. And to this day I don't think she's ever come into the house without Bobby, you know.

Dr. Never by herself?

Pt. No.

Dr. So it's not a very warm relationship for you.

Pt. No.

Dr. Mm-hmmm. And what was their marriage date?

Married May 9, 1966.   *Pt.* May 9, 1966.

Dr. The spring before last.

Grandson, June 27,   *Pt.* Yeah. That would be it. And they've got a little baby 7
1967.   months old. He was 7 months old the 27th of January.

Dr. So he was born in June of '67.

Pt. Yeah.

Interviewer wonders   *Dr.* What is your religious background?
about religious   *Pt.* I'm Protestant.
differences.   *Dr.* You're Protestant. And Judy, I assume, is Catholic?

Pt. Yeah. But that doesn't make any difference, you
Slip of the tongue.   know. My father—my husband is Catholic.

Dr. He is Catholic.

Pt. Mm-hmmm.

Dr. So that wasn't an issue.

Pt. No, no. I think probably because I didn't want him to be married when he was only 20 because he had no job. He had nothing and so I wanted him to wait until he had more to offer. But this girl is—she's very nice. She took it as if we don't like her.

Dr. How old is she?

Pt. She's two years older than he is.

Dr. Two years older than he. What is he doing now?

Pt. He's working for B. Company.

Dr. Doing what?

Pt. He's got a good job. He's some kind of inspector. It isn't anything he wants to do all his life, you know.

Interviewer indicates he   *Dr.* This is kind of a problem mothers have with
appreciates the problem.   children, isn't it?
Patient minimizes.   *Pt.* Yeah. Well, for me, I don't let it bother me.

Dr. You don't let it bother you.

Pt. No.

Return to Past Health.   *Dr.* Now I think I have a pretty good picture of what your health has been. Any other illnesses that . . .

Pt. No.

Dr. You say you have had no operations.

Pt. No.

Allergies, sensitivities.   *Dr.* Do you have any allergies?

Pt. No.

Medication.   *Dr.* Or sensitivities, hay fever, asthma? (shakes head, no) Are you taking any other medication now?

Digitalis.

Pt. I'm taking some digitalis. I can't tell you how much because one day I take three and yesterday I took one. Today I'll take two or something. I don't know.

Dr. When did you start the digitalis?

Pt. When I first entered the hospital in Geneva.

Dr. What else do you take?

Pt. Blood thinner.

Dr. Which blood thinner?

Pt. I don't know.

Coumadin.

Dr. Coumadin?

Pt. Yes, coumadin!

Dr. Coumadin. And how much do you take?

Pt. One five a day.

Dr. One five a day. And how often do you get your blood tested?

Pt. Every day. (laugh) Every day I've had my blood tested every day for 5 weeks in the hospital and for—that week I was home I went every other day to the hospital and I've had it every day, sometimes three times a day since I've been here.

Dr. Uh-huh. Any other medications?

Pt. No.

Asks about other cardiac measures.

Dr. Are you on any diuretics . . .

Pt. No.

Dr. . . . or anything to make you urinate?

Pt. No.

Dr. Have you been at any time since this started?

Pt. No.

Diet.

Dr. Are you on any diet?

Pt. Well, salt free.

Dr. You've been on a salt-free diet since . . . ?

Pt. Since I was in the hospital in September.

Dr. How low is the diet?

Pt. Well, I guess it's pretty rigid.

Dr. Do you take milk?

Pt. No.

Dr. Do you add salt to the cooking?

Pt. No.

Quinidine.

Dr. What about the quinidine? I gather the only time you had it was when you had the pain and palpitations, last August.

Pt. Yeah.

Dr. How many pills a day did the doctor give you then?

Pt. It was about three a day.

Dr. Three a day.

Pt. Yeah.

Dr. And so you took that for a total of how long?

Pt. Well, I was only I would say . . . oh about a week and a half.

Effect of quinidine.

Dr. About a week and a half. During that time did the palpitations change particularly? You said it was better on the first weekend, I remember, but . . .

Pt. It just seemed much better.

Dr. In what way?

Pt. Well, it seemed to calm down.

*Checking detail of
palpitations overlooked
earlier.*

Dr. When these palpitations first started, were they regular or irregular?

Pt. Oh . . .

Dr. Were they very fast like that or . . . jumping around?

Pt. I would say that it was going irregular.

Dr. And as you went out the bank door, did the palpitations start gradually or suddenly?

Pt. Well, suddenly.

Dr. And you had had palpitations before in the summer and . . .

Pt. Yeah.

Dr. Was this different in any way than what you had before? Did it feel different in any way?

Pt. Yes, I could feel it a lot worse.

Dr. In what way?

Pt. Oh, it felt as though it was more than usual, you know, it was unusual.

Dr. More severe?

Pt. Yeah.

*Step 8: Systems Review
(Patient has already
provided sufficient
information about
development and current
situation so that Step 7 is
unnecessary.)*

Dr. Do you have headaches at all?

Pt. No.

Dr. Have you ever had any injuries to your head?

Pt. No.

Dr. You've been wearing glasses for how long?

Pt. Oh, I've worn glasses since I was about 20.

Dr. Mm-hmmm. Are you nearsighted or far . . .

Pt. Nearsighted.

Dr. Nearsighted. Any problems with your eyes other . . .

Pt. No.

Dr. Blurring vision or double vision?

*More information about
stroke.*

*Right homonymous
scotomata.*

Pt. During the stroke I had things wavering in front of my eye like that, you know, if I look up to the light. At first I thought it was something with my glasses, you know.

Dr. On the right side.

Pt. Yeah, the right side. And so I took off my glasses, and gee, it still kept coming so I thought, "Gee, I wonder if it could have been from the stroke?" So I spoke to the doctor and he said, "Sure."

Dr. Uh-huh. Did you notice it when your eyes were closed?

Pt. Yeah. You know, you close 'em like that and the eyelids would flutter so. (laugh)

Dr. Did you have any difficulty closing your eyes with the stroke?

Pt. No, no.

Dr. Any other problems with your eyes?

Pt. No.

Dr. Any blurring of vision after that?

Pt. No.

Dr. Do you get colds, often?

Pt. No, I don't.

Dr. Any trouble with your nose?

Pt. No.

Dr. You mentioned nosebleeds with pregnancy.

Pt. I had that just once during pregnancy.

Dr. The first pregnancy.

Pt. The second one.

Dr. Second pregnancy.

Pt. I had such nosebleeds.

Dr. Any other time?

Pt. No.

Dr. Never again.

Pt. No.

Dr. How about your teeth?

The patient's reference to "so darn much medicine" should have been followed up.

Pt. Well, my teeth aren't too good because I had taken so darn much medicine when I was a kid. This is—these four teeth are capped. And I've only got one, two, four back teeth.

Dr. Any infections?

Pt. No.

Dr. Abscesses, toothaches?

Pt. Every time I had a tooth pulled it was abscessed. I guess it was abscessed. Yeah, I think it was abscessed. . .I kept enough of all these back teeth.

Dr. How about your hearing?

Pt. No trouble.

Dr. No trouble with your ears, earaches? Ringing of the ears?

Pt. No.

Dr. Sore throats?

Pt. No.

Dr. Did you ever have any difficulty swallowing?

Pt. No.

Dr. And did you ever have pneumonia?

Pt. No.

Dr. Ever coughed up blood?

Pt. Well, I have during the pregnancies.

Hemoptysis during pregnancies.

Dr. During the pregnancies. Was that in relationship to the nosebleed or was it separate?

Pt. No, separate.

Dr. So you coughed up blood. Which pregnancy?

Pt. All of 'em.

Dr. All of them. Just during the pregnancy?

Pt. Yeah.

Dr. And what was it like? When you coughed up blood?

Pt. It was just . . . right in with the sputum, and so forth, you know.

Dr. You were coughing at the time?

Pt. I always started coughing before I vomited.

Dr. And how many times did this happen that you coughed up blood?

Pt. Well, I don't know how many times.

Dr. Two or three . . .

Pt. Yeah . . .

Dr. . . . or . . . or a dozen?

Pt. Not every time.

Dr. Did you have x-rays for this?

Pt. No.

Dr. Or a bronchoscope; anybody ever look down your throat?

Pt. No.

Dr. Would it be a little bit of blood or a lot?

Pt. Oh, just a little bit.

Dr. Did you notice shortness of breath?

Pt. I don't remember.

Dr. I neglected to go back to one thing, the pain in the chest that you had . . .

Pt. In August?

Dr. In August. Had you had pain in your chest at any other times?

Pt. No.

Dr. Ever have any pleurisy?

Pt. No.

Dr. Mm-hmmm. What about your digestion?

Pt. Well, they always said that I had nervous indigestion. From the time I was born until I was about 14, I had convulsions. I would have something to eat mostly at night and if it was heavy then I would get sleepy and I'd go and lay down, and I'd have a convulsion. So for years — I can't tell you how many it was — I didn't eat supper. I ate the same thing I ate for breakfast.

Convulsions to age 14.

Dr. What were these convulsions like?

Open-ended question.

Pt. Well, I can only tell you my mother said that she didn't ever know whether I was gonna live or die, your eyes go back and you just — you don't . . .

Specific questions.

Dr. Did you bite your tongue?

Pt. Yeah, well, no, no. I would not. Some people jerk all over, you know, but I didn't.

Dr. You didn't. Did you ever wet yourself?

Pt. No.

Dr. Your eyes would roll back and you would pass out?

Pt. Just pass out.

Dr. And you don't remember anything.

Pt. No. And when I come to, my mother and father would be rubbing my arms and legs.

Dr. You say this disappeared when you were 14.

Pt. Yeah. At 14 I had about three of them in one night and that was the end of it.

Dr. And they gave you medicine for that?

Pt. Yeah. First one and then another. I've taken more medicine than could be lined up on this floor.

Dr. Do you know the names of any of those medicines?

Pt. The only thing I can remember is . . . luminal.

Dr. Luminal? Dilantin ever?

Pt. I don't know. That's the only thing that — that's the only thing that sticks with me.

Dr. Bromides? Do you remember that?

Pt. No, I don't remember anything. But I do remember that my mother used to say that she never was satisfied. At first they gave me medicine for epileptic fits. And my mother said that was not the epileptic fits that I had because she had seen epileptic fits. And so she wouldn't give me any medicine. And then, oh, I've taken so much medicine and then so many doctors.

Dr. What did your mother think the fits were?

Pt. She didn't know what they were. She wouldn't have anybody say they were epileptic fits.

No family history of epilepsy.

Dr. Any history of epilepsy in the family?

Pt. No, no.

Dr. Now any gas or indigestion, or nausea and vomiting, other than during pregnancy?

Pt. No.

Dr. Ever have yellow jaundice?

Pt. No.

Dr. What about your bowels?

Pt. Oh, they're good.

Dr. No trouble there. Have diarrhea?

Pt. No.

Dr. Blood. Hemorrhoids?

Pt. I have hemorrhoids.

Dr. What trouble do they give you?

Pt. They don't give me any problem at all now. But the last time I had trouble I think I had a blood clot. I didn't know what it was. Oh, it was terrible. I tried to doctor myself and I thought it would go away and all of a sudden I saw blood, a great deal of blood from . . .

Dr. When was this?

Pt. This was about five years ago. And so I went to the doctor and he said, "Well, it's a good thing that it happened. Your problem is over with because it had broken." I — he said, "I would have had to lance it." So I haven't had any trouble since.

Dr. And what about your urination?

Pt. Good.

Dr. No trouble. Do you get up at night?

Pt. No.

Dr. Never have. Any pain in your back ever?

Pt. No.

Dr. Ever see blood?

Pt. No.

Dr. No history of kidney trouble?

Pt. No.

Dr. Bed wetting when you were young?

Pt. No.

Dr. High blood pressure?

Pt. No.

Dr. Never had high blood pressure.

Pt. No.

Dr. And what about your menstrual periods?

Pt. I'm still having them.

Dr. Have they been regular?

Menorrhagia.

Pt. Yes. In fact, the first part of January I had a menstruation period, and it just kept carrying on and on and so the doctor gave me a D and C.

Dr. When did you have the D and C?

D and C January 11, 1968.

Pt. About the . . . oh, I'd say about the 11th or 12th, something like that.

Dr. About three weeks ago.

Pt. Yeah.

Dr. And what did they tell you about the D and C?

Pt. They said it was all right.

Dr. It's okay. Have you had any problems with your menstruation over the years?

Menorrhagia, September, 1967.

Pt. Well, in September. It just got awful; it got out of control. I just walked across the floor and I had to clean up the floor afterwards. And so I called the doctor and he said, "Well, if you can come down, you better come down." And so I went down there and he gave me a shot.

Dr. This was after you were here?

Pt. Yes.

Dr. Uh-huh. So you have had several prolonged or profuse periods since September. When did your periods start? How old were you?

Pt. Fourteen.

Menarche, 14.

Dr. You were 14.

Pt. Mm-hmmm.

Interviewer notes menarche and cessation of convulsions both at 14.

Dr. How about the relationship between the start of your periods and your convulsions?

Pt. That's one thing I neglected to say, that it was almost hand and glove. They went—as soon as I had those three, that was the end of them and very soon I started the period.

Dr. You know how long you would be out when you had these convulsions? Did the family say how long you'd be unconscious?

Pt. My mother used to say 3 or 4 minutes to up to an hour.

Dr. Besides the convulsions, were there other times that you passed out? Are there any other times that you've ever had any weakness or paralysis or numbness or tingling or anything such as the stroke for even briefly?

Pt. No, no. Other than that, nothing.

Dr. Any pains in your joints or limbs?

Pt. No.

Dr. Any rashes, itching, or skin trouble?

Pt. No.

Return to Family Health. Grandparents.

Dr. How about the health of your grandparents? Do you know anything about their health?

Pt. My grandmother on my father's side was — she was an old lady. And my grandfather on my father's side, he was only 60 and he died of — something wrong with his heart. I don't know what it was. It was so long ago. And my grandfather on my mother's side was just old and my grandmother was — she had a goiter.

Dr. How old was she when she died?

Pt. Oh, I think she was . . . maybe . . . 50, something like that. She wasn't too old.

Dr. And your mother's father you said was how old?

Pt. He was old; 70 . . . almost close to 80.

Dr. And then your grandfather on your father's side was the one who had the heart trouble in his 60's. And his wife?

Pt. She died of old age.

Dr. She was about how old?

Pt. Oh, she was 70 . . . 5, 6.

Dr. Were there any serious illnesses beside what you've mentioned in — say cousins or aunts and uncles, that you know of, any other heart trouble or . . .

Pt. No.

Dr. . . . .cancer or birth defects?

Pt. No.

Current living situation.

Dr. One other question occurs to me. You live in a house?

Pt. Mm-hmmm.

Dr. Your own house?

Pt. No.

Dr. Rented?

Pt. Mm-hmmm.

Dr. And what is the house like?

Pt. Well, we live in an apartment upstairs. And it's connected with the Church of Reconciliation. My husband takes care of the church in return for the apartment. We get it rent free and heat and so forth.

Dr. So it's an upstairs apartment?

Pt. Yeah.

Dr. So that means you have to go up a flight of stairs to get to your apartment.

Pt. Hmmmm.

Dr. And how much room do you have?

Pt. Oh, we have six rooms.

Dr. And who's downstairs?

Pt. Nobody.

Interviewer rechecks exertional dyspnea.

Dr. Nobody. Have you noticed any difficulty before you were told not to do much, say in last summer or spring, any problem going upstairs?

Pt. The only time I had trouble going up and down stairs was the early part of the summer. It bothered me to go up and down stairs.

Dr. How?

Pt. By the time I'd get up the stairs, I'd have to sit down in a chair 'cause it would make me so . . . breathe so fast.

Dr. How about your breathing at that time?

Pt. Well, you know, you breathe so fast, so rapid . . . that . . .

Dr. This started when?

Pt. Before I had the first episode in the bank, you know.

Dr. About how long . . . in July or June?

Pt. Yeah.

Dr. And how about carrying your groceries upstairs?

Pt. Well, see, I have a very independent streak (laugh) and I have always done it.

Dr. And did you notice any difficulty with that before then?

Pt. Yeah.

Dr. When did you first notice trouble with carrying groceries up?

Pt. Oh, probably a year before that.

Dr. Have you had to stop doing anything in your housework, such as vacuuming or cleaning the walls or anything like that?

Pt. Yeah.

Dr. When did that start?

Pt. Well, maybe a year before that and so forth.

Dr. Two years ago?

Patient now acknowledges she was forced to reduce activity 2 years ago.

Pt. I think approximately that, I'd say. And then I'd wait until I felt like, you know, just for a few minutes and then I'd go right on.

Dr. You could continue then.

Pt. Yeah.

Dr. It's really been about two years then, hasn't it?

Pt. Yes.

Step 9: Completion of interview

Dr. Well fine, I think I've got a pretty good idea of this illness. Is there anything else you would like to say?

Pt. No, I think that's about all.

The next task is to select from the extensive interview material what information should be recorded and how it should be organized. First, the present illness must be identified. Since the story is consistent with valvular heart disease present for at least 25 years, this entire period should be included in the Present Illness. The neurological illness which occurred 7 weeks before admission should also be included, since the symptoms are recent and are probably related to the patient's heart disease. One begins the Present Illness with a description of the abrupt increase in cardiac symptoms starting in August, 1967, describes the course of the illness up to the time of admission, and follows with the sequence of symptoms as they had developed over the preceding years.

The episode reported as "rheumatic fever" at age eight is only briefly mentioned in Present Illness and is described more fully under Past Health, since it was atypical and not necessarily connected with the current illness. The symptoms of edema and dyspnea associated with the pregnancies are handled in a similar way.

In the Personal and Social History, attention is directed to the patient's personality characteristics, which may have direct bearing on the reliability of the history and the course of the illness. The disturbing events in the patient's recent life are emphasized, particularly her unhappiness over the son's marriage and her unresolved grief consequent to the brother's suicide. The temporal relationship of these two events to the increase in the patient's symptoms may be pertinent to both the course and the prognosis of the current illness.

THE CASE WRITE-UP

VIRGINIA CURTIS
UNIT #52-47-81
FEBRUARY 1, 1968

This is the first Strong Memorial Hospital admission of Mrs. Curtis, a 52-year-old married housewife and bank teller, mother of three, who lives with her husband and two younger children in Geneva, New York. She was admitted January 26, 1968, referred by Drs. Robert Jones and James Watson of Geneva for evaluation of her cardiac status and consideration of cardiac surgery.

SOURCE AND RELIABILITY OF THE HISTORY.   The information was obtained from the patient, an intelligent person who tends to minimize symptoms.

PRESENT ILLNESS.   The patient has had a history of rapid heart action since 1943 with gradually increasing dyspnea and ankle edema since 1963 or 1964. A diagnosis of rheumatic fever was made at age 8 and a murmur reported at age 27.

On Friday, August 4, 1967, while walking slowly, she suddenly developed severe aching pain in the left anterior upper chest, radiating to the entire left arm, that was associated with dyspnea and a rapid irregular heart beat. With rest, the arm pain subsided in 10 minutes and the chest pain in 20 minutes. Although the rapid heart action persisted, she remained at work for the rest of the afternoon. That evening her physician advised rest over the weekend and prescribed quinidine three times a day. The tachycardia subsided within two days and she returned to work on August 7. The next day she developed malaise, chilly feelings, fever, and sweats, which lasted a few days but were followed by recurrence of tachycardia, dyspnea, and an increase in ankle edema. Unable to perform light household chores, she remained in bed the rest of that week, sleeping with two pillows and occasionally awakening short of breath. She returned to her job on Monday, August 14, but was admitted to the intensive care unit of St. Jerome's Hospital the next day, where she was started on digoxin, a low salt diet, and warfarin. Although her symptoms had improved at discharge on September 3, some tachycardia and dyspnea persisted. Warfarin was discontinued and digoxin was increased to two a day. The consulting cardiologist, Dr. Watson, raised the question of eventual surgical correction and recommended restriction of activities to light housework. Because of no significant improvement over the next 3 months at home, despite restricted activity, the decision was made on November 7, 1967, that she enter Strong Memorial Hospital in January for consideration of cardiac surgery.

On December 11, 1967, she suddenly developed paresthesias of her fingers and weakness of her right hand and arm that rapidly extended to the right face and right leg. She fell when attempting to stand and was unconscious for approximately 10 minutes. Admitted to the intensive care unit of St. Jerome's Hospital, she was confused for 3 or 4 days, paralyzed on the right side, was unable to see to her right, and had difficulty speaking. After a few days, she began to show progressive improvement except for the right arm, which remained paralyzed. During the 5½-week hospital stay the only cardiac symptom was occasional tachycardia. She was discharged on January 17, 1968.

While at home for 9 days awaiting admission to Strong Memorial Hospital, she was markedly fatigued but attempted to resume her usual household activities.

The patient has had a long history of episodes of rapid heart action, the first in 1943 (age 27), 3 months after her first baby died at birth of a "heart ailment," and 6 months after the death of her mother. At that time, she also had "shortness of breath," which was unrelated to exertion, described as a need to sigh. A BMR was normal and she was told she had a "scar in the heart." Thereafter, she periodically noted rapid heart action, particularly in hot weather. During each of her pregnancies (1943, 1946, 1951, and 1957), she had repeated hemoptyses as well as swelling of her legs, which persisted several months after delivery. During the last two pregnancies she also noted exertional dyspnea. Four or 5 years ago (1963 or 1964), mild exertional dyspnea and swelling of the ankles at the end of the day first developed. Two years ago, she began sleeping with two pillows because her "breathing was easier." In June or July, 1966, she had a sudden, marked increase in leg edema, swelling of the abdomen and a gain of 13 pounds, but no increase in dyspnea. An oral diuretic relieved these symptoms in a few days. During the winter of 1966–1967 she had more persistent edema of her legs by evening and intermittent tachycardia. Exertional dyspnea gradually increased so that by the summer of 1967 she had difficulty climbing one flight of stairs, but there was no increase in orthopnea and no paroxysmal nocturnal dyspnea or cough.

Over these 4 to 5 years she has been distressed by family problems, especially the marriage of her son in 1966 and the death by suicide of her youngest brother in March 1967 (see Personal and Social History).

Currently the patient is on a salt-free diet, digitalis, and warfarin (5 mg. daily).

PAST HEALTH
General Health: In spite of the symptoms noted above, the patient considers herself to have been in good health throughout her life.

Childhood Health: Measles and mumps. No scarlet fever or diphtheria.

At age 8 the patient had an illness diagnosed as "rheumatic fever," characterized by painless swelling of both feet and legs, but no pain or swelling of joints, no fever, sore throat, rash, or chorea. There was no known urinary problem or facial edema. She was kept home at rest for a year.

From early childhood to age 14 she had seizures, characterized by her eyes rolling up, followed by loss of consciousness, but no jerking or incontinence. Age 9, Tonsillectomy.

Adult Health:

MEDICAL ILLNESSES. (See Present Illness.)

SURGICAL PROCEDURES. January 11, 1968, dilatation and curettage for menorrhagia at St. Jerome's Hospital.

PSYCHIATRIC ILLNESSES. None.

OBSTETRICAL HISTORY. 1943 (age 27), first pregnancy: nausea, vomiting, and small hemoptyses throughout the 9 months. The infant died of a "heart ailment" at birth.

1946 (age 30), second pregnancy: nausea, vomiting, epistaxes, occasional small hemoptyses, persistent edema of the legs, and a weight gain of more than 20 pounds. She delivered a full-term, healthy male infant.

1951 (age 35), third pregnancy: nausea, vomiting, hemoptyses, dyspnea, and edema, requiring hospital admission at the third month for intravenous fluids. A healthy male infant was born at term. Dependent edema persisted for 3 months after the delivery.

1957 (age 42), fourth pregnancy: hemorrhage at the second and third months, but she carried the baby, a healthy girl, to term. Again there was nausea, vomiting, edema, hemoptysis, and some dyspnea. This pregnancy was unplanned.

Accidents and Injuries. None.

Allergies. None.

Immunizations. Not asked.

FAMILY HEALTH

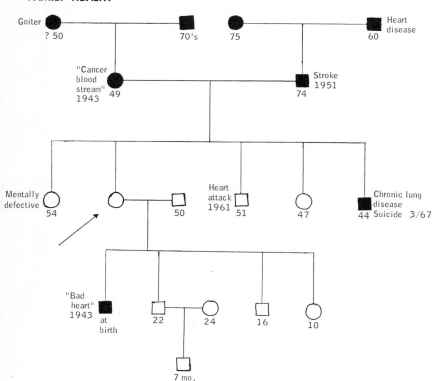

The mother died in 1943, at age 49, during the patient's first pregnancy, with "cancer of the blood," and had been "sickly all the time" with numerous operations. The father had a stroke in March, 1951, and died at home in August, 1951, during the patient's third pregnancy.

Siblings. Bessie, age 54, is living, married, and mentally defective, with two children, one a "Mongolian." John, age 51, had a "heart attack" in 1961, followed by "blood clots." Geraldine, age 47, is in good health except for a hysterectomy a few years ago. Merlin committed suicide by gunshot in March, 1967, age 44. He had chronic lung disease compatible with bronchiectasis, a lobectomy in 1956, and shortly before the suicide a recurrence of pulmonary symptoms.

The patient's three children, Robert, age 22, Mark, 16, Lois, 10, have all been in good health, as has the patient's husband, age 50.

Other than the paternal grandfather and the brother, no one else in the family has had heart disease. There is no family history of cancer, birth defects, or epilepsy. One aunt had a stroke 2 years ago at age 82; she is still living.

PERSONAL AND SOCIAL HISTORY

Current Life Situation. The patient, her husband, and the two younger children occupy a rent-free, six-room apartment on the second floor of a house, in return for which the husband acts as custodian for the church next door. Employed for more than 30 years as a railroad car inspector, he is covered by a company pension and benefits. He works irregular hours, sometimes at night, but he and the children have been able to assist in household chores. The two younger children are in school at appropriate grades. One source of family friction was the engagement and marriage in May, 1966, of the son, Robert, to a girl two years older. The patient opposed the marriage and does not get along with her daughter-in-law, but feels there is nothing further she can do to improve the relationship. She is also still upset about the suicide of Merlin in March, 1967, and did not attend the funeral in Virginia as she feared it would make her sick. She cried when she discussed Merlin's death.

Until August, 1967, the patient had been working for a year as a clerk and bank teller. She has always been a very active, busy person and has found it difficult to be confined to limited activity. Since being ill, she has tried to keep busy by knitting and doing light housework. She needs to present herself as an active, vigorous, and competent person.

Past Development. The patient is the second oldest of five children and was brought up in Geneva, New York, where her father worked as an auto mechanic and truck driver. Because of her mother's chronic ill health and her older sister's mental deficiency, the responsibility for the care of the other children was hers. She finished high school while helping out at home. From 1936 until her first pregnancy in 1943 she worked as a clerk in a paper firm. She married in 1938 but continued to live in the parental home. After her mother's death in 1943, she looked after the mentally deficient sister until she was married and then kept house for her father until his death in 1951, assuming full responsibility for his terminal illness of 6 months.

She is a Protestant and her husband is Catholic.

SYSTEMS REVIEW:[1]

Skin. No rashes or pruritus.

Hematopoietic System. Not asked.

Head and Face. Headaches during pregnancy.

Ears. No difficulty with hearing, tinnitus, or earaches.

Eyes. Glasses for myopia for 20 years; no pain, inflammation, diplopia; visual field defect during stroke (see Present Illness).

Nose and Sinuses. Infrequent colds.

Mouth, Pharynx, and Larynx. A number of teeth have been "abscessed" and extracted. Infrequent sore throats. No dysphagia.

Breasts. Not asked.

Respiratory Tract. No pleurisy. Hemoptysis during pregnancies.

Cardiovascular System. (see Present Illness.)

Gastrointestinal System. Appetite has been good. "Nervous indigestion" as a child. Nausea and vomiting during pregnancies. No jaundice, diarrhea, recent indigestion, or bloody stool. Thrombosed and bleeding hemorrhoids 5 years ago.

Urinary Tract. No history of kidney trouble, back pain, hematuria, nocturia, or enuresis.

Genital Tract. Menarche age 14; last menstrual period, early January 1968. In September 1967, and again in January 1968, she had excessive bleeding.

Skeletal System. No pain in the extremities.

Nervous System. Stroke (see Present Illness). Convulsions (see Past Health).

Endocrine System. In 1943, BMR was normal. Other symptoms not asked.

Psychological Status. (See Personal and Social History.)

PHYSICAL EXAMINATION

RELIABILITY. The patient is cooperative, and the physical examination, done February 1, 1968, is complete.

GENERAL DESCRIPTION. Mrs. Curtis is slight of build, wears glasses, and has graying hair. There is slight hirsutism, including hair on the upper lip and a small amount on her lateral chin. She appears calm, is cheerful, responsive, cooperative, and tries to do things for herself. She is well oriented. Her speech is occasionally hesitant with slight evidence of an expressive aphasia, but she is able to speak her words distinctly. She rises easily from her chair to walk down the corridor without any trace of a limp. There is little motion of her right arm as she walks, and during the examination she frequently holds her right hand with her left.

VITAL SIGNS. Blood pressure 100/62 mm. Hg (recumbent) in both arms. Radial pulse totally irregular at 88 beats/min.; with 10 sit-ups rises to 104. Apical rate 96 beats/min. Respirations normal.

---

[1] The Systems Review is not complete. Those symptoms not inquired about during the first interview, as well as other omissions in the history, would normally be pursued in a subsequent patient visit before writing the case history.

SKIN.   Normal color, a few small angiomata on the anterior chest; an irregular pale 2 × 4 cm. flat, pink hemangioma on the middle of the upper left anterior thigh, and also a similar lesion is present on the midlateral anterior left calf, measuring 4 × 6 cm. There is an old scar 4 cm. long below the right knee cap (from a fall in childhood), and two or three fresh scratch marks on both upper lateral forearms caused by her pet cat.

LYMPHATIC SYSTEM.   Two discrete, soft, 1 cm. right posterior cervical nodes; no other nodes felt.

SKULL.   Normal.

FACE.   Slight flattening of right nasolabial fold. (See neurological examination.)

EYES.   Patient reads 2 mm. print with bifocals at 2 feet. Sclerae and conjunctivae normal. Pupils equal, 4 mm., react to light and accommodation. Extraocular motions normal. Visual fields are full. Right fundus is at −1; left at 0 diopters. Disc margins are sharp. Normal arterioles and veins with no nicking. No hemorrhages or exudates. Maculae normal.

EARS.   Whispered voice is heard equally well in both ears without difficulty. The right canal is occluded with cerumen; the left canal, narrow. Only the anterior part of the left tympanic membrane is seen, which is of normal color.

NOSE.   No lesions, septum slightly deviated to the left but with normal patency.

TEETH.   Gums in good repair. No lesions. Two premolars missing in the right lower jaw; third molars missing on each side of the lower jaw. Teeth filled with amalgam fillings.

PHARYNX.   Not inflamed. No tonsils seen. Tongue coated.

NECK.   Left lobe of thyroid is palpable, not visible, normal in size. Isthmus not felt. No pyramidal lobe.

BREASTS.   Only a small amount of glandular tissue with no masses. Nipples prominent, no abnormalities.

THORAX AND LUNGS.   Slight scoliosis of the middorsal spine to the left; equal expansion of each hemithorax. Breath sounds are normal. Normal tactile and vocal fremitus. Normal percussion. Diaphragms move equally 3 cm. bilaterally. No rales or wheezes.

CARDIOVASCULAR SYSTEM

Heart.   No abnormal pulsations are seen. There is no right ventricular lift. The apical impulse is discrete with a very slight localized thrust 11 cm. to the left of the midsternal line in the fifth intercostal space. The intensity of the first heart sound at the apex is slightly increased and sharp. There is also a slight increase in intensity of the second sound heard in the pulmonic area, which is greater than a normal second sound in the aortic area. There is an opening snap moderately close to the second sound, heard best to the left of the low sternum. No splitting. No basilar murmurs. No left sternal border diastolic murmur. There is a grade 2/6 blowing apical systolic murmur going two-thirds of the way through systole that dies out in the midaxillary line and is also heard to the left of the low sternum. In left lateral position there is a grade 2/6 rumbling diastolic murmur, which occupies all of diastole when the ventricular rate is slow. No gallop.

Peripheral Vascular. No jugular venous distention at 45 degrees. No abnormal venous pulsations. Carotid arteries show normal pulsations of equal intensity, and there are no bruits. The abdominal aorta is normal, easily felt, and measures 3½ cm. in breadth. There is a faint late systolic bruit heard above the umbilicus, that fades out toward the upper abdomen. The peripheral pulses (0-4+) are as follows:

	CAROTID	RADIAL	FEMORAL	POPLITEAL	DORSALIS PEDIS	POSTERIOR TIBIAL
right	+++	+++	+++	+++	+++	+
left	+++	+++	+++	+++	+++	?

There is no pretibial or sacral edema.

ABDOMEN. Scaphoid. No abnormal pulsations or masses. Active peristalsis is heard and is of normal pitch. The liver edge just descends to the costal margin on deep inspiration and is nontender. The span of total liver dullness measures 10 cm. The spleen is not palpable. The lower pole of the right kidney is just felt; the lower pole of the left kidney is not felt. The sigmoid colon is palpable as a soft, cylindrical structure.

GENITAL EXAMINATION. Normal female escutcheon. Labia, urethral meatus, and vaginal introitus appear normal. There is no tenderness and no discharge. The cervix looks normal and is firm, freely movable, and nontender. The uterus is small, firm, without irregularities, and nontender. The ovaries are not palpable. No masses or tenderness in the cul-de-sac.

RECTAL EXAMINATION. Normal sphincter tone. No pain or tenderness. No masses. Brownish stool on examining finger, guaiac negative.

SKELETAL SYSTEM. Normal.

NEUROLOGICAL EXAMINATION

General Status. See above for general description.

Cranial Nerves. I - not tested; II - normal (see above); III, IV, VI - normal (see above); V - normal light touch and pain sensation to pin prick, equal bilaterally; corneal reflexes are equal. Motor V - normal with patient biting down. VII - slight flattening of right nasolabial fold. Symmetrical smile; patient able to wrinkle forehead bilaterally. VIII - gross testing normal. IX, X - uvula moves in midline; slight gag reflex, equal bilaterally. XI - weakness in sternocleidomastoids bilaterally. Slight decrease of strength in right shoulder with elevation. XII - tongue in midline with good force in both cheeks.

Motor System. No abnormality in the strength of the left arm or two lower extremities. Normal gait. The patient is able to rise from a squatting position or from a chair without difficulty, and can stand on toes and heels. The right arm is considerably weak, more so proximally; she can make a fist, but grasp is weak. She can extend and flex wrist against gravity, but there is considerable weakness. Pronation and supination of the forearm are done weakly but can be done against gravity. Twenty per cent limitation of full supination. Full range of motion at elbow, which is able to move against gravity. Marked weakness of the shoulder in all directions. No pain. No fasciculation or atrophy. The skin of the fingers of right hand is slightly shiny, and there is minimal edema.

Coordination: Finger-to-nose on the left is normal and cannot be done on the right. Heel-to-shin bilaterally normal. In putting on her gown, she uses mainly the left arm but is able to lift the right arm enough to direct it into the sleeve. Romberg's test is negative.

Sensory System.   Response to light touch, pin prick, position, and vibration is normal and equal bilaterally. Two point sense is intact on hand and forearm, and there is no extinction phenomenon.

Reflexes.   Note that the right deep tendon reflexes are more active than the left and that the plantar responses are flexor.

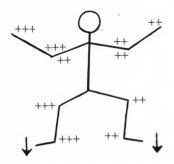

Spinal Nerve Irritation.   Negative.

DIAGNOSIS

The patient, who is 52 years old with possible rheumatic fever at age 8, has had an intermittent cardiac irregularity for 25 years and the gradual progression of dyspnea, orthopnea, and dependent edema over 4 to 5 years. She was hospitalized in August, 1967, for the sudden onset of cardiac irregularity, chest pain, and increased dyspnea. Since then she has been digitalized, placed on a low salt diet, and her activity restricted, without improvement. On December 11, 1967, she was hospitalized with a right hemiplegia of sudden onset, which cleared over 5½ weeks except for weakness of the right arm. She is referred for the consideration of cardiac surgery. On physical examination there is a totally irregular pulse, a grade 2/6 apical systolic murmur, a full length grade 2/6 mitral diastolic rumble, and an opening snap. There are no signs of neck vein distention, pulmonary congestion, or edema. The right arm and face are weak and there is hyperreflexia on the right.

The cardiac findings are classically those of mitral stenosis and mitral regurgitation, the predominant lesion being mitral stenosis. The full length diastolic rumble at a slow ventricular rate means that there is a continuous pressure gradient between the left atrium and left ventricle throughout diastole, that the left atrium cannot empty completely, and consequently the degree of stenosis is severe. The loud mitral first heart sound and opening snap suggest that the valve, though scarred, is still flexible and that mitral stenosis predominates. If there were a severe degree of mitral regurgitation causing valve destruction and allowing rapid ventricular filling, the opening snap would be absent and the intensity of the first mitral sound decreased. The grade 2 mitral systolic murmur, which is not holosystolic, probably represents a minimal degree of mitral regurgitation. Tricuspid regurgitation is an alternative diagnosis since the systolic murmur was also heard at the sternum, but there is no accentuated v wave in the jugular venous pulse and the murmur is also transmitted to the axilla. The history of a "scar" in the heart 25 years ago supports the diagnosis of rheumatic heart disease, although the illness at age 8 is atypical in that the swelling of the legs is reported as painless.

The history of periodic irregular heart action since 1945 is compatible with paroxysmal atrial fibrillation, which is not uncommon in mitral stenosis, but these symptoms could also have been due to intermittent premature beats. The possibility of thyrotoxicosis might be considered, even though the patient volunteers no symptoms of hyperthyroidism, the thyroid gland is not enlarged, and the BMR was normal when palpitations first appeared.

The symptoms of congestive heart failure began 4 or 5 years ago, but may also have been present during the three pregnancies in 1946, 1951, and 1957, precipitated by the increased blood volume of pregnancy. Hemoptysis is not uncommon in the early stages of mitral stenosis resulting from increased pulmonary venous pressure and rupture of pulmonary veins at the time that pulmonary arteriolar resistance is low. Since the edema seemed to be out of proportion to the dyspnea and persisted several months postpartum, one would also have to consider other causes for the edema. Deep leg vein thrombosis would be a possibility; however, the lack of pain, recurrence with each pregnancy, and symmetrical distribution of edema would be against the diagnosis. Edema at age 8 suggests renal disease, but other findings such as hypertension, progressive difficulty with each pregnancy, and urinary findings of residual renal disease are absent.

The gradually developing dyspnea, orthopnea, and more persistent ankle edema 4 to 5 years ago marks the beginning of cardiac decompensation. The sighing type of respiration in 1943 that occurred soon after the death of the patient's mother and infant son "with a heart ailment" is clearly not cardiac dyspnea and more likely represents a conversion symptom.

The episode of cardiac irregularity and transient pain in August, 1967, suggests the sudden onset of atrial fibrillation with a rapid ventricular rate resulting in decreased cardiac output and coronary insufficiency. The patient has continued in atrial fibrillation since August. The absence of effective left atrial contraction and consequent impairment of left ventricular filling as a result of atrial fibrillation, coupled with tight mitral stenosis, has led to a decrease in cardiac output and more congestive heart failure. The psychologic strain of the past 4 or 5 years, to which she has responded by becoming more active and by denying disability, may have led the patient to ignore warning signals and to exert herself beyond her cardiac reserve.

The sudden right hemiparesis, aphasia, and right homonymous hemianopsia of December 11, 1967, suggest an arterial obstruction in the distribution of the left middle cerebral artery. The pyramidal system, the expressive speech areas of the temporal lobe, and the optic radiation were all involved. The abrupt onset without premonitory signs and the relatively rapid improvement in spite of massive involvement is typical of a cerebral embolus. One may postulate vasospasm involving the vascular tree distal to the point of impact and then recovery of function as the spasm relaxed and the embolus moved forward to a smaller vessel. Such a course is unusual with cerebral thrombosis or cerebral hemorrhage. Embolization is common with mitral stenosis and atrial fibrillation where there is stasis of blood in the left atrium and formation of clot. There are no symptoms or signs to invoke the diagnosis of bacterial endocarditis as a cause for the embolism; the history of possible rheumatic fever, as well as the scarred valve 25 years ago, rules against the rare left atrial myxoma, which also is a cause of systemic embolism.

DIAGNOSES

1. Chronic rheumatic heart disease with predominant mitral stenosis and slight mitral regurgitation, Functional Class III.

2. Atrial fibrillation.

3. Congestive heart failure (by history).

4. Right arm paresis, secondary to left middle cerebral artery embolus (6 weeks ago).

5. Depression, occult.

PROGNOSIS

The evidence of slowly developing cardiac decompensation over a 4 or 5 year period with progression over the past 5 months, despite considerable restriction of activity, a low-salt diet, and digitalization, speaks for a very guarded prognosis. Persistent atrial fibrillation and an episode of cerebral embolization with residual neurological deficits also limit the outlook. The problem is further compounded by the patient's proclivity to deny symptoms, which may mean that the degree of failure is even greater than she has reported. On the surface, she seems cheerful enough, but underneath there is evidence of a significant depression, related to the brother's suicide, and also, no doubt, to the consequence of having to restrict her activity because of illness.

If further studies support the impression that the patient has tight mitral stenosis and minimal mitral regurgitation, she should be a reasonable risk for mitral commissurotomy. The recent evidence for clot in the left atrium would favor a commissurotomy done under direct vision, with cardiac bypass rather than a closed procedure, even though the latter operation carries a slightly higher risk. Without surgery, the patient's prognosis is one of a progressively downhill course. Knowing the importance for this woman to be active, one would predict that she would be in favor of commissurotomy. There is no evidence that she exploits symptoms or has accepted chronic illness as a way of life which she would be reluctant to abandon. Hence, any measure which would enhance her range of activity would also be expected to have a favorable psychological impact.

Appendix B

THE COMPLETE CASE WRITE-UP

This case write-up illustrates a complex clinical problem in a 73-year-old man who was interviewed and examined by the authors. A patient was chosen who had mild dementia, a history of several past illnesses, and who presented with a diagnostic neurological problem. Such patients are not uncommon on the wards of a general hospital, and the student is challenged not only in the obtaining of clinical information, but also in the organizing of data into a meaningful written record.

MAX SILBERMAN
UNIT #62-38-95
NOVEMBER 15, 1968

IDENTIFYING DATA. This is the second Strong Memorial Hospital admission of a 73-year-old Polish-born, twice-married, retired barber and pensioned county supervisor, who was transferred from the Genesee Hospital on November 14, 1968, for further evaluation of severe back and leg pain. The patient was interviewed and examined by Randolph C. Palmer, Clinical Clerk, on 11/14/68.

SOURCE AND RELIABILITY OF THE HISTORY. The patient was very cooperative but had a poor memory for dates, details, and past events. Discrepancies were found on reviewing his old Strong Memorial Hospital chart. His wife, interviewed separately, was also vague in her recall of past events but did add information to the Personal and Social History.

PRESENT ILLNESS. The patient had been in excellent health until September 1962, when he suffered a severe myocardial infarction. Two subsequent minor heart attacks followed in 1965 or 1966 and in July 1968, the latter associated with acute gastrointestinal bleeding while on anticoagulants. There is also a history of extensive cutaneous hemangiomas, gout, and a right nephrectomy for hypernephroma in 1964. (See Past Health.)

Approximately 10 months before admission, in January or February, 1968, the patient began to have intermittent pain in the small of his back and posterolateral left thigh. He recalls no specific precipitating event and does not remember the details of his symptoms at this time but believes the pain occurred on and off for about 2 or 3 months. If he sat too long, such as when driving, or if he suddenly put his foot down forcefully, he would not infrequently develop a severe shooting pain into the left thigh "like someone wrenching a nerve." The patient did not take medication or see a physician and was able to walk and sleep without undue discomfort.

Three months before admission in August, 1968, (2 weeks following discharge from the Genesee Hospital after his third heart attack and gastrointestinal bleeding), as he was stepping out from a shower, the patient twisted and suddenly developed severe sharp pain in his mid low back, which radiated down the posterolateral aspect of his left thigh to his knee. This time the pain persisted. Stretching the leg seemed to aggravate the pain, such as when he stepped out of the car. When he was sitting still, driving, or playing cards with his friends, the pain was less severe. Lying down was particularly bad, so he was forced to sleep in a reclining chair most nights up to the time of the current admission. Because of persisting pain, he saw his own physician 2 days after onset, Dr. James Newton on Culver Road. The patient was given pain pills which made him constipated and was told that he had arthritis. After about a week, the pain left his back but persisted in his posterolateral left thigh as intermittent sharp jabs, especially when he lay down. Over the next 2 months the pain was intermittently present day and night.

Two weeks before admission on November 1, 1968, Dr. Newton admitted the patient to the Genesee Hospital because the pain had become more severe and persistent. During this hospitalization, the patient recalls having had several x-ray examinations, and, 5 days before transfer to Strong Memorial Hospital, had a lumbar puncture. Following this procedure, for the first time, he was aware of pain in his right posterior thigh that shot down from his buttocks intermittently "like electricity." Now, when he bent forward or to the right, in addition to pain in the left leg, he would feel "little shocks" around his right hip into the posterolateral right thigh. Because of the progression of his symptoms and the possibility of surgical treatment, the patient was transferred to Dr. Edward Drake at Strong Memorial Hospital on November 14.

Aside from the current illness, the only problem the patient has had is that he has been irritable and depressed for a year or more in relation to family problems. (See Personal and Social History.) In the past month or two, with worsening of his pain, the patient has become more discouraged as he has had to decrease his activities and limit his driving. His wife describes him as depressed, overly concerned about himself, even crying at times, and no longer his usual cheerful self. His cardiac status has been stable with no recent symptoms of congestive heart failure. Retrosternal chest pain occurs only if he overexerts and has remained at the same frequency, approximately two or three times a month. (See Past Health.)

The patient has never experienced an injury to his back. Coughing or sneezing has made no difference in the pain and the patient has had no difficulty voiding or moving his bowels. He has not noted any fever; and there has been no nausea, vomiting, or bone pain. He has continued the medications given him on his first Strong Memorial Hospital admission in 1962, digoxin 0.25 mg. twice daily and chlorothiazide 500 mg. once daily. The patient has rarely taken nitroglycerin pills, and has followed a low salt diet poorly, eating such foods as potato chips and drinking milk with each meal. Before his first heart attack in

1962, he weighed 240 pounds. In the past 2 or 3 years, his weight has been between 185 and 190 pounds. He estimates that he has lost 9 or 10 pounds with the present illness over the past 3 months. With regard to disability, the patient feels life is not worth living if the pain continues at this intensity.

PAST HEALTH

General Health. Even though the patient has had several severe illnesses, he has been in good health between the acute episodes; and he has always been an active, gregarious, and uncomplaining person.

Childhood Health. The patient has had his large "birthmarks" as long as he can remember and has never had associated symptoms. There has been no change in the size or character of the defects. He recalls nothing of childhood illnesses but thinks he may have had typhoid fever in Poland.

Adult Health

MEDICAL ILLNESSES. Acute Anteroseptal Myocardial Infarction was diagnosed on his first Strong Memorial Hospital Admission from September 21, 1962 to October 21, 1962. He had had retrosternal chest pain on exertion for a few months, dyspnea for 2 to 3 weeks, and 2 days of persisting severe retrosternal pain radiating to his left inner upper arm. He entered the Emergency Department in acute pulmonary edema, which persisted 6 hours, despite intensive treatment including venesection. Vasopressor agents had to be given subsequently for 2 days because of hypotension. The remainder of the hospitalization was uncomplicated except that he required a Foley catheter constantly, being unable to void spontaneously. He did develop microscopic hematuria and 3+ guaiac positive stools so that anticoagulant therapy was stopped. At discharge his blood pressure was 130/80 mm. Hg, hematocrit 33 per cent, BUN 24 mg. per cent (which had transiently risen to 64 mg. per cent), and stools were guaiac negative. He had no chest pain or congestive heart failure. His discharge program consisted of a 500 mg. sodium diet, digoxin 0.25 mg. twice daily, chlorothiazide 500 mg. once daily, ferrous sulfate 300 mg. three times a day, and an indwelling Foley catheter with sulfisoxazole 500 mg. four times daily.

In the fall of 1965 or 1966, the patient suffered a second heart attack and was hospitalized at the Genesee Hospital for about a month. He does not remember much about the illness except that the attack was mild, there were no complications, and he was discharged with pink "blood thinning" pills (? warfarin 5 mg.).

In July 1968, he had his third heart attack and gastrointestinal bleeding, for which he was again hospitalized a month at the Genesee Hospital. He was told he was bleeding from an ulcer and required a total of seven units of blood. At first, Dr. Newton told him that he did not have a heart attack, but later electrocardiograms apparently showed some change. The patient states that gastrointestinal x-ray studies were negative and that anticoagulants were discontinued. He experienced no shortness of breath or chest pain in the hospital.

Since discharge, perhaps once a week, if he overexerts, such as walking quickly, he might develop a retrosternal sensation of pressure, also felt in the left anterior shoulder, immediately subsiding with rest. This distress has been present at about the same frequency since the second heart attack.

In July 1968, during the Genesee Hospital admission, the patient also had an attack of gout in his right big toe. He was given colchicine. One previous episode occurred 4 years ago in one of his great toes.

Surgical procedures.   1920: Tonsillectomy in Poland.

1951 (age 56): Cholecystectomy at the Park Avenue Hospital. He remembers pain and that there were many small stones. Reoperation was done 6 months later by Dr. Russell at the Highland Hospital "because all the stones had not been removed."

December 1962: Transurethral prostatectomy by Dr. Edwin Walzer at the Genesee Hospital. In the 3 months following his first heart attack, he had continued to be unable to void without an indwelling catheter.

November 1964: Right nephrectomy by Dr. Walzer at the Genesee Hospital The patient's old chart documents that he was seen in the Strong Memorial Hospital Urology Clinic July 18, 1964, for an intravenous pyelogram because of gross hematuria. A 10 cm. diameter mass was found in the lower pole of the right kidney, compatible with a renal cell carcinoma. A letter from Dr. Walzer, dated December 9, 1964, is also included in the old record that confirms the pathological diagnosis of hypernephroma.

Psychiatric illnesses.   There is no past history of illness, but the patient has been depressed recently. (See Present Illness.)

Accidents and Injuries.   At age seven or eight, he fell and broke a wrist.

Allergies and Immunizations.   The only allergy known to the patient occurred in 1962 when he developed a rash while taking sulfisoxazole. His doctor told him to never take sulfa again. He does not recall if he ever had any immunizations.

FAMILY HEALTH

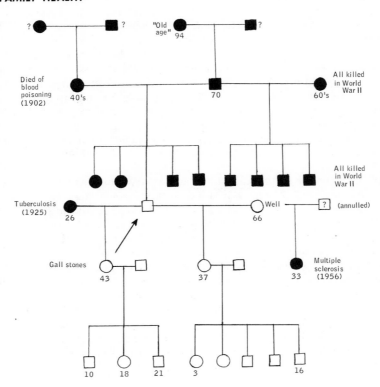

The patient knows of no family illnesses, including heart attacks, diabetes, gout, or hypertension. His father, stepmother, and eight siblings were killed by Hitler in Poland during World War II.

PERSONAL AND SOCIAL HISTORY

Current Life Situation.   The patient has been retired since 1962, following his first heart attack. A year ago, he moved to a single, one story home on Seneca Avenue. His wife had insisted they move from their home of 50 years on Clinton Avenue because the neighborhood was deteriorating. Although the present neighborhood is more pleasant, the patient misses his former friends and neighbors. He is financially comfortable, with money in the bank, social security, and a state pension from the Board of Supervisors. He likes to keep busy and, up to the time of the current illness, had no significant physical limitations. He had worked as a barber before retirement in a shop attached to his home and was a local ward supervisor for 10 years until 1962, enjoying considerable influence and popularity. Despite the move to a new neighborhood, he still manages to visit and cut hair for friends, shop for groceries, and play cards at least once a week. The patient smokes two to three cigars a day, has an occasional beer, and, up to the time of the current illness, slept well 7 or 8 hours a night.

Past Development.   The patient was born in Breslau, Poland and has worked as a barber since the age of 14. His father was a musician. The patient's mother died in 1902 when he was 7 years old. At the age of 26 in 1920, the patient emigrated to Rochester, New York. The patient's first wife of one year's duration came with him to the United States. She was found to have pulmonary tuberculosis and was hospitalized at Iola Hospital for 2 years before dying in 1925 at age 26. A daughter, Rachael, by this first marriage is now 43 and lives in Detroit, Michigan.

The patient remarried in 1926. His second wife, Clara, states that she too had been married 4 years previously, and that the marriage had been annulled because she was too young. Her daughter, Gloria, by her first marriage was raised by the patient, developed multiple sclerosis, was hospitalized at the County Home for 7 years, and died 12 years ago. The patient's second daughter, Martha, is 37, born in 1931. She is married to an insurance salesman, lives only a few blocks away from the patient, and has five children, three boys and two girls, whose ages range from 3 to 16 years. In December 1967, the son-in-law went to live with an older woman, which hit the patient hard, "leaving him speechless." Since the separation, the patient's daughter and children have visited frequently, but in the past few months, the daughter has taken a job and a neighbor baby-sits.

SYSTEMS REVIEW

Skin.   No lesions other than the birthmarks.

Hematopoietic System.   Negative.

Head and Face.   No headache or trauma.

Eyes, Ears, Nose, Mouth, Pharynx.   Glasses worn 20 years, last checked 5 years ago. No epistaxis or sinus trouble. Upper and lower dentures for 20 to 30 years.

Breasts.   Negative.

Respiratory Tract.   No chronic cough, wheeze, or hemoptysis.

Cardiovascular System. (See Past Health for heart attacks and chest distress with exertion.) The patient sleeps on two small pillows without nocturnal dyspnea. He has had no difficulty climbing one flight of stairs at a normal pace; there has been no ankle edema or phlebitis. His blood pressure is normal as far as he knows but was said to be 240 before his first heart attack.

Gastrointestinal System. Appetite is fair, and since 1962 he has tended to bring up excessive gas, for which he takes antacids. He may develop heartburn after greasy or spicy foods. There has been no nausea, vomiting, or jaundice. Bowels move regularly once a day without blood or known hemorrhoids. He has had a "rupture" on the right for 30 or 40 years without symptoms, and he wears no truss.

Urinary Tract. There have been no kidney stones or known infections. He gets up once a night to void and has had no difficulty with his stream, hematuria, or burning since his nephrectomy (1964).

Genital Tract. Negative.

Skeletal System. No joint or back pain other than that of the present illness.

Nervous System. No dizziness, syncope, or tremor.

Endocrine System. Negative.

Psychological Status. Depression. (See Present Illness.) The patient also feels his memory has not been too good in the past 5 years.

PHYSICAL EXAMINATION

RELIABILITY. The examination is reliable and complete, done with the patient in bed. He is very cooperative and able to ambulate but insists on lying with his hips slightly flexed for fear of inducing pain.

GENERAL DESCRIPTION. The patient looks cheerful, is balding with a fringe of gray hair, and shows definite flattening of his right nasolabial fold. He speaks with a slight accent, but his speech is clear and coherent. He is perfectly comfortable, except on rising from a sitting position when he is stopped by a transient pain, which he says is sharp and radiates laterally under his right buttock. When he moves to a sitting position in bed, the patient invariably turns to his left and pulls himself up by the side rails. Striking are large areas of hemangiomas covering his trunk and extremities. (See Skin, hair, and nails.)

VITAL SIGNS. BP_R (sitting): 150/70 mm. Hg, BP_L :144/70 mm. Hg, P = 72 with 8 to 10 premature beats/min. R = 16 per min. and regular.

SKIN, HAIR, AND NAILS. There are multiple hemangiomas varying from relatively smooth, deep pink patches to elevated, slightly warmer, rough, purple port wine stains (as on his right anterior thorax and right arm). The borders are irregular. (See diagram.)

The patient has a few small cherry angiomata on his upper anterior and posterior thorax. Medial to his cholecystectomy scar, he has a reducible 4 cm. epigastric hernia; and laterally, a 2 cm. incisional hernia. The hair is normal, as are the nails, except for thick, opaque yellow nails of the great toes.

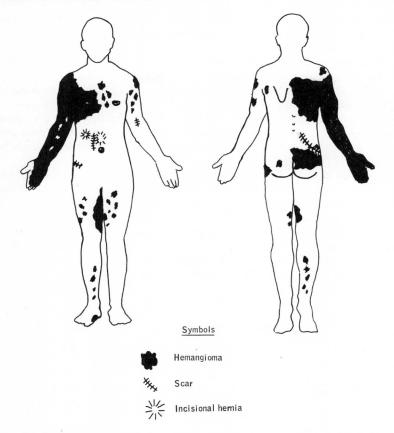

Symbols

Hemangioma

Scar

Incisional hernia

LYMPHATIC SYSTEM.   No enlarged or tender lymph nodes.

SKULL.   No hemangiomas, scars, or tenderness.

EARS.   Whispered voice is heard equally well bilaterally, no tophi, and the drums are not seen because of cerumen.

EYES.   Vision: 1 cm. print easily read at 3 feet with glasses. Sclerae and conjunctivae are normal. Funduscopic: faint lenticular opacity in left lens, disc margins flat, normal vessels with slightly increased light reflex; no hemorrhages or exudates. (See remainder of eye examination described under neurologic examination.)

NOSE.   Patent, with septum slightly deviated to the left.

MOUTH AND PHARYNX.   Edentulous with no lesions seen, including under the dentures. No tonsils are visualized. Tongue papillated but slightly smooth.

NECK.   Normal mobility. No masses. Thyroid cartilage low and the trachea is deviated slightly to the left. The right lobe of the thyroid, felt with swallowing, is normal.

BREASTS.   Normal.

THORAX AND LUNGS.   There is normal equal expansion of the thorax and a slight scoliosis appears to the left in the lower dorsal spine. No abnormal dullness; diaphragms descend 4 cm. bilaterally. Normal vesicular breath sounds posteriorly, and there is a slight decrease in the intensity of breath sounds in the left anterior chest. No rales.

CARDIOVASCULAR SYSTEM. Heart. Diffuse apical impulse in the fifth intercostal space, 11 cm. to the left of the midsternal line with a palpable and audible S_4 gallop in the left lateral position. Sounds are slightly distant with the pulmonic component of the second sound louder than the aortic. Normal splitting with respiration. There is a short slightly harsh Grade 2/6 ejection systolic murmur in the aortic area, which is grade 1/6 in the mitral area and is not transmitted to the neck; the murmur is also accentuated following a premature beat.

Peripheral Vascular System. <u>Neck</u>. Jugular venous pulse shows normal a and v waves, with venous distention 2 cm. above the sternal angle. Normal carotid pulses without bruit. <u>The abdominal aorta</u> measures 4 cm. in diameter, and there is no epigastric bruit.

<u>Extremities</u>. The patient has moderately prominent varicosities of both lower extremities, more marked on the right. There is no redness or calf tenderness, but when ace bandages are removed, imprints are left in both slightly edematous lower legs. Arterial pulsations (0-4+) are as follows:

	CAROTID	RADIAL	FEMORAL	POPLITEAL	DORSALIS PEDIS	POSTERIOR TIBIAL
right	++	+++	+++	+++	+	++
left	++	+++	+++	+++	?	++

ABDOMEN. There are two large abdominal scars from previous surgery. (See diagram above.) The abdomen is soft and nontender. No masses are felt. On deep inspiration a rounded, nontender liver edge descends 2 cm. below the costal margin in the midclavicular line, with total dullness measuring 12 cm. No palpable left kidney or spleen. Normal peristalsis.

GENITAL EXAMINATION. The penis is circumcised. Normal, slightly atrophic testes are present with a moderately large hernia filling the right scrotum. No hernia is in the left inguinal canal.

RECTAL EXAMINATION. No perianal lesions. Sphincter tone normal, slightly lax. The prostate is of normal consistency, with a median furrow. The right lobe is slightly bigger than the left and nontender. No rectal masses. Stool specimen, guaiac negative.

SKELETAL SYSTEM. (See description of leg muscles under neurologic examination.) The joints appear normal. The patient is able to move his extremities through their normal range without discomfort. (Extension of the hips is not tested because the patient is fearful that this will produce thigh pain.) There is no spasm of back muscles and no localized tenderness of any of the vertebrae.

THE NEUROLOGIC EXAMINATION

General Status. The patient's behavior is appropriate and speech normal. As noted, he has difficulty recalling dates and sequences, frequently contradicting himself. His gait is slightly shuffling as he walks with short steps, keeping his hips slightly flexed. There is no difficulty in walking. Romberg's test is normal.

Cranial Nerves.

I-Not tested.

II-Normal. Gross visual fields normal.

III, IV, VI-Pupils regular, 4 mm., and equal, reacting to light and accommodation. Extraocular motions normal.

V-Normal corneal reflexes, normal facial sensation to light touch and pain. Motor strength normal.

VII-Definite flattening of the <u>right</u> nasolabial fold, although the crease appears when he is asked to smile.

VIII-Normal.

IX, X-Normal gag and uvula midline.

XI-Normal.

XII-Normal.

Motor System. The patient is right handed. No tremor or muscle fasciculations are seen. The patient is able to rise from a sitting position without difficulty but does assist himself with his arms. He is able to stand briefly on his heels and toes. There is wasting of the anterior lateral left thigh muscles, the circumference of the left thigh measuring 41 cm. as compared to 48 cm. for the right thigh (12 cm. above the knee cap). There is questionable decreased strength of abduction of the left hip. Tone is normal, as is coordination, including the finger-to-nose and heel-to-shin tests.

Sensory System. No definite sensory deficit is found when testing with light touch and pin. He inconsistently says that there is increased pain sensation to pin prick in the left lateral thigh (L2) and a slight decrease to light touch in the left lateral calf (L5). Position and vibration sense in the toes and fingers are normal, with perhaps a slight decrease in vibration at the base of the left great toe compared to the right. Stereognosis with coins and tactile localizations are normal.

Reflexes.

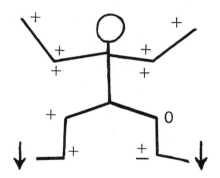

All deep tendon reflexes are difficult to obtain, requiring distraction and reinforcement, but the left knee jerk is definitely absent. The left ankle jerk is questionably present.

Spinal Nerve Irritation. There is no localized tenderness over the sciatic nerve or over either thigh. Straight leg raising is 70 degrees on the right and 50 degrees on the left, limited by a drawing sensation in the posterior thighs.

ADMISSION LABORATORY DATA

Hematocrit: 37 per cent; white blood count 6600 per ccm.; differential count: 70 per cent polymorphonuclear leukocytes, 19 per cent lymphocytes, 7 per cent monocytes, 3 per cent eosinophils, 1 per cent basophils; blood smear: platelets are normal in number and morphology. The red blood cells appear slightly hypochromic and are normal in size, with slight variation in size and shape. Urinalysis: specific gravity: 1.018, pH 5, 1+ protein, no sugar, and the sediment shows a rare white blood cell per high powered field. Stool specimen is guaiac negative.

DIAGNOSIS

This 73-year-old patient has suffered three coronary occlusions since 1962 and had a right nephrectomy for hypernephroma in 1964. He has had low back and left thigh pain for 10 months, becoming more severe and persistent the 3 months prior to admission. He has also been somewhat depressed for a year, more so the last 3 months as the pain has become worse. Physical examination shows slight cardiac enlargement and an aortic systolic murmur but no congestive heart failure. He has extensive cutaneous hemangiomas. The patient prefers to keep his hips slightly flexed; there is atrophy of the left thigh, limited straight leg raising on the left, and an absent left knee jerk. The admission hematocrit is 37 per cent, and the urinalysis reveals 1+ protein and an occasional white blood cell in the sediment.

The primary diagnostic problem is left posterolateral thigh and low back pain that has more recently extended to the right side. A neurologic disorder best explains the findings, with the lesion most likely localized to the lumbar spinal cord or to one or more of its nerve roots. The absent left knee jerk, the location of the thigh pain, and the atrophy of the thigh muscles correspond with the distribution of the second to fourth lumbar roots. This localized distribution, coupled with the absence of other neurological findings, locates the pathological process to the extradural space. The recent development of similar but milder pain on the right side indicates an asymmetrical process, which first involved the roots on the left and which now also involves the same roots on the right.

The differential diagnosis to be considered that would explain the proposed extramedullary extradural lesion would include four major possibilities: degeneration of a lumbar intervertebral disc, metastatic hypernephroma, nerve root compression by a congenital hemangioma, and a primary extradural tumor.

The best diagnosis appears to be a <u>ruptured intervertebral disc</u>. The long course of symptoms, their intermittency, and the radiation of pain all appear typical. The location of pain in the L2, L3 dermatome is less common, however, than rupture of a disc between the L4 and L5, or the L5 and S1 vertebrae. The absence of a history of trauma is not unusual. The past history of hypernephroma and the not uncommon extradural location of metastatic disease make <u>metastatic hypernephroma</u> a definite possibility. A localized lesion in a lumbar vertebra could slowly enlarge and press against a motor root; indeed, aggravation of pain when lying down at night is not uncommon. Slight evidence against the diagnosis is that there are no other signs of metastatic disease and no localized vertebral tenderness. Nerve root compression by a <u>congenital hemangioma</u> must be considered in a patient who has extensive skin lesions. One would have to postulate an increase in size of an extradural plexus of congenital vessels due to bleeding or thrombosis. The fact that the neurologic deficit is so discrete, that there is no sensory deficit, and that the lesion appears to be slowly progressive would be evidence against such a diagnosis. A <u>primary extradural tumor</u>, such as a nerve sheath tumor or meningioma, would also be possible, even though both are usually located in the intradural space. Such slow growing neoplasms could give the clinical picture seen in this patient but would be statistically less common than a ruptured intervertebral disc or metastatic implant.

The patient's <u>coronary heart disease</u> appears stable with only occasional angina pectoris and no congestive heart failure. The aortic systolic murmur appears to be hemodynamically insignificant, since there have been no progressive symptoms, no left ventricular hypertrophy on physical examination, and the murmur is faint without radiation to the neck. The murmur may be caused by atherosclerosis at the base of the valve cusps or dilation of the aorta beyond. The memory defect suggests a <u>mild dementia</u>, probably secondary to cerebral atherosclerosis. Brain damage incurred during his coronary attacks and gastrointestinal hemorrhage is possible but less likely. In the absence of other evidence, metastatic hypernephroma to the central nervous system is unlikely. The patient's <u>depression</u> appears to be related to his move a year ago to a new home and to his daughter's marital difficulties; it is compounded by the discouraging course of his present illness, which restricts his activities and interferes with his sleep. His attacks of <u>gout</u> may have been aggravated by the daily dosage of thiazide drugs which can raise the blood uric acid. The hematocrit and urinalysis should be repeated to confirm the mild anemia and proteinuria.

The admitting diagnoses are:
1. Herniated intervertebral disc, L2-L3.
2. Coronary heart disease with angina pectoris and three former myocardial infarctions.
3. Reactive depression.
4. Sulfisoxazole allergy (by history).
5. Mild dementia due to cerebral atherosclerosis.
6. Gout.
7. Congenital cutaneous hemangiomas.
8. Indirect right inguinal hernia and incisional hernias.
9. Varicose veins.
10. Anemia and proteinuria of uncertain significance.

PROGNOSIS

The disease underlying the patient's present illness appears to be severe and advanced. The pain has required him to sleep sitting up and has necessitated hospitalization. Objective evidence of the chronicity of the illness is wasting of the left thigh muscles. If the diagnosis of rupture of an intervertebral disc is confirmed, there is a possibility of surgical therapy which is usually highly successful. On the other hand, operation for a metastatic implant or hemangioma would be only palliative. The predicted outcome of the patient's illness is guarded. Even should a herniated disc be confirmed by diagnostic studies, surgery carries a higher than normal risk in a 73-year-old man with a history of three myocardial infarctions. The outcome of his depression is also difficult to predict. Although relief of pain may well lead to improvement, there are also situational factors, such as his daughter's marital difficulties and his recent move, which may act to sustain the depression.

PLAN OF STUDY

HERNIATED DISC
1. Obtain a transcript of the patient's record at the Genesee Hospital to review previous hospitalizations and recent studies.
2. Serum glutamic pyruvic transaminase, alkaline phosphatase, and bromsulphthalein clearance for possible metastatic hypernephroma to the liver.
3. Lumbosacral films.
4. Myelography.
5. Neurological consultation.

CARDIOVASCULAR DISEASE
1. Cholesterol, 2 hour postprandial blood sugar.
2. PA and lateral chest films.
3. Electrocardiogram.

DEPRESSION
Note fluctuations of mood and behavior in relationship to pain, disability, and visitors.

DEMENTIA
Mental status examination. Watch for nocturnal confusion.

GOUT
Serum uric acid.

ANEMIA AND PROTEINURIA
Repeat hematocrit and urinalysis. If abnormal, consider the following:
1. Repeat stool guaiac examinations, reticulocyte count, and serum iron. Serum protein electrophoresis for the possibility of multiple myeloma.
2. Urine culture, blood urea nitrogen, intravenous pyelogram.

PLAN OF MANAGEMENT

HERNIATED DISC
1. Ambulate as tolerated; bedboard.

2. Give propóxyphene regularly and narcotics as needed.

3. Physiotherapy: passive exercises to legs.

4. Surgical intervention, if studies confirm the diagnosis. Although there is an increased risk in this patient who has severe cardiovascular disease, the definitive nature of the operation, the severity of his pain, and his present stable cardiac status outweigh conservative management.

CORONARY HEART DISEASE

1. No added salt diet.

2. Continue maintenance digoxin and nitroglycerin as needed.

DEPRESSION

Discuss the patient's problem with his wife to gain her support and understanding. Also encourage visits by the patient's friends. Consider the use of an antidepressant drug.

DEMENTIA

Avoid sedation. Apply side rails at night if necessary.

GOUT

1. Consider long-term probenecid therapy.

2. Discontinue thiazide diuretics as a trial.

Randolph C. Palmer
Clinical Clerk

Index

Note: Page numbers in *italic* type refer to illustrations.
Page numbers followed by (T) refer to tables.

Σ